LEADERSHIP
& NURSING

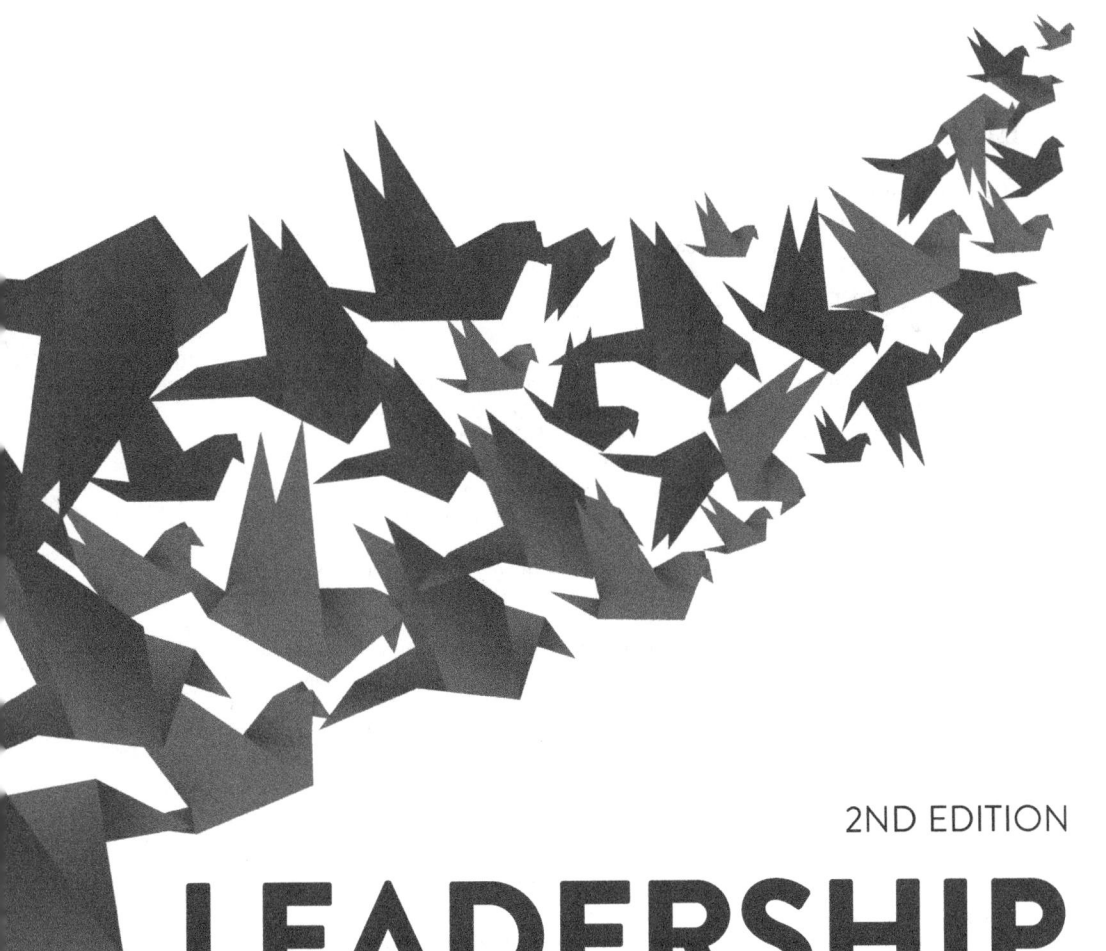

2ND EDITION

LEADERSHIP & NURSING

CONTEMPORARY PERSPECTIVES

John Daly

Sandra Speedy

Debra Jackson

ELSEVIER

ELSEVIER

Elsevier Australia. ACN 001 002 357
(a division of Reed International Books Australia Pty Ltd)
Tower 1, 475 Victoria Avenue, Chatswood, NSW 2067

This publication has been carefully reviewed and checked to ensure that the content is as
accurate and current as possible at time of publication. We would recommend, however, that
the reader verify any procedures, treatments, drug dosages or legal content described in this
book. Neither the author, the contributors, nor the publisher assume any liability for injury
and/or damage to persons or property arising from any error in or omission from this
publication.

National Library of Australia Cataloguing-in-Publication Data

---

Daly, John, 1958- author.
Leadership & nursing : contemporary perspectives / John Daly, Sandra Speedy, Debra Jackson.
2nd edition.
9780729541534 (paperback)
Includes index.
For young adults.
1. Nursing–Australia–Management. 2. Nurse administrators–Australia. 3. Leadership–
Australia–Textbooks.   I. Speedy, Sandra, author.   II. Jackson, Debra, 1959- author.
362.173068

Senior Content Strategist: Libby Houston
Content Development Specialist: Tamsin Curtis and Vicky Spichopoulos
Project Manager: Karthikeyan Murthy
Edited by Jo Crichton
Proofread by Annabel Adair
Cover and internal design by Georgette Hall
Index by Robert Swanson
Typeset by Toppan Best-set Premedia Limited
Printed by 1010 Printing International Ltd

CONTENTS

CONTRIBUTORS

Nourah Alsadaan RN, MSN, PhD candidate
Faculty of Health, University of Technology, Sydney, NSW, Australia

Jen Bichel-Findlay HScD, MN, MPH, RN, FACN, FACHI, AFCHSM, CHIA
Director of Studies, Health Services Management, Faculty of Health, University of Technology, Sydney, NSW, Australia

Marion E. Broome PhD, RN, FAAN
Dean and Vice-Chancellor for Nursing Affairs, Duke University Durham, North Carolina, USA
Associate Vice-President for Academic Affairs, Duke University Health System, Durham, North Carolina, USA

Rosemary Bryant BA, RN, Grad Dip Hlth Admin, DUniv, FACN
Chief Nurse and Midwifery Officer, Department of Health, Canberra, ACT, Australia

Mary Casey RN, RM, RNT, BNS, MSc Med Science (Nursing), PhD
Associate Dean for Taught Graduate and Continuous Professional Development Programmes, University College Dublin, Dublin, Ireland

Mary Courtney RN, PhD
National Head, School of Nursing, Midwifery and Paramedicine, Australian Catholic University, Brisbane, QLD, Australia

John Daly PhD, RN, FACN, FAAN
Dean and Professor of Nursing, Faculty of Health; Head of the WHO Collaborating Centre for Nursing, Midwifery and Health Development, University of Technology, Sydney, NSW, Australia

Patricia M. Davidson PhD, RN, FAHA, FACN, FAAN
Professor and Dean, Johns Hopkins University School of Nursing, Baltimore, Maryland, USA

Cheryl Dennison-Himmelfarb RN, PhD, FAAN, FAHA, FPCNA
Associate Professor, Johns Hopkins University School of Nursing, Baltimore, Maryland, USA

Cathy Doran MHSc (Health Informatics), MSc (Health Policy and Management), RN, FACHI, AFCHSM
Senior Business Analyst Clinical Applications (ICT), Justice Health and Forensic Mental Health Network, NSW, Australia

Christine Duffield RN, PhD, FACN, FAAN
Director, Centre for Health Services Management; Professor of Nursing and Health Services Management, University of Technology, Sydney, NSW, Australia
Professor of Nursing and Health Services Management, Edith Cowan University, Perth, WA, Australia

Gerard Fealy BNS, MEd, PhD
Associate Professor, School of Nursing, Midwifery and Health Systems, University College Dublin, Dublin, Ireland

Philip Furspan PhD
Senior Research Associate, School of Nursing, University of Michigan, Ann Arbor, Michigan, USA

Lynore K. Geia PhD, MPH&TM, BN, RN, RM
Senior Lecturer, Indigenous Futures Research Lead, James Cook University, Townsville, QLD, Australia

Lisa Giallonardo RN, BScN, MScN, PhD Candidate
Bachelor of Nursing Program, University of New Brunswick, Fredericton, New Brunswick, Canada

Jason H. Gilbert RN, BSN, MBA
Director, Nursing Operations, Indiana University Health Methodist Hospital, Indianapolis, Indiana, USA
PhD Student, Indiana University School of Nursing, Indianapolis, Indiana, USA

John H. V. Gilbert CM, PhD, FCAHS
Principal and Professor Emeritus, College of Health Disciplines, University of British Columbia, Vancouver, British Columbia, Canada

Martha N. Hill PhD, RN, FAAN
Dean Emerita, Professor of Nursing, Medicine and Public Health, Johns Hopkins University School of Nursing, Baltimore, Maryland, USA

Marie Hutchinson RN, RM, BapSci, Grad Cert HA, MHSc, PhD
Associate Professor, School of Health, Southern Cross University, Lismore, NSW, Australia

Debra Jackson RN, PhD
Professor of Nursing, Faculty of Health, University of Technology, Sydney, NSW, Australia

Heather K. Spence Laschinger RN, PhD, FAAN, FCAHS
Distinguished University Professor and Arthur Labatt Family Nursing Research Chair in Health Human Resource Optimization, Arthur Labatt Family School of Nursing, Western University, London, Ontario, Canada

Hugh McKenna CBE, PhD, BSc(Hons), RMN, RGN, RNT, DipN(Lond), AdvDipEd, FRCSI, FEANS, FRCN, FAAN
Pro Vice Chancellor, Research and Innovation, University of Ulster, Londonderry, UK

Martin McNamara EdD, DSc(hc), MA, MEd, MSc, BSc, RNT, RGN, RMN
Dean of Nursing and Head, School of Nursing, Midwifery and Health Systems, University College Dublin, Dublin, Ireland

Robyn Nash RN, PhD
Associate Dean (Learning and Teaching), Faculty of Health Sciences, Queensland University of Technology, Brisbane, QLD, Australia

Daniel J. Pesut PhD, RN, PMHCNS-BC, FAAN, ACC
Professor of Nursing Population Health and Systems Cooperative Unit, Director of the Katharine J. Densford International Center for Nursing Leadership, Katherine R. and C. Walton Lillehei Chair in Nursing Leadership, University of Minnesota School of Nursing, Minneapolis, Minnesota, USA

Kathleen Potempa RN, PhD, FAAN
Professor and Dean, School of Nursing, University of Michigan, Ann Arbor, Michigan, USA

Ingrid Potgieter BA, MA (International Studies)
Faculty of Health, University of Technology, Sydney, NSW, Australia

Tamara Power RN, PhD
Lecturer in Nursing, Faculty of Health, University of Technology, Sydney, NSW, Australia

Emily Read RN, MSc, PhD Candidate
Arthur Labatt Family School of Nursing, Western University, London, Ontario, Canada

Juanita Sherwood RN, DipTeach, PGCert Research, PhD
Professor of Australian Indigenous Education, Faculty of Health and Arts and Social Science, University of Technology, Sydney, NSW, Australia
Adjunct Professor, James Cook University, Townsville, QLD, Australia

Sandra Speedy RN, BA(Hons), DipEd (Adelaide), MURP, EdD, MAPS
Emeritus Professor, Southern Cross University, Lismore, NSW, Australia

Debra Thoms RN, RM, BA, MNA, Grad Cert Bioethics, Adv Dip Arts, FACN(DLF), FCHSM(Hon)
Adjunct Professor, University of Technology, Sydney, NSW, Australia
Adjunct Professor, University of Sydney, NSW, Australia
Chief Executive Officer, Australian College of Nursing, Australia

Robert Thornton RN, PhD
Former Senior Lecturer, School of Nursing, Queensland University of Technology, Brisbane, QLD, Australia

Joanne Travaglia BSocStuds(Hons), GradDipAdEd, MEd, PhD
Director, Health Management, School of Public Health and Community Medicine, Faculty of Medicine, University of New South Wales, Sydney, NSW, Australia

Roianne West PhD, MMHN, RN, BN
Professor of Indigenous Health and Workforce Development, Griffith University, Nathan, QLD, Australia

Carol A. Wong RN, PhD
Associate Professor, Arthur Labatt Family School of Nursing, Western University, London, Ontario, Canada

REVIEWERS

Associate Professor John Hurley PhD
School of Health and Human Science, Southern Cross University, Lismore, NSW, Australia

Professor Brendan McCormack DPhil(Oxon), BSc(Hons), FEANS, PGCEA, RMN, RGN
Head of the Division of Nursing, Queen Margaret University, Edinburgh, UK
Professor II, Buskerud University College, Drammen, Norway
Adjunct Professor of Nursing, University of Technology, Sydney, NSW, Australia
Visiting Professor, School of Medicine and Dentistry, University of Aberdeen, Aberdeen, UK
Extraordinary Professor, Department of Nursing, University of Pretoria, Pretoria, South Africa

Dr Sonia Allen RN, RM, PhD, MACS, Grad DipHlthSc (Community) BHSM, GCPHE, FCHSE
Associate Honorary, University of Tasmania, Hobart, TAS, Australia

Professor Bridie Kent PhD, BSc(Hons), RN
Plymouth University, Plymouth, UK; FHEA

Professor Shake Ketefian EdD, RN, FAAN
Professor and Interim Director, Bronson School of Nursing, Kalamazoo, Michigan, USA
Professor Emerita, University of Michigan, Ann Arbor, Michigan, USA

FOREWORD

It is an honour to write the foreword of the second edition of *Leadership and Nursing: Contemporary Perspectives*, edited by John Daly, Sandra Speedy and Debra Jackson. Leadership is probably one of the themes most written about across many spheres of human endeavour; for example, in the literature on the professions, politics, the military, to name a few—not surprisingly it has also received considerable attention in nursing. Leadership influences all spheres of nursing—practice, teaching, research and professional development. We can therefore identify with the interest in leadership. With reference to practice, evidence indicates that good leaders have a positive influence on the work environment. As John C. Maxwell stated eloquently, 'a leader is one who knows the way, goes the way, and shows the way'. In knowing, going and showing the way, it is thus timely that the authors unpack the concept and challenges of leadership in relation to the practice in Chapter 1. The authors give due recognition to the position of practice, and continue to focus on important aspects related to practice in, for example, Chapter 4: Leadership, ethics and the nursing work environments, Chapter 9: Leading contemporary approaches to nursing practice, Chapter 10: Governance of nursing practice: Steps for the quality and safety of healthcare and Chapter 12: Leadership and its influence on patient outcomes.

Long gone are the days that research is conducted for the sake of research. Nursing research is focused at improving the practice of nursing, to ensure quality patient care, to improve patient outcomes and, therefore, nursing decisions based on evidence are critical. Throughout the book it is evident that the authors support these aspects. In Chapter 7 the authors articulate the overlap between leadership, research and practice coherently and describe leading research to enhance nursing practice.

Wendell L. Wilkie stated that 'education is the mother of leadership' and Nelson Mandela echoes that 'education is the most powerful weapon which you can use to change the world'. Nursing professionals realise the importance of education, yet we are increasingly aware of the changing landscape of education. This century asks for transformation of education of healthcare professionals to strengthen health systems. The authors give due attention to interprofessional education practice and leading nursing in the Academy in Chapters 16 and 18, respectively, and highlight the challenges faced by leaders.

Leaders and managers are aware of the concepts of 'empowerment', 'change management', 'identity' and 'legacy management'. The description of these concepts in various chapters provides useful explanations and simplifies the complexities of how these concepts are related to leadership. Bill Gates so rightly states that 'as we look ahead into the next century, leaders will be those who empower others'—an element that is embraced throughout the book. Of particular note is the structure of the chapters: each starts with learning objectives and keywords, and concludes with reflective exercises as well as a recommended list for reading.

I believe that this edition of *Leadership and Nursing: Contemporary Perspectives* is a timely revision and addresses all of the important aspects of leadership and the related concepts of equal importance. This book is a resource for the leaders and managers in various contexts and will be useful across the career span. The book is inspiring and provides valuable information that is not freely available in the literature. It makes an important contribution to leadership and nursing, and will be a resource as we continuously renew ourselves through personal and professional development. I strongly recommend this book as a most valuable resource.

Prof Dr Hester Klopper PhD, MBA, FANSA
President of Sigma That Tau International (2013–2015)

PREFACE

This second edition, of what was a timely book first published in 2004 to fill a vital need in the nursing profession and in nursing practice, has been radically revised and improved. It represents a diverse range of scholarly voices who interrogate the current condition of nursing leadership as practised in a diverse range of settings, and indicates the challenges that nurse leaders face in ethically fulfilling their various leadership roles, both now and in the future. It points to a future for nursing that is dependent on skilled and informed leadership from within its ranks, whether this be formal or informal leadership. The book rests on the premise that leadership is the responsibility of health professionals in all settings. It is not just for the person authorised to hold a position of leadership within the organisation. Equally, we believe that effective leadership is not possible until one has an understanding of self, what motivates others and what systems can facilitate or frustrate leaders. A major feature of this edition is the inclusion of carefully selected global nurse leaders whose expertise will be apparent to readers.

A number of individuals provided vital assistance and support during the preparation of this book. First and foremost, gratitude must go to our families and loved ones for their patience, tolerance and sacrifice of lost time with us. Our sincere thanks go to Libby Houston, Tamsin Curtis, Vicky Spichopoulos and Karthikeyan Murthy of Elsevier for seeing us through the project and providing support along the way, and especially to Jo Crichton for her diligent editorial work.

John Daly
Sandra Speedy
Debra Jackson
Sydney
June 2014

CHAPTER ONE

Leading and managing in nursing practice: Concepts, processes and challenges

Mary Courtney, Robyn Nash,
Robert Thornton & Ingrid Potgieter

LEARNING OBJECTIVES

At the completion of this chapter, the reader will be able to:

▲ describe the principles of leadership and management theories;

▲ describe old and new paradigms in the management of nursing practice;

▲ discuss challenges and issues in nursing practice;

▲ describe four factors that are essential for transforming and leading change in nursing practice;

▲ understand the essential requirements to become effective leaders and managers; and

▲ understand the leadership role within the health context and describe essential aspects for nurse leaders.

KEY WORDS

Leadership, management, theories, creativity, modelling

INTRODUCTION

This chapter explores leadership and management theories, as well as concepts that underpin current understandings of complex organisations such as healthcare systems. We give an overview of how such organisations interact with their environments and discuss the challenges and issues that impact upon these organisations. Four factors essential for transforming and leading change in nursing practice are examined. Finally, we look at essential requirements in becoming effective leaders and managers and how to understand the leadership role within the healthcare context.

PRINCIPLES OF LEADERSHIP AND MANAGEMENT THEORY

Differences between leadership and management

Theorists continue to debate the relationship between leadership and management. Some theorists argue that leadership is simply one of the many functions of management (Tranbarger, 1988), while others assert that leadership requires an extended range of complex skills and that management is simply one role of leadership (Hersey, Blanchard, & Johnson, 2013).

When examining the literature on both leadership and management it is evident that both concepts have a symbiotic or synergistic relationship with each other. That is, in order for managers and leaders to function effectively, the two concepts must be integrated (Marquis & Huston, 2012). Traditionally, strong management skills have been highly valued within healthcare organisations. However, more recently the demand for leadership skills has gained prominence. We will return to the difference between leadership and management later in this chapter.

Development of management theory

Like nursing science, management science has developed a theoretical base from a wide range of other disciplines, such as business, psychology, sociology and anthropology. Over the past 100 years, theorists' views of what constitutes successful management practices have evolved because of the ever-changing nature of healthcare organisations and the external and internal environment in which they are located.

In order to understand healthcare organisations, it is necessary to clarify some of the different theoretical approaches used to describe organisations in general. Systems theory offers a range of insights into the functions of organisations. Sampson and Marthas (1990) describe systems theory as having specialised components that work together interdependently to form an overall balanced framework.

Organisations conduct their everyday activities by taking either an open systems or a closed systems approach (see Table 1.1). The open systems approach places

Table 1.1 Open and closed systems functions

Type of system	Function
Open systems	Links between organisations Adaptable Innovative Flexible
Closed systems	Organisation functions independently of external environment

importance on the links between organisations, emphasising the need for ensuring open lines of communication. They must also be adaptive, innovative and flexible (Shortell & Kaluzny, 1997). Organisations operating under an open systems approach acknowledge the impact of the world around them, upon which they must draw for resources, support and legitimacy (Burns, Bradley, & Weiner, 2012). On the other hand, organisations with a closed systems approach tend to function independently from the external environment and have processes and procedures set in place to ensure that the organisation's internal efficiency reaches its full potential.

A brief summary of the various theoretical approaches undertaken during the development of management theory is presented on the following pages.

Scientific management

In the late nineteenth century, Frederick W. Taylor was working as a mechanical engineer in a steel plant in Pennsylvania. At the time, 'systematic soldiering' was rife—workers would undertake the least amount of work possible to achieve minimum standards. Taylor (1911) believed that the introduction of 'one best way to accomplish a task' would ensure workers achieved an agreed-upon standard, which in turn would lead to increased productivity.

Did scientific management achieve results? Yes. Indeed, productivity and profits increased dramatically. However, from a closed systems perspective on organisations, scientific management saw puritan work ethics prevail and indeed some have argued that Taylor was ahumanistic.

Bureaucratic theory

In 1922, Weber expanded upon Taylor's theories and wrote an essay entitled 'Bureaucracy', which espoused the need for more rules, regulations and structure within organisations to further improve efficiency and productivity (Weber, 1978 (1922)). This closed systems approach encouraged the establishment of an internal hierarchy with clear lines of responsibility and authority. Professional bureaucratic management strategies have traditionally dominated healthcare organisations. Indeed, Weber's theories and design for bureaucratic organisation are still largely used today in the majority of healthcare organisations around the world. The structure includes parallel professional and administrative hierarchies with specific lines of responsibilities and operating rules and procedures.

Identification of management functions

In 1925, Fayol described the management functions of planning, organisation, command, coordination and control. Gulick (1937) extended this work by introducing the 'seven activities of management'—planning, organising, staffing, directing, coordinating, reporting and budgeting. These theorists also took a closed systems perspective on organisations.

Human relations theory

In the 1920s the introduction of the assembly line meant that great numbers of relatively unskilled workers were working in large, complex factories on specific tasks. There was great worker unrest, causing human relations theorists to examine what motivated workers to work. M. P. Follett (1926), in her essay entitled 'The Giving of Orders', asserted that managers should have authority with, rather than over, employees.

Follett was one of the first theorists in this era to argue for what is known today as 'participative decision-making'.

Other human relations theorists such as Mayo (1953), McGregor (1960) and Argyris (1964) all expanded upon her work. Mayo identified the 'Hawthorne effect'. He found that employees increased their productivity levels when special attention was paid to them, regardless of any other changes in their working environment. He noted that people responded to the fact that attention was being paid to them and that they would continue to display the behaviour needed to continue to gain the attention. McGregor (1960) extended upon these concepts by labelling managers as either Theory X or Theory Y managers, depending upon their views of how employees performed their activities (see Table 1.2). Argyris (1964) reinforced the theories of Mayo and McGregor by arguing that managerial domination leads workers to become discouraged and passive, therefore creating low productivity levels and reduced profits. He believed this would subsequently lead to troublesome employees, and eventually an increased turnover of staff.

Although human relations theory seeks to empower individuals, it still adopts a closed system approach to improving the workplace. Individual worker motivation and involvement are recognised by the organisation; however, to encourage harmonious social relations, appropriate structures are usually institutionalised to suit the type of workforce employed. Managers often espouse the importance of developing interpersonal communication and collaboration with individuals to improve workplace relations, while commonly using systems of performance management to motivate workers.

The human relations theory of organisations is based upon a static environment where structures are organised around the professional disciplines. On its own it is not sufficient to describe complex healthcare organisational structures. Nor does it adequately provide a means of understanding and managing the changes that are taking place in today's healthcare organisations (Lloyd & Boyce, 1998).

Institutional theory

Institutional theory takes an open systems perspective of organisations. It examines how organisations succeed by ensuring they fit together with the external environment (DiMaggio & Powell, 1983; Powell & DiMaggio, 1991). Powell and DiMaggio (1991) argued that organisations gain legitimacy from key external stakeholders as they adopt norms, rules and values that reflect the stakeholders' belief systems. By adapting to the external stakeholder environment, organisations signal their congruency with the expectations of stakeholders, such as funding agencies, governments, professional bodies and customers (Daft, 1998).

Population ecology theory

Population ecology theory is another open systems approach to organisation theory and is founded on the notion that an organisation's success depends on its relationship to competitors in its external environment (Hannan & Freeman, 1977). The theory is similar to that of natural selection in biology, whereby as pressures increase on a population within a similar environment, the stronger and more dominant will survive while the weak will suffer and become extinct. Thus, in organisations subject to similar external environments that are under pressure, the more powerful will survive and prosper and the weaker will not.

Subsequently, a gradual evolution of organisational structural changes will occur within the organisation in order to accommodate the complexities of the external

Table 1.2 Historical development of management theory

Systems perspective	Theory	Explanation	Theorist
Closed	Scientific management	Workers could be taught the 'one best way to accomplish a task'	Taylor (1911) 'father of scientific management'
Closed	Bureaucracy of organisations	A need to provide rules, regulations and structure within organisations to increase efficiency	Weber (1922 (1978))
Closed	Management functions	Planning, organisation, command, coordination and control	Fayol (1925)
Closed	Seven activities of management	Planning, organising, staffing, directing, coordinating, reporting and budgeting	Gulick (1937)
Closed	Participative management	Authority with, rather than over, employees	Follett (1926)
Closed	'Hawthorne effect'	People respond to the fact they are being studied	Mayo (1953)
Closed	Theory X and Theory Y	How managers treat employees directly correlated with employee satisfaction Theory X managers believe employees are basically lazy, need constant supervision and direction, and are indifferent to organisational needs Theory Y managers believe workers enjoy work, are self-motivated and willing to work hard to meet personal and organisational goals	McGregor (1960)
Closed	Employee participation	Managerial domination causes workers to become discouraged and passive Flexibility in workplace requires employee participation in decision making	Argyris (1964)
Open	Institutional theory	Success depends on ensuring an organisation and its external environment fit together Adaptive and congruent with expectations of external stakeholders	DiMaggio & Powell (1983)
Open	Population ecology theory	Success depends upon relationship with competitors in external environment Stronger and more dominant survive Weak become extinct	Hannan & Freeman (1977)
Open	Strategic management theory	Success depends upon following logical process to meet chosen goals and objectives Adaptive to internal and external environment	Ellis & Brockbank (1993) Biscoe & Lewis (1996)

environment. Daft (1998) notes that niche markets are often left open in unexploited environments.

Within healthcare organisations, unresolved social dilemmas concerning inadequate service provision can become the subject of media campaigns and taken up in the political arena. Organisations that are able to adapt their organisational structures to address the complexity of change will therefore be more likely to survive.

Strategic management theory

Strategic management theory is yet another open systems approach to organisations. The organisations that use this theory seek to incorporate the internal and external environment into their planning process as they strive to meet targeted objectives. Strategic management theory is commonly used in healthcare organisations because of the need to try and balance limited resources while ensuring that patient care is not threatened. Healthcare organisations must respond to the changing political, economic, technological and demographic environments, all the while maintaining their competitive advantage (Walston & Chou, 2012).

An overview of these various theoretical approaches is presented in Table 1.2. More recently, we have seen organisations moving towards more open systems perspectives in an endeavour to adapt to the ever-changing environment. This paradigm shift will be discussed in the following section.

OLD AND NEW PARADIGMS IN MANAGEMENT OF NURSING PRACTICE

In examining the functions of leadership within an organisation, Stout-Shaffer and Larrabee (1992) identified five paradigm shifts to transform healthcare organisations into the new millennium (see Table 1.3). In the past, organisations were characterised by centralised hierarchies, with power vested in the management. Employees were sceptical of management and distrusted it. Healthcare organisations undertook strategic planning activities in isolation from patients and set benchmarks for planned productivity and efficiency within their own organisations in isolation from the external environment.

In contrast, the future scenario sees a move away from centralised hierarchies to semi-autonomous work units where all employees are empowered to work intuitively and creatively—where strategic planning is undertaken in partnership with patients and where employee scepticism is replaced by trust of management.

Table 1.3 Paradigm shifts transforming healthcare organisations

Past	Future
Centralised hierarchies	Semi-autonomous work units
Power resting with management	Empowerment of all employees
Distrust of management	Trust
Planning for patients	Planning with patients
Quantitative productivity	Intuition and creativity

Source: Stout-Shaffer & Larrabee, 1992, pp. 54–58.

CHALLENGES AND ISSUES FOR NURSE LEADERS AND MANAGERS

The world of healthcare continues to change rapidly. Today's healthcare system presents challenges to administrators and clinicians that have few or no precedents, and there is no indication that it will be any different in the future. Some years ago, Vaill (1989) coined the term 'permanent white water' to describe the phenomenon of change as a constant rather than discontinuous state. Taking this as an accurate statement about the nature of our current and future environments raises an important question about the factors that are influencing such change. Given the increasing complexity of our personal and professional worlds, it is perhaps not surprising that the answers are to be found in multiple arenas—technological, social, political, economic and scientific—each contributing significantly and cumulatively to the impetus for change (Alderman, 2001).

Economic and political issues

The term 'doing more with less' has become familiar to clinicians and administrators alike, both at 'ground level' as well as at 'the top'. The challenges associated with delivering quality patient care within an environment of rising consumer expectations and increasingly constrained human and financial resources are everyday realities for many nurses (Gantz et al., 2012). Continued downsizing of healthcare facilities/services, increased acuity and decreasing lengths of stay—the 'high-tech short stay' phenomenon—and increased pressures on community-based service provision, add further pressures to the day-to-day delivery of appropriate patient care. Other responses related to this issue include the maintenance of financial viability with increased government and managed care constraints, and declining reimbursement. In Australia, government plans to privatise hospital services and possible changes to the country's universal healthcare Medicare system are further issues of concern (Collyer & White, 2011).

Social and demographic issues

Social changes, both within and outside of the nursing profession, also present contemporary challenges for nursing leadership and management. Governments must provide healthcare services to culturally and linguistically diverse populations. In Australia, the 2011 census revealed that more than one quarter of Australians were born overseas, and that more than 300 languages and 100 religions are spoken and practised (ABS, 2013). Homelessness, unemployment, the widening gap between rich and poor, and the increase in prevalence of 'lifestyle' diseases are further social challenges to healthcare. Advances in medicine and technology have resulted in issues related to organ donation, assisted suicide, euthanasia and genetic engineering that will continue to challenge nurses' beliefs and ethics.

Professional issues

Within nursing there are several contemporary issues that present significant challenges for nursing leadership and management. Foremost among these are the changing demographics of the nursing workforce and the shortages of nursing staff being experienced in many areas of clinical practice. In Australia, nursing workers (including registered and enrolled nurses, assistants in nursing and personal care assistants) are older than they were just over a decade ago.

The proportion of workers aged 50 years and over increased by 6.1% to 39.1% between 2007 and 2012, consolidating the overall trend of more workers in the older age categories and fewer in the younger age categories (AIHW 2012, 2013). It is expected that the ageing of this workforce will continue for some time, resulting in a significant impact as the numbers of retirements increase (Graham & Duffield, 2010) and as reports of nurse dissatisfaction emerge. In a recent survey of Australian nurses, 15% stated their intention to leave the nursing profession completely in the next 12 months, due to burnout, job dissatisfaction, workload and unhappiness with management (Holland, Allen, & Cooper, 2012). In addition, there has been a shift towards part-time work, particularly among registered nurses and midwives and, for nurse workers in general, a trend towards working shorter hours per week (AIHW, 2013). It is clear that these changes are not confined to the Australian context, with registered nurse shortages, or predictions of shortages, in many countries around the world, including Australia, New Zealand, the United Kingdom, the United States and Europe (Aiken, Sloane, Bruyneel, Van den Heede, & Sermeus, 2013; Chan, Tam, Lung, Wong, & Chau, 2013; Gantz et al., 2012). Although shortages of registered nurses are not new, the pervasive nature of the current phenomenon suggests that the current situation is going to be difficult to turn around. These issues raise critical questions for nurse leaders and managers with respect to the deployment of scarce resources and the recruitment and retention of competent staff. How effectively these and other questions are addressed affects nurses, nursing and the delivery of patient care.

TRANSFORMING AND LEADING CHANGE IN NURSING PRACTICE

Like other health professionals, nurses are shaped to some extent by changes in the healthcare system, but as the single largest group of healthcare workers, they also have considerable opportunity to shape the system itself. It is suggested that to effectively negotiate these increasingly dynamic healthcare environments several imperatives will be critical for nurse leaders and managers. These can be seen in Figure 1.1 and are discussed briefly in the following section.

Building shared visions

As put so aptly by Tornabeni (2001), 'to create a new world order in anything that you do, you've got to dare to dream' (p. 1). Visioning has long been considered a key element of leadership, particularly transformational leadership (Bass, 1985; Bennis & Nanus, 1985). Visioning is about making an assessment of current reality, determining what a desired state would be, and managing the resultant tension between these two states in a manner that is constructive and productive (Yoder-Wise, 1999). A vision communicates strategic intent; it inspires, clarifies and focuses (Cartwright & Baldwin, 2007). The ability to conceptualise a vision and communicate it to others is a critical issue for nurse leaders and managers. A clear visualisation of a better or more ideal future state is a powerful means of providing staff with a sense of direction and common purpose (Capowski, 1994), guiding and focusing decision making (Ireland & Hill, 1992), creating a balance between the competing interests of various stakeholders (Goffee, Scheele, & Pitman, 2000), and creating forward momentum towards desired goals. Well-communicated visions are more likely to be incorporated by staff, and this vision integration has been shown to be positively related to organisational commitment, job satisfaction and group and individual performances (Kohles, Bligh, & Carsten, 2012).

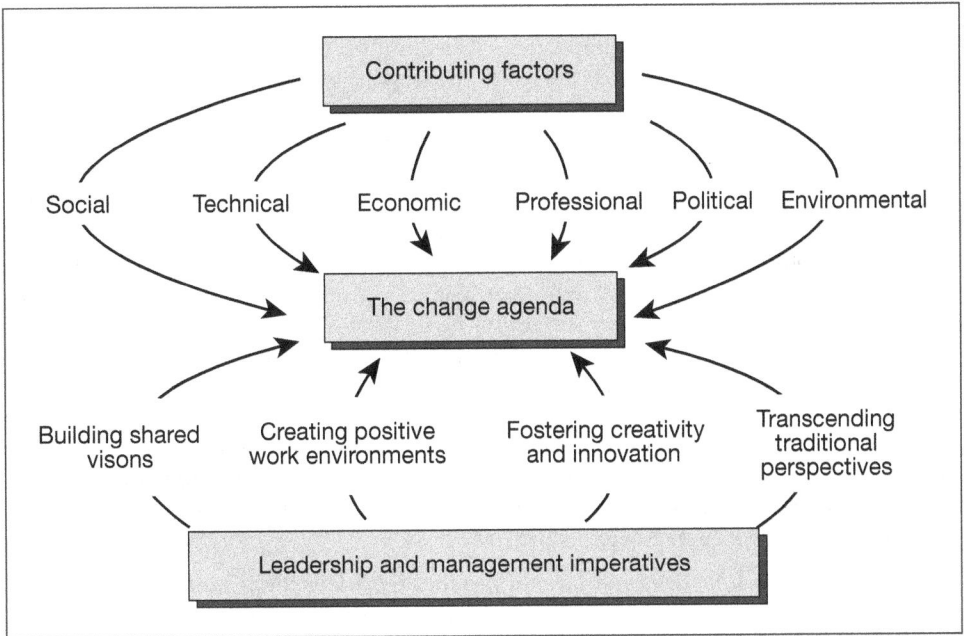

FIGURE 1.1

Critical leadership and management imperatives

However, it is suggested here that one of the most important elements of visioning is the building of shared visions; that is, creating a 'common mental model' (Pearce & Ensley, 2004) of future states that have 'buy-in' from all relevant staff and/or external stakeholders. Senge (1990) suggests that leadership is really about people working at their best to create the future. Without 'buy-in' even the best vision may never become reality. Shared visions facilitate 'buy-in' and are linked to team potency, teamwork behaviours, and team performance, staff satisfaction and staff performance (Gang, In-Sue, Stephen, & Amy, 2011; Jing, Avery, & Bergsteiner, in press; Pearce & Ensley, 2004). Thus a crucial challenge for nurse leaders and managers is to be able to work 'top down' as well as 'bottom up' to define the way forward. Being able to foster an 'our' attitude; for example, 'our' reputation, 'our' organisation, 'our' service, will be an important part of creating and maintaining system-wide continuity of quality care in the face of significant challenges.

Creating positive work environments

From the above discussion it is clear that the creation and maintenance of positive work environments, as characterised by the Bennis and Nanus (1985) concept of a social architecture that provides meaning for employees, will be another significant challenge for nurse leaders and managers. Among other things, this will require, indeed demand, a deep understanding of and abiding respect for others. Respect is often treated as a vague and implied characteristic of leadership, but Clarke (2011) describes it as 'A set of judgments relating to the perceived worthiness, ethical behaviors and shared values that exist between leader and follower'. According to Tornabeni (2001), this is what empowers the building of teams, in her view 'the essential task faced by leaders' (p. 9). Barbara Perra (2001) echoes this sentiment and goes further to highlight the importance of the leader's reflection on their own personal and professional values and sense of self. She puts the view that leaders and managers will only be able to 'reach out to develop trusting and respectful relationships with staff, peers and administrators' (p. 70) when they are working from a firm base of personal values that are not in conflict with those of the organisation.

Leadership can be seen as the practice of 'small actions that can engage or alienate, or nourish or deplete those around us' (Kerfoot, 2001, p. 42). Jack Welch said, 'What we are building is fragile. It's built on trust. The process can be set back in a heartbeat by people at any level who see leadership as a process of intimidation, whose own lack of esteem makes them unable to trust and let go' (cited in Lewin & Regine, 2000, p. 305). Leaders and managers need to actively cultivate and finely hone the skills of 'listening more, asking more and talking less' (Tornabeni, 2001, p. 10), thereby allowing leaders to add value to their followers (Maxwell, 2007 cited in Boone & Makhani, 2012). Human beings do not react like machines. With the ever-increasing pace of change in our personal and professional lives, staff are likely to be more demanding in terms of work environments that meet their needs efficiently and effectively. In the words of Kerfoot (2001):

> We are leading a journey, not an end product. This journey is better led by a structure that allows everyone to contribute his/her talents to the fullest rather than the leader providing all the direction. The ability to connect with people and to engage their spirit in the noble adventure of patient care is what really matters (p. 74).

Fostering creativity and innovation

Creativity is essential for the generation of ideas, options and solutions. According to Bunkers (1999, p. 28), the capacity to 'create new order' is one of the four major capacities that are the hallmarks of futuristic leaders. This capacity encompasses the ability to see relationships between unrelated parts or, in other words, relevance and fit between things that have not previously been connected together. Implicit within this is the capacity for systems thinking, described by Senge (1990) as the ability to see the big picture and analyse how things work from a systems perspective. Having a systems understanding facilitates the anticipation and identification of unintended consequences from changes in one or more parts of the system. An important and related skill is that of critical thinking and analysis. Critical analysis enables an individual to see patterns and trends in seemingly unrelated heterogeneous events, thus bringing order to the decision-making process (Alderman, 2001, p. 47). Not accepting things at face value, being prepared to ask critical questions, challenging assumptions, clarifying conflicting ideas and pursuing the 'what if?' possibilities are essential skills for leaders and managers to develop.

From a nursing perspective, Gilmartin (1999) makes the point that, although a common wisdom exists that nurses are creative when it comes to finding solutions for patient care problems, nursing service has been delivered historically within bureaucratic structures characterised by conformity and regimentation designed to support production efficiency. She comments further that 'in the new era of knowledge-based organisations, responsive strategic actions are driven by imaginative yet feasible solutions that are driven by those who carry out the organisation's primary work' (p. 4). There is a natural tendency for people to continue to do things in older, more traditional and comfortable ways, especially as increasing energy is required to deal with the ongoing pace of the change agenda. However, the ability to see challenges and opportunities in doing old things in new ways can be a path to personal success, as well as a means to contribute to improved methods of care (Tushman & O'Reilly, 1997). A significant challenge for nursing leaders and managers will be to capitalise effectively on the opportunities to 'tap into' the collective wisdom that exists among staff members and promote an environment where new ideas and fresh approaches are valued. This will require risk taking as well as creativity. But without the courage to take risks, to 'push the envelope' or try new things, organisational change will not occur and visions will not be realised. The willingness to take risks requires courage and the willingness to persist, particularly in the face of adversity or lack of progress. This will never be easy, but 'entering courageously life's turning points' (Bunkers, 1999, p. 28) is an essential attribute for contemporary nurse leaders and managers to cultivate and promote.

Transcending traditional perspectives

According to Kerfoot (2001):

> *Effective leaders do not engage themselves in struggles with others. They move out of the control mode and into one of adaptation and change. Their success lies in the ability to clearly specify the outcomes needed, and to nourish and coach others to achieve these outcomes . . . Effective leaders do not try to force people into roles in which they don't fit. They know when to let go (p. 42).*

One of the issues highlighted by this statement is what can, arguably, be seen as a fundamental distinction between transformational and transactional leadership. Theories of transformational leadership became popular during the 1980s and 1990s as a result of work by people such as Bass (1985), Bennis and Nanus (1985), Kouzes and Posner (1987) and Tichy (1986). In essence, the transformational leader is someone who can motivate others to perform to their full capacity by influencing a change in perceptions and by providing a sense of direction. The notion of performance beyond expectations is a hallmark of transformational leadership. Transactional leadership, on the other hand, is about 'getting the job done'. Transactional leaders identify what needs to be done, and work within the existing culture to ensure that it gets done. Expectations of performance, performance outcomes, contingent reward and management by exception are hallmarks of transactional leadership (Hargis, Watt, & Piotrowski, 2011).

In a similar fashion, Fedoruk and Pincombe (2000) distinguish between the traditional views of leadership and management, and make the point that the 'old (managerialist, bureaucratically oriented) competencies required of a nurse executive are no longer appropriate for a constantly changing environment driven by competing demands' (p. 6). They go on to suggest that 'the nurse executive has to coalesce the technical demands of a management with the visionary dimensions of leadership if nursing is to survive into the next century as a discrete entity' (p. 7).

There is increasing evidence that highlights the role of transformational leadership in terms of achieving positive outcomes (Cummings et al., 2010; Jacobs et al., 2013). However, in a brief overview of transformational and transactional leadership, Huber (2014) states that 'the transactional leader is more common' (p. 14). The healthcare organisation of the future will be very different from the institutional models in existence today. It is likely that, in the future, healthcare service delivery will be described within vertically integrated systems embracing primary care, home health, long-term health and related components of the healthcare continuum (Shortell,

Gillies, Anderson, Mitchell, & Morgan, 1993). These and other changes will provide important windows of opportunity for nurses in terms of leadership and management. However, in capitalising on these opportunities, a significant challenge for nurse leaders and managers of the future will be to transcend traditional, perhaps more comfortable, ways of thinking and doing in order to move forward with a reflective understanding about what will work best and the courage to make it happen. 'Letting go' is never easy, but the rewards that can potentially be realised through reconfiguring old leadership and management practices to more contemporary integrated approaches will make it worthwhile.

BECOMING A LEADER AND MANAGER

Understanding the difference between leading and managing

The terms 'leader' and 'manager' are often seen as synonymous and used interchangeably in role descriptions. This concept conveys the notion that if one is managing, then one is leading, and vice versa. The popular literature and some conference speakers often use a rather simplistic description by referring to leadership as dealing with people and management as dealing with paper. Although not critical in its approach, this paradigm is a beginning point from which to understand the differences between the two terms.

In the nursing context, the leader is a visionary with a concentration of time and effort who looks outward to how the unit, organisation or profession can go forward. The day-to-day organisation therefore becomes the domain of the manager. Excellence in leadership requires one to see above the plethora of paper, policies and procedures required to maintain the functionality of the workplace. A leader needs to be a negotiator with a broader worldview about how the area of responsibility will grow and develop within overall bureaucratic influences. Often the two roles must be complementary, depending on the size of an organisation. However, without a clear focus, a potential leader can end up spending valuable time dealing with details that should really be delegated. This means that they can never break free of day-to-day responsibilities to provide the staff with the vision and direction essential to maintain a high quality of patient care.

To further emphasise this point, Tappen, Weiss, and Whitehead (2001) indicate that one does not need to be a manager to be a leader—even the most novice practitioner, given the right opportunities, can assume this role.

Knowing oneself as a leader and manager

Paramount to the attainment of any leadership or management role is the ability to be in tune with oneself, or, as stated by Goleman (1998, p. 318), to have 'emotional self-awareness'. Despite the above simplistic view of 'paper versus people', all our business involves dealing with people, to a greater or lesser extent. It can be argued that if a role requires you to organise staff and deal with people with a plurality of values, then one firstly needs to have developed an insight into one's emotions and feelings—especially in a conflict situation. This is not to imply the need to undertake psychoanalysis, but rather the need to have a sense of one's strengths and shortcomings. This insight will foster a proactive approach, rather than being reactive to differing opinions as policies and programs are implemented.

The demands of managers and leaders are ever-increasing and self-knowledge about the issues that drive you, and how you respond to others, is important. It is erroneous to think that you have two personas—one for your personal life and the other for your professional life. While many nurses in leadership and management roles claim that they are different people at work compared with at home, one needs to recognise the basic constructs of one's make-up and use this self-awareness to manage situations and lead people. The attainment of 'emotional intelligence' has become an important issue. It refers to 'the capacity for recognising our own feelings and those of others, for motivating ourselves and for managing emotions well in ourselves and in our relationships' (Goleman, 1998, p. 317). This concept applies equally in one's personal and professional life.

Essential knowledge for leaders and managers

To be effective in either a leadership or managerial role one needs to look beyond the pragmatics of nursing care delivery. Effective nurse leaders and managers need to move from a comfort zone of what one has acquired and learned through education and clinical experience. They need to be able to deal with high technology changes, rapid throughput of patients, high intensity environments and ever-changing government policy. It is essential to the role for managers and leaders to be able to make good business decisions based on an understanding of bureaucratic structures. Effective nurse leaders and managers need to be able to internalise and practise skilled application of 'knowledge work'—cognitive activity, analysis of information and application of specialised expertise in problem solving, teaching and creation of new ideas or products (Huber, 2000, p. 144).

Skill elements for leaders and managers

While it is necessary to acquire a base level of operational knowledge as described above, it is also paramount to acquire or enhance skills to convey management and leadership concepts. Three essential skills include:

- ▲ an ability to communicate decisions and visions to individuals and groups. This is a hallmark of being able to influence peers and others (Huber, 2000, p. 202);
- ▲ an ability to discipline oneself regarding time management—working at a fast pace may not equate to achieving a great deal (Tappen et al., 2001, p. 76); and
- ▲ an ability to deal with stress by setting personal and professional goals, establishing priorities, practising good health habits and relaxation techniques, improving self-esteem by obtaining necessary skills and using support systems (Marriner Tomey, 2000, p. 27).

Personality traits of leaders and managers

Ineffective managers and leaders are a composite of their habits. Habits are unconscious patterns that express our character, and in the demanding role of quality management, negative traits will not inspire others to follow or be directed. To become effective within and outside an organisation one needs to develop or acquire traits that will result in positive outcomes. Personal traits that others need to acquire will enable one to demonstrate mutual respect, connection, praise and public acknowledgement of colleagues' contributions. In a five-year study of successful leaders and their followers, Bennis (1984, quoted in Hersey et al., 2013) identified four traits found in all the leaders: management of attention, meaning, trust and self.

THE LEADERSHIP ROLE

The function of leadership

In nursing today it is becoming evident that autocratic leadership no longer brings staff together to share a common vision. Nursing leaders need to build and develop others to realise their greatest achievement. Grossman and Valiga (2000) argue that leaders need to focus on people, have a long-range perspective, develop innovative ideas and be able to generate a power base from knowledge and credibility to motivate others.

Developing leadership potential

As outlined by Covey (1992), many people live their lives with unused potential and are thus not as effective as they might be. Leaders need to develop the full potential in others, looking for approaches to assist people to improve themselves. Developing potential in others in a nursing context entails building self-directed working teams and mentoring others (Bower, 2000).

Modelling leadership behaviour

Nurse leaders need to model behaviour that others wish to emulate. Displayed behaviour that is deemed to be negative or that lacks credibility will cause others to withdraw. Behaviour and reputation clearly demonstrating that one is supportive and willing to listen, will attract people to you and assist them to grow and develop. Decision-making behaviour is a common expectation of nursing leadership, along with the personal qualities of approachability. Leaders who appear unable to make decisions can look ineffective in a situation where an organisation or set of circumstances demands attention. Wheeler (cited in Bower, 2000, p. 207) suggests further that leaders demonstrating proactive decision-making behaviour are more effective when possessing 'the ability to anticipate the "event" so they act before'. A final recommendation for a potential leader is to avoid becoming known as someone who managed everything, but led nothing.

Encouraging self-assessment for leadership

Self-assessment can be used to monitor one's own actions or behaviour and those of others. In the previous section, the issue of knowing oneself was discussed and remains an important consideration when asking others to undertake self-assessment. Leaders must be confident enough to disclose their own personal weaknesses. Staff will also be less defensive if they are allowed to express their feelings and concerns regarding their own performance, rather than being told of any shortcomings they may have. Leaders in nursing need to also assist others to recognise any perceived weakness when they lack insight. Credibility when facilitating this process will be enhanced if you are prepared to share how you have overcome difficulties in similar circumstances. This approach will not only enhance the development of others but also create an environment that fosters self-assessment.

Delegation to develop leadership potential

Leaders within nursing need to take opportunities to practise delegation. A common reaction to the notion of delegation is to assume that the leader cannot do, or does not want to do, a particular activity. As stated by Arnold (in Bower, 2000, p. 291), 'Delegation is another form of letting go—it means passing a task from yourself to another'. The manner in which this 'passing' is conducted is very important. A model that creates a positive response can be summarised as follows: when delegating, a leader needs to demonstrate that they have the ability to do the task themselves. The person to whom the activity is delegated needs to be able to undertake this responsibility knowing that the leader is available for support. Once the delegate feels confident in the activity, then they only need to report the outcomes to the leader. This approach can only strengthen the leadership role.

CASE STUDY

Building trust and confidence

Deborah was a senior nurse with a long track record of successful management in an intensive care unit. A new staff member, Jeanette, had noticed that a nursing student on clinical placement from the local university was acting in an unprofessional manner towards a patient. Jeanette raised the issue with Deborah and they agreed that the manner of the nursing student was inappropriate. They both counselled the student, the behaviour was recognised and undertakings were made by the student not to repeat the behaviour.

When Deborah and Jeanette met after the meeting with the student, Jeanette expressed admiration that the issue had been resolved and thanked Deborah for her support in dealing with this difficult situation.

A week later Deborah was summoned to the Director of Clinical Services' office to be informed that Jeanette had made a complaint about her regarding the manner in which she had dealt with the nursing student incident. Deborah was discouraged by this event, wondering why Jeanette had not brought this issue to her directly and why the Director of Clinical Services had not, at the very least, held a three-way meeting to discuss this issue in person.

CONCLUSION

This chapter has presented an overview of leadership and management theories and concepts underpinning current understandings of complex organisations. It has provided an overview of how such organisations interact with their environments and examined some of the challenges and issues impacting upon healthcare organisations. Finally, we looked at some of the essential requirements needed to become an effective leader and manager.

We argued it is important for organisations to clearly understand and evaluate both their internal and external social, economic, political, technological and professional environments. Because of the pace and complexity of change experienced by healthcare organisations, these issues raise critical questions for nurse leaders and managers with respect to the deployment of scarce resources, and the recruitment and retention of competent staff.

REFLECTIVE EXERCISE

1. Reflect on leaders and managers that have had a positive influence on your nursing practice or your nursing career.
   a. Reflect on why and how they influenced you.
   b. Consider these attributes and compare them with your own.

   The exercise will help you to develop a template to further develop additional skills, attitudes and knowledge and to recognise potential areas for development in the leadership and management role.

2. Discuss the leadership issues and concerns in the case study above regarding the way in which the Director of Clinical Services dealt with this situation.

3. Comment on the appropriateness of a new staff member, Jeanette, going directly to the Director and circumventing Deborah.

4. If you were Deborah describe how you would react in a similar situation.

5. Reconstruct the case study to result in a more positive leadership outcome.

6. Outline what can be learned from this case study regarding leadership behaviour.

Recommended Readings

Bower, F. (2000). *Nurses taking the lead: Personal qualities of effective leadership.* Philadelphia: W. B. Saunders.

Covey, S. (1992). *Principle-centered leadership: Strategies for personal and professional effectiveness.* New York: Simon & Schuster.

Porter-O'Grady, T. (1997). Quantum mechanics and the future of healthcare leadership. *Journal of Nursing Administration, 27,* 15–20.

References

ABS. (2013). *4102.0—Australian social trends.* Canberra: Australian Bureau of Statistics.

AIHW. (2012). *Nursing and midwifery workforce, 2011.* National health workforce series no. 2. Cat. no. HWL 48. Canberra: Australian Institute of Health and Welfare.

AIHW. (2013). *Nursing and midwifery workforce, 2012.* National health workforce series. Canberra: Australian Institute of Health and Welfare.

Aiken, L. H., Sloane, D. M., Bruyneel, L., Van den Heede, K., & Sermeus, W. (2013). Nurses' reports of working conditions and hospital quality of care in 12 countries in Europe. *International Journal of Nursing Studies, 50*(2), 143–153.

Alderman, M. C. (2001). Nursing in the new millennium: Challenges and opportunities. *Dermatology Nursing, 13*(1), 44–49.

Argyris, C. (1964). *Integrating the individual and the organization.* New York: John Wiley and Sons.

Bass, B. M. (1985). *Leadership and performance beyond expectations.* New York: Free Press.

Bennis, W., & Nanus, B. (1985). *Leaders: The strategies for taking charge.* New York: Harper & Row.

Biscoe, G., & Lewis, B. (1996). *Strategic planning.* Geneva: World Health Organization.

Boone, L. W., & Makhani, S. (2012). Five necessary attitudes of a servant leader. *Review of Business, 33*(1), 83–96.

Bower, F. (2000). *Nurses taking the lead: Personal qualities of effective leadership.* Philadelphia: W. B. Saunders.

Bunkers, S. S. (1999). Emerging discoveries and possibilities in nursing. *Nursing Science Quarterly, 12*(1), 26–31.

Burns, L., Bradley, E., & Weiner, B. (2012). The management challenge of delivering value in health care: Global and U.S. perspectives. In L. Burns, E. Bradley, & B. Weiner (Eds.), *Shortell and Kaluzny's health care management: Organization design and behavior* (6th ed.). New York: Delmar Cengage Learning.

Capowski, G. (1994). Where are the leaders of tomorrow? *Management Review, 83*(3), 10–17.

Cartwright, T., & Baldwin, D. (2007). Seeing your way: Why leaders must communicate their visions. *Leadership in Action, 27*(3), 15–24.

Chan, Z. C. Y., Tam, W. S., Lung, M. K. Y., Wong, W. Y., & Chau, C. W. (2013). A systematic literature review of nurse shortage and the intention to leave. *Journal of Nursing Management, 21*(4), 605–613.

Clarke, N. (2011). An integrated conceptual model of respect in leadership. *Leadership Quarterly, 22*(2), 316–327.

Collyer, F., & White, K. (2011). The privatisation of Medicare and the National Health Service, and the global marketisation of healthcare systems. *Health Sociology Review, 20*(3), 238–244.

Covey, S. (1992). *Principle-centered leadership: Strategies for personal and professional effectiveness.* New York: Simon & Schuster.

Cummings, G. G., MacGregor, T., Davey, M., Lee, H., Wong, C. A., Lo, E., et al. (2010). Leadership styles and outcome patterns for the nursing workforce and work environment: A systematic review. *International Journal of Nursing Studies, 47*(3), 363–385.

Daft, R. L. (1998). *Organisational theory and design* (6th ed.). Ohio: South-Western.

DiMaggio, P., & Powell, W. W. (1983). The iron cage revisited; Institutional isomorphism and collective rationality in organizational fields. *American Sociological Review, 48*, 147–160.

Ellis, B., & Brockbank, B. K. (1993). Changing competition in health care marketing: A method for analysis and strategic planning. *Health Marketing Quarterly, 10*, 5–22.

Fayol, H. (1925). *General and industrial management.* London: Pittman and Sons.

Fedoruk, M., & Pincombe, J. (2000). The nurse executive: Challenges for the 21st century. *Journal of Nursing Management, 8*(1), 13–20.

Follett, M. P. (1926). The giving of orders. In H. C. Metcalf (Ed.), *Scientific foundations of business administration.* Baltimore: William and Wilkins.

Gang, W., In-Sue, O., Stephen, C., & Amy, C. (2011). Transformational leadership and performance across criteria and levels: A meta-analytic review of 25 years of research. *Group & Organization Management, 36*(2), 223–270.

Gantz, N. R., Sherman, R., Jasper, M., Choo, C. G., Herrin-Griffith, D., & Harris, K. (2012). Global nurse leader perspectives on health systems and workforce challenges. *Journal of Nursing Management, 20*(4), 433–443.

Gilmartin, M. J. (1999). Creativity: The fuel of innovation. *Nursing Administration Quarterly, 23*(2), 1–8.

Goffee, R., Scheele, N., & Pitman, B. (2000). Send out the right signals. *People Management, 8*(21), 32–36.

Goleman, D. (1998). *Working with emotional intelligence.* London: Bloomsbury.

Graham, E., & Duffield, C. (2010). An ageing nursing workforce. *Australian Health Review, 34*(1), 44–48.

Grossman, S., & Valiga, T. (2000). *The new leadership challenge: Creating the future of nursing.* Philadelphia: F.A. Davis.

Gulick, L. (1937). Notes on the theory of the organization. In L. Gulick & L. Urwick (Eds.), *Papers on the science of administration* (pp. 3–13). New York: Institute of Public Administration.

Hannan, M., & Freeman, J. (1977). The population ecology of organisations. *American Journal of Sociology, 82,* 929–964.

Hargis, M. B., Watt, J. D., & Piotrowski, C. (2011). Developing leaders: Examining the role of transactional and transformational leadership across business contexts. *Organization Development Journal, 29*(3), 51–66.

Hersey, P., Blanchard, K., & Johnson, D. (2013). *Management of organizational behavior: Leading human resources* (10th ed.). Boston: Pearson.

Holland, P., Allen, B., & Cooper, B. (2012). *What nurses want: Analysis of the first national survey on nurses' attitudes to work and work conditions in Australia.* Melbourne, Vic: Department of Management, Monash University.

Huber, D. (2000). *Leadership and nursing care management* (2nd ed.). Philadelphia: W. B. Saunders.

Huber, D. (2014). Leadership and management principles. In D. Huber (Ed.), *Leadership and nursing care management* (pp. 1–36). Missouri: Elsevier.

Ireland, R., & Hill, M. A. (1992). Achieving and maintaining strategic competitiveness in the 21st century: The role of strategic leadership. *Academy of Management Executive, 13*(1), 43–57.

Jacobs, C., Pfaff, H., Lehner, B., Driller, E., Nitzsche, A., Stieler-Lorenz, B., et al. (2013). The influence of transformational leadership on employee well-being. *Journal of Occupational & Environmental Medicine, 55*(7), 772–778.

Jing, F., Avery, G., & Bergsteiner, H. (in press). Enhancing performance in small professional firms through vision communication and sharing. *Asia Pacific Journal of Management, 30*(1).

Kerfoot, K. (2001). Leading from the inside out. *Dermatology Nursing, 13*(1), 42–43.

Kohles, J. C., Bligh, M. C., & Carsten, M. K. (2012). A follower-centric approach to the vision integration process. *The Leadership Quarterly, 23*(3), 476–487.

Kouzes, J. M., & Posner, B. Z. (1987). *The leadership challenge: How to get extraordinary things done in organisations.* San Francisco: Jossey-Bass.

Lewin, R., & Regine, B. (2000). *The soul at work. Listen. Respond. Let go.* New York: Simon and Schuster.

Lloyd, P., & Boyce, R. A. (1998). Management theory and practice. In M. Clinton & D. Scheiwe (Eds.), *Management in the Australian health care industry* (2nd ed., pp. 140–171). Melbourne: Longman.

Marquis, B., & Huston, C. (2012). *Leadership roles and management functions in nursing: Theory and application.* Philadelphia: Wolters Kluwer Health/Lippincott Williams & Wilkins.

Marriner Tomey, A. (2000). *Guide to nursing management and leadership* (6th ed.). St. Louis: Mosby.

Mayo, E. (1953). *The human problems of an industrialized civilization.* New York: MacMillan.

McGregor, D. (1960). *The human side of enterprise.* New York: McGraw-Hill.

Pearce, C. L., & Ensley, M. D. (2004). A reciprocal and longitudinal investigation of the innovation process: The central role of shared vision in product and process innovation teams (PPITs). *Journal of Organizational Behavior, 25*(2), 259–278.

Perra, B. (2001). Leadership: The key to quality outcomes. *Journal of Nursing Care Quality, 15*(2), 68.

Powell, W. W., & DiMaggio, P. (1991). *The new institutionalism in organisational analysis.* Chicago: Chicago University Press.

Sampson, E. E., & Marthas, M. (1990). *Group process for the health professions* (3rd ed.). New York: Delmar.

Senge, P. (1990). *The fifth discipline: The art and practice of the learning organization.* New York: Doubleday.

Shortell, S. M., Gillies, R. R., Anderson, D. A., Mitchell, J. B., & Morgan, K. L. (1993). Creating organised delivery systems: The barriers and the facilitators. *Hospital and Health Services Administration, 38*(4), 447–466.

Shortell, S. M., & Kaluzny, A. D. (1997). Organization theory and health services management. In S. M. Shortell & A. D. Kaluzny (Eds.), *Essentials of health care management*. New York: Delmar.

Stout-Shaffer, S., & Larrabee, J. (1992). Everyone can be a visionary leader. *Nursing Management, 23*(12), 54–58.

Tappen, R., Weiss, S., & Whitehead, D. (2001). *Essentials of nursing leadership and management* (2nd ed.). Philadelphia: F.A. Davis.

Taylor, F. W. (1911). *The principles of scientific management*. New York: Harper & Row.

Tichy, N. M., & Devanna, M. A. (1986). *The transformational leader*. New York: Wiley & Sons.

Tornabeni, J. (2001). The competency game: My take on what it really takes to lead. *Nursing Administration Quarterly, 25*(4), 1–13.

Tranbarger, R. (1988). The nurse executive in a community hospital. In M. Johnson (Ed.), *Series on Nursing Administration* (Vol. 1). Menlo Park, CA: Addison-Wesley.

Tushman, M. L., & O'Reilly, C. A., III (1997). *Winning through innovation: A practical guide to leading organisational change and renewal*. Boston: Harvard Business Press.

Vaill, P. (1989). *Management as a performing art*. San Francisco: Jossey Bass.

Walston, S., & Chou, A. (2012). Strategic thinking and achieving competitive advantage. In L. Burns, E. Bradley, & B. Weiner (Eds.), *Shortell & Kaluzny's health care management: Organization design and behavior* (6th ed.). New York: Delmar Cengage Learning.

Weber, M. (1978). *Wirtschaft und Gesellschaft (Economy and society: an outline of interpretive sociology)* (G. Roth & C. Wittich, Trans.) Berkeley: University of California Press. (Original work published 1922).

Yoder-Wise, P. S. (1999). *Leading and managing in nursing* (2nd ed.). St Louis: Mosby.

CHAPTER TWO

Psychological influences on leadership style

Sandra Speedy

LEARNING OBJECTIVES

At the completion of this chapter, the reader will be able to:

▲ gain an overview of the research literature relating to personality as it influences leadership;

▲ be aware of the various factors which influence personality style in relation to leadership behaviour;

▲ consider the role of social, emotional and spiritual intelligence as it impacts on leadership capacity;

▲ understand the role conflict plays in the workplace, and strategies leaders can employ to effectively deal with these; and

▲ consider the potential for gender differences in leadership.

KEY WORDS

Personality, self-efficacy, introversion-extroversion, locus of control, Machiavellianism, self-monitoring, emotional competence

INTRODUCTION

Leadership in professional situations requires a foundation of knowledge and skills that is influenced by a diverse range of factors. These factors include the personalities of leaders, their psychological characteristics and make-up, and the situation or context in which leadership and managerial style is manifest. The type of leadership style adopted by the leader will be influential in determining how effective the leader is. Thus, this chapter examines, in some detail, a range of these characteristics and their influence. It also considers how such characteristics will determine how leaders deal with conflict, and how leaders can enhance their communication techniques to be maximally effective. Finally, the question of differing styles of leadership according to gender is briefly explored. Readers are also referred to Chapter 3 of this text, which addresses gender, politics and power in the context of leadership.

A historical review of the leadership literature can be found in general management texts and will not be provided here (see, for example, Daft, 2008; McShane & Glinow, 2012; Robbins & Coulter, 2013; Robbins & Judge, 2010). Generally, however, researchers have constructed a range of theories to explain their views of leadership, including trait theory, behavioural theories, reward and punishment theory, situational contingency theories, path–goal theory, and attribution theory, to name just a few (Scouller, 2011).

Some theorists have questioned whether leadership itself is a useful concept at all. This has arisen from the question of whether 'followership' explains leadership effectiveness, suggesting that the relationship between the follower and leader impacts on both and has enduring effects (Bass & Bass, 2009; Hughes, Ginnett, & Curphy, 2011; Grossman & Valiga, 2008). Kupers (2007) adds that 'integral' wise leadership and followers can enhance the development of individuals, teams and organisations (and their various dimensions) (p. 213). Whatever explanations for effective leadership are provided, two vital factors require our focus: the people interacting and being, and the situation or context in which behaviour occurs. This is why this chapter focuses on the role of personality and intelligence, and the way in which personality influences a leader's capacity to handle conflict constructively in the professional setting.

First let us consider a typology of leadership styles that takes a macro-view of leader characteristics within particular contexts. These leadership styles have been described as autocratic, bureaucratic, participative and laissez-faire (Mullins, 2010; Oforchukwu, 2011). In the autocratic style, leader behaviours range from the 'do as I say or else' style to the paternalistic style of 'father/mother knows best'. When leaders have this style, subordinates are left with little freedom and autonomy and no opportunity to participate in problem solving or decision making. The advantages of this style are its appropriateness in emergency or crisis situations, since it is the most efficient way to get action. It is also useful when subordinates have low tolerance for ambiguity, are immature or insecure. The disadvantages include the lack of allowance for personal growth and development of potential because it assumes there is no likelihood of this happening; it places great responsibility on the leader, who must be competent and knowledgeable in every situation.

The bureaucratic style, on the other hand, requires the leader to tell subordinates what to do, but in a way that is 'by the book'. Procedure and policy manuals, rules and regulations support the bureaucrat. There are certain advantages in this style because technically it guarantees consistency in the performance of procedures, in the treatment of personnel and in setting standards. The disadvantages include the lack of recourse when common sense dictates that there should be an exception to the rule. This can result in a feeling of frustration because of what some people refer to as 'red tape'. Furthermore, if rules are ambiguous, productivity decreases, morale drops and subordinates may become frustrated and resentful.

The participative leadership style allows subordinates to take part in problem solving and decision making. This style can range from democratic involvement to simple consultation. Its advantage is that it allows staff to feel committed to implementing a decision they help to make, and provides the opportunity for creativity. The disadvantages include that decision making can take a long time; it may not result in effective and efficient attainment of goals; and that participation may be compromised by group pressures and dynamics so that the decision is 'watered down' to the lowest common denominator (Mullins, 2010; Robbins & Judge, 2010).

Typically, a leader who uses the laissez-faire style sets the goal to be achieved, provides the rules of the game, and becomes accessible to the group for guidance and clarification if and when required. The advantages of this style are that it allows for full utilisation of the talents and energies of group members who have been delegated full responsibility for decision making and problem solving. The disadvantages include a high level of risk because the leader must have thorough knowledge of the level of competence and personal integrity of group members in order for this mode of leadership to be successful. Note that there is no recognition of the potential for followership within these leadership styles (Mullins, 2010).

PERSONALITY AND LEADERSHIP

There are several factors considered to shape leadership functioning and style. Researchers have established relationships between personality and key aspects of organisational behaviour, including leadership and managerial style (Robbins & Judge, 2010). While different situations may require different styles of leadership (as indicated above), there are also other influential factors, including age, heredity, social conditioning, gender, marital status, ethical principles, moral perspective, seniority in the organisation, intellectual abilities, values, physical abilities, the ability/job fit and the culture of the organisation.

Personality refers to the unique and relatively stable patterns of behaviour, thoughts and emotions shown by individuals; that is, their profile, which creates the uniqueness of a person. These are responsible for how we behave in our professional settings, because they affect the way we interact with others, and the situations encountered. While personality is generally persistent and resistant to change, it can be shaped by external pressures and may therefore vary across situations. Behaviour, however, is the result of personality and the nature of the situation experienced, known as an interactionist perspective of organisational behaviour (Ivancevich, Konopaske, & Matteson, 2008).

Personality traits

Much research has gone into what determines personality and how it is expressed (Furnham, 2012). This includes personality traits such as being shy, aggressive, lazy or ambitious. Research suggests that personality traits must be considered in their situational context (Vroom & Jago, 2007). A whole range of personality traits is said to exist; for example, in charismatic or transformational leaders, or effective managers. Another aspect is the personality type, such as extroversion, in which people attend to the world of objects, people or external ideas, or introversion, when people focus on inner thoughts, feelings and ideas. Extroverts are generally considered effective salespeople, public relations professionals and teachers, while introverts are more likely to be research scientists, academics or librarians (Robbins & Coulter, 2012).

The 'Big Five' personality dimensions

Another theory is that there are five dimensions of personality, sometimes referred to as the 'Big Five' personality dimensions (Greenberg & Baron, 2008; Hughes et al., 2011; McAdams & Pals, 2006; McCrae & Costa, 2008). These include: introversion and extroversion, agreeableness, conscientiousness, emotional stability and openness to experience.

Research has found that conscientiousness is a good predictor of work performance in all types of jobs; emotional stability, however, is not related to performance and extroversion is highly related to job success for people in managerial and sales positions (Robbins & Coulter, 2013). The history of research, the development of theory and studies which seek to clarify all aspects of personality (including the Big Five dimensions) makes fascinating reading (see Barrick, Parks, & Mount, 2005; Block, 2010; McCrae & Costa, 2005; Wiggins, 1996). Readers are encouraged to explore these.

As a predictor of behaviours at work, the 'Big Five' model has received some endorsement from researchers in recent years, although some disagreement exists. The research literature suggests that while the 'Big Five' structure has created remarkable consensus among psychologists, there is no particular theory to account for or support its existence. Some suggest that the 'Big Five' model needs to be expanded to include an increase of factors to adequately describe all aspects of personality. The debate continues.

Myers-Briggs personality types

Another theoretical approach, known as the Myers-Briggs approach, is derived from the work of analyst Carl Jung, as well as Myers and Briggs. It is a system that describes different patterns of behaviour based on personality differences, all of which affect and determine how we function in the world. This approach suggests that we are born with four preferred ways of behaving, each having an opposite 'preference'. These include:

▲ extraversion/introversion (E) and (I), which refers to how we focus our attention and what gives us energy;

▲ 'becoming aware', which refers to sensing (S) and intuition (N), and indicates how we prefer to take in the information around us;

▲ ways of deciding, thinking (T) and feeling (F), which refers to how we evaluate information and make decisions; and

▲ the amount of control, judgement (J) and perception (P) we have, which refers to our lifestyle orientation (Robbins & Coulter, 2013).

With respect to this theory, personality 'style' has been shown to be a significant factor in the strategic decision making of leaders and managers. For example, 'sensing-feeling' types want hard data and are less willing to take risks; 'intuitive-feeling' types are more likely to make a decision without considering all facts in the situation; and 'intuitive-thinking' types test the logic of the decision and often require more hard data on which to base their decisions. As a leader with a preferred style, it is important to be aware of the strengths and limitations of that style, and take into account the needs of your followers in order that they work most effectively with you and you with them.

Exploration of the Myers-Briggs typology as an explanation of your personality can be an insightful exercise for those who hold nursing leadership positions, or who aspire to them (McGuiness, 2004; Tieger & Barron-Tieger, 2007).

Locus of control

Locus of control refers to the degree to which leaders believe they are in charge of their own fate and are able to affect their own lives. Leaders who believe they can control their own lives or their fate are said to have an 'internal orientation', as they demonstrate internal control. Those who believe that what happens to them is out of their control, or controlled by outside forces, are labelled as 'externals', having an external orientation.

Some interesting findings about the two types are that those who have an external locus of control are:

▲   less satisfied with their jobs;

▲   alienated and/or absent more often from work;

▲   less involved with work (due to the fact that they perceive they have less control over the organisation and their work life in general);

▲   more compliant and willing to follow directions; and

▲   need structure and routine (Robbins & Coulter, 2013).

Those who have an internal locus of control:

▲   are more likely to take responsibility for their behaviour;

▲   have lower absenteeism rates;

▲   can cope with higher levels of stress;

▲   hold higher-level jobs;

▲   are promoted more quickly; and

▲   are motivated to achieve and make greater attempts to control their environment (Robbins & Coulter, 2013).

It is important to note that if you want to be an effective nursing leader or want to develop others for nursing leadership roles, locus of control can be modified over time by individuals, and can be significantly enhanced by a supportive organisation. This can be done by using rewards and recognition for individual initiatives and performance, which can be related to individual performance.

Machiavellianism

Another personality attribute reputed to influence leadership style is Machiavellianism, named after Niccolo Machiavelli, an Italian philosopher, who wrote *The Prince* (1513), which addressed the acquisition and manipulation of power. He outlined a ruthless strategy for seizing and holding political power, which has been translated into a personality attribute useful for leaders who seek to control others. Machiavelli believed that people could be readily used or manipulated by applying a few basic rules, including:

▲   never show humility;

▲   be arrogant, as it is far more effective when dealing with others;

▲   moral values and ethics are for the weak;

▲   being free to lie, cheat and deceive, whenever it suits your purpose; and

▲   it is better to be feared than loved (Greenberg & Baron, 2008).

Machiavellianism is a measure of the degree to which people are pragmatic, maintain emotional distance and believe that 'the end justifies the means'; 'if it works, use it' is the approach, and may often be of questionable ethics and moral beliefs. So leaders who are high in Machiavellianism (known as 'high Machs') tend to manipulate others and 'win' more, are less persuaded by others, are pragmatic and emotionally distant, and have a greater influence over others than do 'low Machs'. They work best when there are a minimum number of rules and regulations, as they can improvise and be less constrained by existing rules (Ivancevich et al., 2008). Low Machs, on the other hand, tend to accept direction imposed by others in loosely structured situations, and work hard to perform well in highly structured situations.

High Machs can be very difficult to contend with in the work setting. It is wise to protect yourself and others from them by exposing them to others wherever possible, since they often get away with breaking promises or lying because their victims remain silent (typically because they may be too embarrassed to confess that they have been manipulated or cheated). Another strategy is to pay attention to what they do, not what they say: high Machs excel at deception. They often succeed in convincing others that they have others' best interests at heart, and are at their most convincing when they are busy cutting the ground out from under the unsuspecting person. If their actions suggest that they are cold-bloodedly manipulating the people around them, even while they loudly proclaim commitment to such principles as loyalty and fair play, chances are that they are Machiavellian in orientation and should be carefully avoided. Avoid situations that give high Machs an advantage; they prefer to operate in situations where emotions run high, in which others are uncertain of how to proceed. They know that under these conditions many people will be distracted and less likely to recognise that they are being manipulated for someone else's gain (Robbins & Coulter, 2013).

Rubin (1997) was one of the first researchers to take an interesting gender lens to Machiavellianism. She stated that women who are struggling to succeed in a man's world must learn that men and women are not equal, but that this difference should be viewed as a strength. They are encouraged to embrace conflict, establish their authority and vigorously pursue their own goals. In summary, women should claim what they want and deserve using passion, intuition, sensitivity and cunning—subtle weapons that women are reputed to have in abundance (Buchanan & Badham, 2008). This is in contrast to 'playing by the rules of the game'. Princessas, the female variant of the male, the Prince, therefore have to mark themselves as different from others (Rubin, 1997, pp. 12–17).

Self-esteem

Another factor that impacts on leadership style is level of self-esteem—the degree to which you like or dislike yourself, or the extent to which you have a positive or negative view of self. Those with low self-esteem are more likely to need others' approval, are less successful in job searches, and more likely to be dissatisfied with their job because they are not confident at solving problems that confront them (Robbins & Coulter, 2013).

Low self-esteem can be minimised by making people feel uniquely valuable, so that they recognise everyone has a special contribution to make. This encourages constructive ideas and behaviours. When people are appropriately praised and credited with their ideas and achievements they feel more competent, appreciated and accepted. This enhances feelings of empowerment, connectedness and belonging (Robbins & Coulter, 2013; Stern, 2010). Building and maintaining the self-esteem of nurses and patients can provide enormous pay-offs.

Self-monitoring

Self-monitoring refers to the ability to adjust behaviour to external, situational factors, thus requiring social perceptiveness. It has also been defined as sensitivity to social cues (Pierce & Newstrom, 2010). Those who are described as 'high self-monitors' are sensitive to external cues; they pay close attention to the behaviour of others and can modify their own behaviour readily if necessary (Barrick et al., 2005). In this way, they can present a public persona quite different from their private image of self.

High self-monitors are more successful in leadership and managerial roles when this requires a subset of multiple and even contradictory roles (Robbins & Coulter, 2013). High self-monitors are often very good communicators and effective in jobs that require 'boundary spanning'—communicating and interacting with different groups of people from different professional or occupational groups. They are also more likely to be effective at creating a favourable impression, having the capacity to conceal their true feelings when they consider it inappropriate to reveal them.

In addition, high self-monitors are often more concerned with others' feelings (Ivancevich et al., 2008). In conflict situations they therefore tend to find resolution through collaboration or compromise rather than through avoidance or competition. They tend to be more conciliatory in their approach, and more concerned with long-range solutions.

Low self-monitors cannot disguise their behaviour; they 'let it all hang out' and therefore will not conform to the situation in which they find themselves. They use their own moods and preferences to decide how to behave in any situation. Low self-monitors are more tolerant of unsatisfactory working conditions and less likely to think of resigning. In general, low self-monitors are less aware of, or less concerned about, their impact on others; they just act according to their inner feelings without changing them in each new context. This makes their behaviour quite predictable within specified situations (Robbins & Coulter, 2013).

Self-efficacy

Self-efficacy is the belief in one's own ability to perform a specific task well and can thus influence leadership style. It is a learned belief and is derived from life experiences, socialisation within the family group and/or treatment in the work setting (Ng, Sang, & Chan, 2008). High self-efficacy develops when specific tasks are performed with subsequent positive feedback on performance (Robbins & Coulter, 2013). People with high self-efficacy will respond to negative feedback with increased motivation and effort, while those with low self-efficacy will give up and reduce their efforts (Ivancevich et al., 2008). Nursing leaders need to be aware that training, constructive feedback, coaching and rewards for gradual improvement all increase levels of self-efficacy, while destructive feedback can reduce feelings of self-efficacy (Paglis, 2010).

Risk taking

Risk taking or willingness to gamble is another personality characteristic that is usually demonstrated in rapid decision making when all the information is not available to make that decision. This is probably not a characteristic that should be in abundance in leaders in certain types of organisations, such as nursing organisations. Share-broking firms, on the other hand, benefit from employing people comfortable with a high degree of risk taking.

THE ROLE OF MULTIPLE INTELLIGENCES

Emotional intelligence

An extensive review of the management and leadership literature reveals that intelligence and task competency is insufficient for optimal performance as a leader. Consequently, the concepts of emotional intelligence (EQ), and emotional capital were developed. In 1998, Goleman asserted that emotional competence mattered twice as much as cognitive ability (Goleman, 1998, p. 36). This is particularly so in the 'new workplace', with its emphasis on flexibility, teamwork and strong 'client' or service orientation. Goleman suggested that the higher one goes in the hierarchy of the organisation, the more important it is to have a high emotional intelligence score (Goleman, 1998, p. 39). Subsequent research using factor analysis calls into question Goleman's initial research (see Cherniss, 2010; Cherniss, Extein, Goleman, & Weissberg, 2006; Mayer, Salovey, & Caruso, 2004). Further research demonstrates the imperative for high-level emotional intelligence in nursing leaders to ensure safe environments exist (Hutchinson & Hurley, 2013). The implications for leaders in nursing and healthcare are obvious (Barron & Hurley, 2012).

Emotional competence has been defined as a learned capability based on emotional intelligence, which results in outstanding performance (Goleman, 1998). Our emotional competence indicates how much of our potential we translate into on-the-job capabilities. EQ, on the other hand, determines our potential for learning the practical skills that are based on its five elements, including self-awareness, motivation, self-regulation, empathy and adeptness in relationships.

In acknowledging the importance of EQ to managerial and leadership success, Goleman (1998) developed an emotional competence framework, comprising personal, cognitive and social competence (pp. 32–34), which has guided subsequent research. In terms of leadership, which results in inspiring and guiding individuals and groups, Goleman suggested that leaders with these competencies share a range of characteristics, including empathy, vision, a sense of mission, strategic thinking, proactive behaviour to guide others and leading by example (p. 217). Goleman also uses the term 'emotional incontinence' to refer to the leakage of destructive emotions from the top down, which results in sapping people's energy, often making them anxious, depressed and angry (1998, p. 221).

Later research has brought its detractors, claiming that the concept of emotional intelligence does not have adequate empirical support and is not consistent with cognitive neuroscience findings (Waterhouse, 2006). Nor has it met its initial promised potential in explaining aspects of personality (Locke, 2005; Matthews, Zeidner, & Roberts, 2012). However, this conclusion has been strongly refuted (Ashkanasy & Daus, 2005; Cherniss et al., 2006; Modassir & Singh, 2008). What this demonstrates is that emotional intelligence is still a developing theory and that further research is required.

Social intelligence

Gardner (1999) first mooted the notion of social intelligence, which has led to a focus on the role of biology in intelligence as a significant variable. This work was supported by Albrecht (2006), who extended the research with a focus on neurological structures within the brain. Goleman and Boyatzis (2008) suggested that 'effective leadership is about having powerful social circuits in the brain' (p. 76). They further progressed the concept of social intelligence, defined as 'a set of interpersonal competencies built on specific neural circuits (and related endocrine systems) that inspire others to be effective' (p. 76). This research also suggested that social intelligence is important in crisis situations and there may also be gender differences in levels of social intelligence, with women tending to have higher levels than men.

Spiritual intelligence

In 2000, Zohar and Marshall suggested the existence of a third type of intelligence (human and emotional intelligence being the other two), known as spiritual intelligence (SQ), which they claimed was essential for leadership success. They define spiritual intelligence as:

> *the intelligence with which we address and solve problems of meaning and value,*
> *the intelligence with which we can place our actions and our lives in a wider,*
> *richer, meaning-giving context, the intelligence with which we can assess*
> *that one course of action or one life-path is more meaningful than another.*
> *SQ is the necessary foundation for the effective functioning of both*
> *IQ and EQ. It is our ultimate intelligence (pp. 3–4).*

Zohar and Marshall argued that IQ and EQ, either separately or in combination, did not explain the full complexity that is potentially human intelligence. They suggested that, while Goleman's emotional intelligence concept allows us to judge the situation in which we work, and hence how to behave appropriately within its boundaries, our spiritual intelligence allows us to ask if we want to be in this situation at all. The question for nurse leaders then becomes, would I rather change the situation to create a better one? Here we are working with boundaries, so that we guide the situation rather than be guided by it. Zohar and Marshall refer to this as the transformation of SQ (p. 5). For them, SQ provides:

> *an understanding of who we are and what things mean to us, and have these*
> *give others and their meanings a place in the world . . . it helps us live life*
> *at a deeper level of meaning (p. 14).*

Individuals with high SQ tend to be servant leaders who bring vision and values to others, and show them how to use it. Such leadership is inspirational and includes, for example, Mahatma Gandhi, Nelson Mandela and the Dalai Lama. Leaders with highly developed SQ exhibit flexibility, self-awareness and a capacity to face and use suffering and pain. They are inspired by vision and values, eschew unnecessary harm, are holistic, tend to ask 'why' or 'what if' questions and are 'field independent'; that is, they readily work against convention.

More recently, Wigglesworth (2012) has reinvigorated and updated the concept of spiritual intelligence, outlining the skills required for spiritual intelligence, which are crucial for leaders. These skills enable nursing leaders to make decisions on a higher level, when there is stress, complexity and rapid change in their organisations.

Cultural intelligence

The concept of cultural intelligence is a relatively recent addition to the multiple intelligences examined so far. Cultural intelligence (CI), defined as 'the capability to be effective across cultural settings' (Ng & Earley, 2006, p. 4), is considered crucial for leadership, particularly in organisations that have a global outreach, or those that have a multicultural environment. Interested readers will find the views of Crowne (2013), Rockstuhl, Seiler, Ang, Dynes, and Annen (2011) and Triandis (2006) useful in developing a broader understanding of cultural intelligence. However, as with all the 'intelligences', there are critiques of cultural intelligence (see in particular Blasco, Feldt, and Jakobsen, 2012).

LEADERSHIP AND CONFLICT

A significant challenge to leaders is that of managing conflict, an inevitable event in workplace settings. Without its management, destructive relationships can develop, impacting on the quality of healthcare delivery. This is not to say that some conflict is not of value, as it can lead to positive benefits for the organisation, generating productive, mutually beneficial and shared decisions. Conflict is a process that begins when one party perceives that another party has negatively affected, or is about to negatively affect, something that the first party cares about (Robbins & Judge, 2010). This definition acknowledges that there must be an awareness or perception that there is conflict; two or more parties whose interests or goals appear to be incompatible; and limited resources, be they money, power or prestige. Scarcity of resources often creates blocking behaviour. When one party is perceived to block the goal achievement of another, a conflict state exists. And because we all have differing views and priorities, this can lead to conflict in many situations.

Levels of conflict

There are four identified levels of workplace conflict: intrapersonal (conflict within the individual), interpersonal (individual-to-individual conflict), intergroup conflict and inter-organisational conflict.

Intrapersonal conflict occurs within the individual due to actual or perceived pressures from incompatible goals or expectations. This can result in an approach conflict, when a person must choose between two positive and equally attractive alternatives (a promotion or a new job); avoidance conflict occurs when a person must choose between two negative and equally unattractive alternatives, such as accepting a transfer to an undesirable location or having one's position terminated; while an approach-avoidance conflict occurs when a person must decide to do something that has both positive and negative consequences, such as being offered a higher-paying job (positive consequence), but which is potentially very stressful (negative consequence).

Interpersonal conflict occurs between two or more individuals who are in opposition to each other, while intergroup conflict occurs among groups in an organisation. Inter-organisational conflict occurs between organisations, when competition and rivalry are manifested as a result.

Managing conflict

Different individuals have different and preferred ways of handling conflict. In 1994, Pace and Faules developed a model that focused on the individual's management of conflict, according to personality type. They postulated the following management styles: the competitive or tough battler, the collaborator or problem solver, the compromiser or manoeuvring conciliator, the accommodator or friendly helper, and the avoider or impersonal complier.

Competitive or tough battlers pursue their own concerns ruthlessly and often at the expense of others in the group. Losing is viewed as a serious weakness, giving reduced status and a negative self-image. Winning is seen as the only worthwhile goal. The strategy here is clearly 'win-lose'.

Collaborators or problem solvers, on the other hand, seek to create a situation in which the goals of all parties can be accomplished. They examine mutually acceptable solutions and work with a strategy for 'win-win'.

Compromisers or manoeuvring conciliators begin from the premise that everyone stands to lose, so it is best to work out a desirable solution to the conflict. This may mean that there is only partial satisfaction of everyone's concerns, resulting in acceptable rather than optimal outcomes. Using this strategy, no one totally wins or loses.

Accommodators or friendly helpers are usually non-assertive, neglecting their own concerns in favour of those of others. They feel that harmony is vital and that anger and confrontation are bad. Unfortunately they may later wish that the outcome was different, and they may harbour resentment, which is bound to find expression at a later time.

Avoiders or impersonal compliers view conflict as unproductive and punitive, so they will try to move away from the situation. There is usually no commitment to future actions, so this strategy may be self-defeating (Pace & Faules, 1994). Despite its datedness, this description retains its usefulness in understanding the various ways that individuals manage conflict.

Quite clearly, it may be more productive in the long term to adopt the collaborative 'win-win' style of approaching conflict. However, this requires effective communication and assertive behaviours, which the avoider or complier may not have. Furthermore, different individuals have different views of what is important, creating another source of conflict.

Effective communication with others is something we all seek, as it provides us with the potential to meet basic human needs. Such communication may develop self-understanding and self-acceptance, and develop qualities for effective relationships, such as trust vs. defensiveness, empowerment vs. control, understanding vs. judging, genuineness vs. dishonesty. Part of effective communication is being able to deal with conflict. For some of us this is easy; for others it is much more difficult. Often we have learned through our socialisation to fear, or at least avoid, conflict. Sometimes we have had ineffective behaviour patterns modelled for us, and we use these as unsuccessfully as those we seek to imitate. Or we may have been taught a range of messages about conflict and our reactions to it, such as: 'If you can't say anything nice, don't say anything at all', which can be a way of controlling anger, and is a message to which women, in particular, are exposed. There are many interesting gender lessons here: women in conflict situations may be intimidated into submission by being told that they are 'aggressive', 'bitchy', 'castrating' and the like. Being described in this way can be intensely insulting to some women, often resulting in rapid compliance.

There is a range of responses to conflict situations. These include: avoidance, defusion (which involves delaying action and/or keeping issues unclear), confrontation, use of power, whether it be covert or overt, and negotiation. There is also a range of individual styles to cope with conflict. These include an assertive interpersonal style, confrontive assertion, and I-language assertion, all of which are constructive. Less constructive styles include non-assertion and aggression. Readers who wish to pursue these concepts in greater depth and the relationship to leadership are referred to Ames (2009).

Indirect approaches to conflict management

Assertive leaders use direct conflict management techniques. There are also indirect approaches, including:

▲ appealing to common goals, which requires focusing the attention of conflicting parties on mutually desirable solutions;

▲ using 'hierarchical referral', which requires the use of the chain of command, usually upwards, for conflict resolution; and

▲ organisational redesign, in order to avoid the conflict or reduce its intensity. This can involve what is known as 'decoupling', separating groups, reducing contact or having two people act as 'link pins' within the conflict situation (Robbins & Judge, 2010).

Goleman (1998) also suggested that emotionally intelligent leaders who are adept at negotiating and resolving disagreements are typically able to manage difficult people and tense situations with diplomacy and tact. They have the competence to identify potential conflict and bring disagreements into the open before too much damage is done. This assists in de-escalating the situation, encourages debate and open discussion and facilitates the potential for 'win-win' solutions.

LEADERSHIP STYLE: A GENDER DIFFERENCE?

Of continuing interest within the research literature is the question of differing styles of leadership for women and men, which in itself has led to conflicting views. Some researchers find that leadership style does vary between women and men, while others can find few or no differences (Gurian & Annis, 2010; Klenke, 2011; Northouse, 2010; O'Connor, 2010; Paludi & Coates, 2011; Valerio, 2009; Werhane & Painter-Moreland, 2011). The reason for this may have little to do with leadership style, but might be explained by the context of the research, the methodology and the complexity of measuring leadership itself. There are also cultural stereotypes that permeate gender relationships, as they can obscure real individual differences, but these can become self-fulfilling. Gender stereotypes typically are generalisations and are often over-inclusive (Paludi, 2008).

However, some research finds that there are crucial gender differences, including degrees of cooperativeness, collaboration and style of problem solving (Avolio, 2011; Klenke, 2011; Paludi & Coates, 2011). It was also suggested that female leaders are more likely to structure flatter organisations and to emphasise frequent contact and sharing of information in 'webs of inclusion' (Rosener, 1990). She asserted that women's leadership style is highly interactive, participative, shares power and information, enhances the self-worth of others and energises others, in contrast to a more traditional style of 'command and control' (p. 120).

One of the major differences between women and men that has also been established is in the area of communication (DeFrancisco & Pakzewski, 2007; Dindia & Canary, 2012) after groundbreaking work by Tannen (2007, 2011). In a 1995 publication, Reardon suggested that women tend to talk about what they feel, while men talk about what they do. Further, she suggested that women process information differently, and therefore, gender based language remains problematic in the workplace.

Interesting recent research that investigated female and male constructs of leadership and empowerment found that women's descriptors related directly to transformational leadership, while men's related directly to transactional leadership (Alimo-Metcalfe, 2010a). Alimo-Metcalfe (2010b) also made the case for a more inclusive model, entitled 'engaging leadership', which has empowerment at its centre. This type of leadership facilitates organisations coping with change, but also importantly, being proactive in shaping their future.

More recently, research has called for a shift in focus, suggesting that male leaders develop their expressive dimension and take on more stereotypical 'feminine' characteristics in order to lead effectively (Gartzia & van Engen, 2012). This is a novel and fresh approach that is certainly worthy of further research.

Given the lack of agreement regarding differences (if any) of leadership styles between and among women and men, it is probably most prudent to keep an open mind on the question. However, it might be useful to reflect for a moment on your observations of leadership style as expressed by both women and men. Have you found any generalisable differences?

CONCLUSION

This chapter has established that distinctive aspects of individuals, referred to as personality attributes, the 'intelligences', genetic make-up and socialisation practices, have important effects on the way they behave in organisations. The situation in which leaders find themselves also plays a vital part in influencing leadership style. Therefore, it is obviously important to develop an awareness of the impact of these factors and variables if nursing leadership is to be optimally effective. Otherwise, such leadership can fail to produce desired outcomes.

Failure in leadership can occur because of rigidity within the individual leader, resulting in an inability to adapt leadership style to changes in the organisational culture. To be adaptive, nursing leaders need to take in or respond to feedback about the traits they need in order to change or improve their leadership style. They need to listen and learn, and be agile in working with different styles and with people at all levels of the organisation. This demands empathy and emotional self-management of leaders.

Another frequently mentioned reason for failed leadership is poor relationships with others, especially followers. Being too harshly critical, insensitive and demanding can alienate followers. These are fatal handicaps that nursing cannot afford. High levels of insight and awareness of one's psychological make-up are essential. Additionally, knowledge of values and meanings within diverse cultural groupings can provide sensitivity to others that can only enhance leadership behaviour. To be a most effective leader, we need to know and understand ourselves as thinking, feeling beings; to be aware of our fears, values, principles and aspirations (Whitehead, Weiss, & Tappen, 2010).

REFLECTIVE EXERCISE

1. Consider the characteristics listed for individuals with both external and internal loci of control.
    a. Can you identify your own orientation?
    b. How does this orientation affect your leadership style?
    c. Can you identify the orientation of nursing staff you lead or manage?
    d. Now turn your sights in a different direction. Can you identify the orientation of nursing (and other) leaders within your organisation, and how this orientation affects their leadership?
2. Can you identify your mode of reaction to conflict?
3. Are there differences in your dealing with conflict in personal situations with your friends and family?
    a. Do these differ from your reactions within the clinical setting?
    b. Why do you think there are differences, if any?

Recommended Readings

Ames, D. (2009). Pushing up to a point: Assertiveness and effectiveness in leadership and interpersonal dynamics. *Research in Organizational Behavior, 29,* 111–133.

Blasco, M., Feldt, L. E., & Jakobsen, M. (2012). If only cultural chameleons could fly too: A critical discussion of the concept of cultural intelligence. *International Journal of Cross-Cultural Management, 12*(2), 229.

Buchanan, D. A., & Badham, R. (2008). *Power, politics and organizational change: Winning the turf game* (2nd ed.). London: Sage.

Buchanan, D. A., & Huczynski, A. (2013). *Organizational behaviour* (8th ed.). Harlow, Great Britain: Pearson Education.

Dubrin, A. J., Dalglish, C., & Miller, P. (2012). *Leadership* (2nd ed.). South Melbourne, Australia: Cengage Learning.

Goleman, D. (1998). *Working with emotional intelligence.* New York: Bantam Books.

References

Ames, D. (2009). Pushing up to a point: Assertiveness and effectiveness in leadership and interpersonal dynamics. *Research in Organizational Behavior, 29,* 111–133.

Albrecht, K. (2006). *Social intelligence: The new science of success.* San Francisco: Jossey-Bass.

Alimo-Metcalfe, B. (2010a). An investigation of female and male constructs of leadership and empowerment. *Gender in Management: An International Journal, 25*(8), 640–680.

Alimo-Metcalfe, B. (2010b). Developments in gender and leadership: Introducing a new 'inclusive' model. *Gender in Management: An International Journal, 25*(8), 630–639.

Ashkanasy, N. M., & Daus, C. S. (2005). Rumours of the death of emotional intelligence in organizational behaviour are vastly exaggerated. *Journal of Organizational Behaviour, 26,* 444–452.

Avolio, B. J. (2011). *Full range leadership development* (2nd ed.). London: Sage.

Barrick, M. R., Parks, L., & Mount, M. K. (2005). Self-monitoring as a moderator of the relationships between personality traits and performance. *Personnel Psychology, 58,* 745–767.

Barron, D., & Hurley, J. (2012). Emotional intelligence and leadership. In J. Hurley & P. Linsley (Eds.), *Emotional intelligence for health and social care professionals: A guide for improving human relationships.* Oxford: Radcliffe Publishing.

Bass, B. M., & Bass, R. (2009). *The Bass handbook of leadership: Theory, research and managerial applications.* New York: Simon and Schuster.

Blasco, M., Feldt, L. E., & Jakobsen, M. (2012). If only cultural chameleons could fly too: A critical discussion of the concept of cultural intelligence. *International Journal of Cross-Cultural Management, 12*(2), 229–245.

Block, J. (2010). The five-factor framing of personality and beyond: Some ruminations. *Psychological Inquiry: An International Journal for the Advancement of Psychological Theory, 21*(1), 2–25.

Buchanan, D., & Badham, R. (2008). *Power, politics and organizational change: Winning the turf game* (2nd ed.). London: Sage.

Cherniss, C. (2010). Emotional intelligence: Toward clarification of a concept. *Industrial and Organizational Psychology, 3*(2), 110–126.

Cherniss, C., Extein, M., Goleman, D., & Weissberg, R. P. (2006). Emotional intelligence: What does the research really indicate? *Educational Psychologist, 41*(4), 239–245.

Crowne, K. A. (2013). Cultural exposure, emotional intelligence, and cultural intelligence: An exploratory study. *International Journal of Cross-Cultural Management, 13,* 5–22.

Daft, R. L. (2008). *The leadership experience.* South Melbourne: Cengage Learning.

DeFrancisco, V. P., & Pakzewski, C. H. (2007). *Communicating gender diversity: A critical approach.* London: Sage.

Dindia, K., & Canary, D. J. (Eds.), (2012). *Sex differences and similarities in communicating.* New York: Routledge.

Furnham, A. (2012). *The psychology of behaviour at work: The individual in the organization* (2nd ed.). London: Psychology Press.

Gardner, H. (1999). *Intelligence reframed: Multiple intelligences for the 21st Century.* New York: Basic Books.

Gartzia, L., & van Engen, M. (2012). Are (male) leaders 'feminine' enough? Gendered traits of identity as mediators of sex differences in leadership styles. *Gender in Management: An International Journal, 27*(5), 296–314.

Goleman, D. (1998). *Working with emotional intelligence.* London: Bloomsbury.

Goleman, D., & Boyatzis, R. (2008). Social intelligence and the biology of leadership. *Harvard Business Review, 86*(9), 74–81.

Greenberg, J., & Baron, R. A. (2008). *Behaviour in organizations* (9th ed.). New Jersey: Prentice-Hall.

Grossman, S. C., & Valiga, T. M. (2008). *The new leadership challenge: Creating the future of nursing* (3rd ed.). Philadelphia: F. A. Davis.

Gurian, M., & Annis, B. (2010). *Leadership and the sexes: Using gender science to create success in business.* Washington: John-Wiley.

Hughes, R. L., Ginnett, R. C., & Curphy, G. J. (2011). *Leadership: Enhancing the lessons of experience.* New York: Irwin/McGraw-Hill.

Hutchinson, M., & Hurley, J. (2013). Exploring leadership capability and emotional intelligence as moderators of workplace bullying. *Journal of Nursing Management, 21*(3), 553–562.

Ivancevich, J. M., Konopaske, J. M., & Matteson, M. T. (2008). *Organizational behaviour and management* (8th ed.). Boston: McGraw Hill.

Klenke, K. (2011). *Women in leadership: Contextual dynamics and boundaries.* Bingley, U.K.: Emerald Group Publishing.

Kupers, W. (2007). Perspectives on integrating leadership and followership. *International Journal of Leadership Studies, 2*(3), 194–221.

Locke, E. A. (2005). Why emotional intelligence is an invalid concept. *Journal of Organizational Behaviour, 26,* 425–431.

Matthews, G., Zeidner, M., & Roberts, B. D. (2012). Emotional intelligence: A promise fulfilled? *Japanese Psychological Research, 54*(2), 105–127.

Mayer, J. D., Salovey, P., & Caruso, D. R. (2004). Emotional intelligence: Theory, findings and implications. *Psychological Inquiry, 15*(3), 197–215.

McAdams, D. P., & Pals, L. (2006). The new Big Five: Fundamental principles for an integrative science of personality. *American Psychologist, 61*(3), 204–217.

McCrae, R. R., & Costa, P. T. (2008). The five-factor theory of personality. In O. P. John, W. W. Robins, & L. A. Pervin (Eds.), *Handbook of personality, theory and research* (3rd ed.). New York: Guilford Press.

McGuiness, M. (2004). *You've got personality: An introduction to the personality types described by Carl Jung and Isabel Myers.* Sydney: MaryMac Books.

McShane, S., & Glinow, M. V. (2012). *Organizational behaviour* (6th ed.). New York: McGraw-Hill.

Modassir, A., & Singh, T. (2008). Relationship of emotional intelligence with transformational leadership and organizational citizenship behaviour. *International Journal of Leadership Studies, 4*(1), 3–21.

Mullins, L. J. (2010). *Management and organizational behaviour.* Essex: Pearson Education.

Ng, K.-Y., & Earley, P. C. (2006). Culture + Intelligence: Old constructs, new frontiers. *Group and Organizational Management, 31*(1), 4–19.

Ng, K.-Y., Sang, S., & Chan, K. Y. (2008). Personality and leader effectiveness: A moderated mediation model of leadership, self-efficacy, job demands, and job autonomy. *Journal of Applied Psychology, 93*(4), 733–743.

Northouse, P. G. (Ed.), (2010). *Leadership: Theory and practice* (5th ed.). London: Sage.

O'Connor, K. (2010). *Gender and women's leadership: A reference handbook*. London: Sage.

Oforchukwu, J. I. (2011). *Perspectives on leadership: A synthesis of types and theories*. Bloomington, Indiana: Author House.

Pace, R. W., & Faules, D. F. (1994). *Organizational communication*. Englewood Cliffs, New Jersey: Prentice-Hall.

Paglis, L. (2010). Leadership self-efficacy: Research findings and practical applications. *Journal of Management Development, 29*(9), 771–782.

Paludi, M. A. (2008). *The psychology of women at work: Challenges and solutions for our female workforce*. Connecticut: Greenwood Publishing.

Paludi, M. A., & Coates, B. E. (2011). *Women as transformational leaders: From grassroots to global interests. Vol: 1, Cultural and organizational stereotypes, prejudice and discrimination*. California: Praeger.

Pierce, J. L., & Newstrom, J. W. (2010). *Leaders and the leadership process: Readings, self-assessment and application* (6th ed.). New York: McGraw-Hill/Irwin.

Robbins, S. P., & Coulter, M. (2013). *Management* (11th ed.). New Jersey: Prentice Hall.

Robbins, S. P., & Judge, T. A. (2010). *Organizational behaviour* (14th ed.). New Jersey: Prentice-Hall.

Rockstuhl, T., Seiler, S., Ang, S., Dynes, L. V., & Annen, H. (2011). Beyond general intelligence (IQ) and emotional intelligence (EQ): The role of cultural intelligence (CQ) on cross-border leadership effectiveness in a globalized world. *Journal of Social Issues, 67*(4), 825–840.

Rosener, J. B. (1990). Ways women lead. *Harvard Business Review*, (Nov–Dec), 119–125.

Rubin, H. (1997). *The Princessa: Machiavelli for women*. New York: Dell Books.

Scouller, J. (2011). *The three levels of leadership: How to develop your leadership presence, knowhow and skill*. Oxford: Management Books.

Stern, T. (2010). Self-esteem and high-achieving women. In M. A. Paludi (Ed.), *The psychology of women at work*. Connecticut: Greenwood Publishing.

Tannen, D. (2007). *You just don't understand: Women and men in conversation*. New York: Harper.

Tannen, D. (2011). *That's not what I meant! How conversational style makes or breaks relationships*. New York: Harper Perennial.

Tieger, P. D., & Barron-Tieger, B. (2007). *Do what you are: Perfect career for you through the secrets of personality type*. London: Sphere.

Triandis, H. C. (2006). Some dimensions of intercultural variation and their implications for community psychology. *Journal of Community Psychology, 11*(4), 285–302.

Valerio, M. A. (2009). *Developing women leaders: A guide for men and women in organizations*. West Sussex: Wiley-Blackwell.

Vroom, V. H., & Jago, A. G. (2007). The role of situation in leadership. *American Psychologist, 62*(1), 17–24.

Waterhouse, L. (2006). Inadequate evidence for multiple intelligences, the Mozart effect and emotional intelligence theories. *Educational Psychologist, 4*(4), 247–255.

Werhane, P. H., & Painter-Moreland, M. (Eds.), (2011). *Leadership, gender and organization*. New York: Springer Science.

Whitehead, D. K., Weiss, S. A., & Tappen, R. M. (2010). *Essentials of nursing leadership and management* (5th ed.). Philadelphia, PA: F. A. Davis Company.

Wiggins, J. S. (Ed.), (1996). *Five-Factor model of personality: Theoretical perspectives*. New York: Guilford Press.

Wigglesworth, C. (2012). *SQ21: The twenty-one skills of spiritual intelligence*. New York: Select Books.

Zohar, D., & Marshall, I. (2000). *Spiritual intelligence: The ultimate intelligence*. London: Bloomsbury.

CHAPTER THREE

Power, politics and gender: Issues for nurse leaders and managers

Sandra Speedy & Debra Jackson

LEARNING OBJECTIVES

At the completion of this chapter, the reader will be able to:

▲ describe how gender polarisation of the workplace affects nurses;

▲ list sources of power and describe where they come from;

▲ discuss the misuse of power and how it can affect the work environment;

▲ describe the role that language plays in perpetuating images of nursing and nursing leaders; and

▲ list the traits that will enhance political effectiveness of nurse leaders.

KEY WORDS

Power, language, gender polarisation, empowerment, political effectiveness

INTRODUCTION

Nursing is the most strongly gender segregated of all occupational groups. The beginnings of modern nursing were strongly feminine and the traditional view of nursing work has been that it is women's work, and that the knowledge associated with it is somehow innate to women (Evans, 2004a). Though nursing has also attracted men, it remains strongly female dominated (Loughrey, 2008). This means that one of the key features of the healthcare industry is its strongly polarised occupational segregation (Snyder & Green, 2008). This polarisation positions gender, politics and power as central to nurses and nursing. The effects of this polarity are seen in aspects of workplace culture, such as occupational violence, workplace oppression, and in current debates such as those addressing the education of nurses and recruitment into the profession. Occupational segregation also has an effect on nurses' pay and potential for career advancement, especially for female nurses (Hakim, 2006; Maher, Lindsay, Bardoel, & Advocat, 2008). Men are greatly over-represented in leadership positions (Wolfenden, 2011). This means that gender, particularly aspects pertaining to disadvantage and privilege, needs to remain firmly on the nursing agenda.

If we consider the structure of healthcare organisations such as hospitals, it is evident that nurses represent a high proportion of employees. However, this dominance does not transform into significant organisational power (Carter & Silva, 2010). Nurses are not necessarily appropriately represented in political processes, decision making and authoritative committees, all of which can impose change (Porter-O'Grady, 2011). One of the effects of this is that nurses are subject to imposed change, as important decisions may be made with little regard for their effects on nurses and nursing. Imposed change is recognised as a contributing factor to nurses' job dissatisfaction, retention of nurses and emotional burnout, especially where the change impacts on nurses' workloads (Buerhaus, 2010; Kowalski et al., 2010).

This chapter considers the concepts of power, politics and gender within the context of nursing practice, management and leadership. There is a broad literature around some of these concepts that spans approximately 30 years. However, despite having raised awareness and scholarly scrutiny, these areas are dynamic and continue to evolve.

GENDER AND LEADERSHIP IN NURSING

Female nurse leaders are confronted with many barriers including the glass ceiling (Hewlett, Peraino, Sherbin, & Sunberg, 2011), the glass cliff (Bruckmuller & Branscombe, 2011; Sabharwal, 2013) and the inability to internalise a leadership identity (Ibarra, Ely, & Kolb, 2013). Notwithstanding the influence of feminism on nursing, female nurses still earn less than male nurses (Lalanne & Seabright, 2011; World Bank, 2012), and are still under-represented in leadership positions in nursing (Evans, 2004b), which results in fewer role models and mentoring opportunities. Despite the female-dominated nature of nursing, the managerial playing field is tilted in favour of men and behaviours associated with the masculine gender stereotype (Powell, 2012). It is noteworthy that women have slower rates of achieving promotion than men (Blau & DeVaro, 2007; Yap, 2010), with some findings suggesting that attainment of a senior position in nursing takes longer for women than it does for men.

As previously noted, the literature suggests that feminine characteristics are seen as undesirable and inappropriate in leaders, while male characteristics are highly valued (Evans, 2004a; Heilman & Parks-Stamm, 2007; Powell, 2012). The general management literature indicates that leadership is most commonly slanted to 'think leadership, think male' (Linstead, Fulop, & Lilley, 2009; Robbins & Coulter, 2013; Sinclair, 2005, 2007) and specific reports (Husu, Hearn, Lamsa, & Vanhala, 2010) suggest that these male characteristics include aggression, competition, dominance, ambition, decisiveness, rationalness, responsibility and logic, whereas women supposedly value quite different qualities, including connectedness, inclusivity and relationships (Hoss, Bobrowski, McDonagh, & Paris, 2011). Discrimination against women as leaders can be subtle, with stereotypes and insinuation being used to devalue women and make it more difficult for them to move to leadership positions (Chamorro-Premuzic, 2013). Furthermore, some women may feel it inappropriate to be openly ambitious.

Evans (2004b) suggested that although men represent a minority in nursing, they do not experience the hostility and lack of support that women can encounter in male-dominated professions. Rather, she suggests that men are advantaged, with their minority status according them special power and privileges. A contrary view is asserted by Wolfenden (2011), which is that men in nursing are marginalised by the use of gender-biased language and sex-based discrimination within the education of nurses. For this reason, Wolfenden concludes that men will never be accepted in nursing. This view is reinforced by the work of the Ministry of Women's Affairs (2013), O'Lynn and Tranbarger (2006) and Pham (2013). Though it is sometimes postulated that attracting greater numbers of men into nursing would elevate the prestige and status of nursing, Evans (2004b) suggests that there is the possibility that female nurses might become increasingly subordinate to yet another layer of male dominance. Pham (2013) asserts that men do not pursue nursing as a career, as they believe there are higher expectations of them, they are outnumbered, treated differently in a negative way and are ridiculed for being male.

Ryan and Haslam (2007) postulate that women are more often appointed to precarious leadership positions; that is, those in which failure is more likely. This identifies the concept of the 'glass cliff' as a form of gender discrimination and often occurs when an organisation is in crisis (Ryan, Haslam, & Kulich, 2010).

In addition to stereotype advantages, social institutions such as heterosexual marriage also represent career advantage to men (Eagly & Carli, 2007; Evans, 2004b; Hakim, 2006), and there is evidence that women who reach leadership positions are more likely to be single and not responsible for the care of children. This suggests that women who have family responsibilities are disadvantaged when aspiring to leadership positions, which is supported by evidence that women consider family responsibilities a barrier to career progression (LaPierre & Zimmerman, 2012). Female leaders are under scrutiny as there may be doubts in some quarters about women's capacity to lead; thus gender politics means that women need to cultivate particular leadership traits (Toegel & Barsoux, 2012). Many women are quite used to having aspects of their appearance commented on (including dress, accessories, make-up and hair style) and criticised in their professional lives, whereas male managers are not subjected to the same level of personal scrutiny (Committee for Economic Development of Australia, 2013). Women's ways of interacting with others may also be the subject of comment in the workplace; for example, women may be accused of being flirtatious or using their femininity to unfair advantage (Sinclair, 2005).

POWER

Power is a necessary aspect of management and leadership (Bal, Campbell, Steed, & Meddings, 2008), and can be defined as the capacity to produce effects on others, change their behaviour, or influence others. There is a difference between power and influence, in that power has the capacity to cause change, whereas influence is the degree of actual change that occurs in the person over whom we have either power or influence. Power can exist in leaders, followers and in situations, and is an important aspect of the working landscape, although the literature suggests women may be ambivalent about power (Ernst, 2008; Inam, 2013; Pfeffer, 2010). Feldt (2012), however, does point out that women are becoming less ambivalent about holding power, as they gain greater experience in leadership positions. Leaders can influence their followers, and, conversely, followers can affect the leaders' behaviours, as well as their attitudes.

Power may hold negative associations for women, and certainly has been viewed as a dominance/submission issue; that is, associated with personal inadequacies and physical attributes, rather than skill (Feldt, 2012; Painter-Morland, 2011). Thus, many of the attributes associated with holding and using legitimate power—for example, assertiveness, decisiveness and autonomy—are more commonly associated with male than female socialisation (Feldt, 2012).

Knowledge is also associated with power. To be informed is necessarily to be empowered and essential to the maintenance of professional credibility—no one would argue with the assertion that effective leadership requires a sound knowledge base. To be uninformed is to necessarily be disempowered and threatens professional credibility. Lack of knowledge of the total context in which nursing occurs will jeopardise decision making, planning and service delivery. Despite the time pressures nurse leaders and managers face, the importance of remaining well-informed and cognisant of current policies and relevant research cannot be overstated. Strategies for knowledge enhancement may include membership and participation in professional organisations, reading current relevant journals, regular involvement in professional development activities and a commitment to lifelong learning. Such strategies are not only crucial to enhance current knowledge, but also provide opportunities for networking and support.

Sources of power

While there has long been an assumption that leaders have power, the question is now being asked: do leaders have power or do followers give it to them? This is an interesting question because the answer is yes on both counts. Power is not evenly distributed among individuals or groups; everyone has some power that originates from varying sources.

Power relationships can be observed between individuals by non-verbal behaviours or what is called 'dominance/submission' behaviour (Painter-Morland, 2011). These behaviours consist of stylised rituals, including staring, which typically dominant individuals do, while submissive individuals do not; pointing, where again, powerful individuals point, while those without power do not; touching is often done by the more powerful to demonstrate the power differential; and interrupting is more often done by powerful individuals, while less powerful individuals are those who are interrupted. Significant research has established that women tend to be interrupted more often than men (Holmes, 2006; Tannen, 2007). Does this mean that men are more powerful, generally speaking, than women?

Other rituals or non-verbal messages of power in the workplace include placement of furniture, size of office space and displaying symbols of achievement or power, such as diplomas or awards. Choice of clothing can also affect power and influence. Uniforms are a classic example, as they have been shown to influence people who are in crisis, which results in instructions being more likely to be followed. A person's appearance is an important aspect of leadership, and has led to the 'power dressing' phenomenon that is evident, especially in the business world (Goodall, 2013; Young, 2011). Technology has created the capacity of 'virtual politicking' within organisations—political players increasingly use email for political means, creating significant new challenges and risks for organisations (Waterford Technologies, 2013). Other sources of power by which an individual can potentially influence others are expert, referent, legitimate, reward and coercive power (after French & Raven (1959) who established these categories in what is now considered pioneering work. This model has subsequently gone through significant developments, see Raven (1993, 2008)).

Note that leaders and followers can use all of these types of power and that effective leaders generally work to increase their sources of power. In addition, Choi (2006) describes charismatic power, which, as the name suggests, comes from personal dynamism and charisma; information power, which comes from having information needed by others; and feminist or self-power, which comes from personal maturity and self-confidence (Allen, 2013). Leaders vary in the degree to which they share power with subordinates. Some leaders view power as fixed in amount, meaning they consider the more they give away, the less they have (Allen, 2013; Martin, 2006). However, there is an argument for increasing one's power by delegating it to others and encouraging more participative approaches in the work setting.

Empowerment of others is an essential aspect of leadership and gives responsibility, accountability and authority to others to undertake the work that needs to be done. It also has the effect of increasing job satisfaction, affective commitment and retention of staff (Dewettinck & Ameijde, 2011). Empowerment is thus an abstract concept that is fundamentally positive, referring to solutions rather than to problems. Empowerment of staff also helps to develop them and build their skill base, which, in providing wellbeing at both the individual and organisational level, will reinforce staff self-image and cooperation networks. Nevertheless, empowerment will not work in every setting, as it requires the professional to have capability, initiative, commitment and independence in decision making, which organisational structures may impede. Using empowerment as a leadership strategy is more democratic and participative than using power-based strategies (Whitehead, Weiss, & Tappen, 2010). However, Alimo-Metcalf (2010) warns that if the 'masculine' version of empowerment is adopted, then empowered 'individuals are being seen as "recipients of power" rather than "sharers of power" and that it is in the power of the leader to remove the gift' (p. 645). In effect, those empowered are held more accountable for failures of matters that were previously the responsibility of the manager.

Leaders who rely on power-based strategies to achieve their own ends will generally work to increase their sources of power, be they referent, expert, reward or legitimate. Leaders who rely most on referent and expert power have teams that are more motivated and satisfied and perform better (Wood et al., 2012). In general, this suggests that leaders who take advantage of all their sources of power and influence are the most effective; the type of power they use depends on the situation in which they are placed. Further, while leaders have strong influence and power over their staff, those who are in turn influenced by their team tend to be most successful (Hughes, Ginnett, & Curphy, 2008). This type of reciprocity provides opportunities for optimum functioning of their organisation because it requires participation based on empowerment.

Individual personality and power

Research conducted in the 1970s and 1980s suggested that there are other forms of power, which are derived from the personalities of individuals. Individuals vary in their motivation to control or influence others. This is known as the 'need for power' (n Power). Those with high 'n Power' derive psychological satisfaction from influencing others (McClelland, 1975). They seek positions where they can influence others.

Two ways of expressing 'n Power' have been identified: personalised power and socialised power (McClelland & Boyatzis, 1982).

Individuals who have a high need for personalised power are said to be selfish, impulsive, uninhibited and lacking in self-control. They aim to exercise power for their own ends and needs. Individuals who have a high need for socialised power demonstrate service of higher goals to others or to organisations, which may involve self-sacrifice towards those ends. This often requires an empowering rather than an autocratic style of management and leadership. Note, too, that some followers also have high needs for power. This can lead to tension between leaders and followers when followers are directed to do something they may not wish to do—one of the reasons why it is useful for each of us to be aware of our own power needs, and further, whether our preference is to be a leader or a follower (Hughes et al., 2008).

People with high needs for power often demonstrate a number of capacities and attributes, including the maintenance of good relationships with authority figures; competition for recognition and advancement; enhanced knowledge and information; personal charisma, such as pleasant personality characteristics, agreeable behaviour, creativity, honesty and integrity and appropriate personal appearance (Greenberg, 2010). They also tend to demonstrate a capacity for sheer hard work; active and assertive behaviours; readiness to exercise influence over subordinates; are visibly different from followers; and are willing to do routine administrative tasks (Hughes et al., 2008; Wood et al., 2012).

It is important to understand the dynamics of power because power can be used inappropriately, and can become abusive and oppressive. Power implies physical force, such as may be used to restrain patients who are in danger of harming themselves. Inappropriate use and abuse of power is relatively commonplace in the nursing workforce, and this is evidenced by the alarmingly high incidence of work-related violence and harassment experienced by nurses. This important issue and that of bullying and horizontal violence between nurses is addressed in detail elsewhere in this text, and will not be repeated here.

STRATEGIES TO ENHANCE POWER AND INFLUENCE

Individuals who acquire managerial power seek to maintain or enhance their power by using a number of strategies. These may include:

▲ increasing their centrality and criticality to the organisation;

▲ augmenting their personal discretion and flexibility in their job;

▲ building into their job tasks that are difficult to evaluate; and

▲ expanding the visibility of their job performance, resulting in increased contact with the senior people they seek to impress (Wood et al., 2012).

There are a number of other common strategies used to enhance one's power and influence. These include:

▲ building and developing personal resources;

▲ the use of reason (using facts and data to support a logical argument);

▲ being friendly and flattering in order to create favourable impressions;

▲ developing coalitions in which relationships with other people are used for gaining support;

▲ bargaining with others, which involves using the exchange of benefits as a basis for negotiation;

▲ assertiveness, which requires a direct and forceful personal approach;

▲ appealing to a higher authority, which results in high-level support for requests;

▲ continually increasing one's own skills and knowledge; and

▲ the use of sanctions, which are organisationally derived rewards and punishments (Wood et al., 2012).

POLITICS IN NURSING PRACTICE ORGANISATIONS

Politics in organisations refers to political behaviour that is used to affect decision making. Political behaviour involves those activities that are not required as part of one's formal role in the organisation but that influence or attempt to influence the distribution of advantages and disadvantages within the organisation. Organisational politics is the management of influence to obtain ends not sanctioned by the organisation or to obtain sanctioned ends through non-sanctioned means of influence (Wood et al., 2012).

Nursing has a history of political activism (Mason, Isaacs, & Colby, 2011; Sanford, 2012; Simon, 2012), and politics is a fact of life for nurses, nursing and healthcare organisations. Politics occurs because organisations are made up of individuals who have different needs, values, goals, interests and where there is competition for finite resources. Furthermore, the 'facts' that are used for decision making are often open to interpretation and there can be many interpretations of these 'facts'. Politics also occurs because organisations exist in a climate of ambiguity, leading to uncertainty, conflict and concern for one's wellbeing in the organisation (Robbins, Judge, Millett, & Waters-Marsh, 2008).

Political behaviour

Any organisational chart you examine will indicate who the boss is and who reports to whom. It will not, however, reveal the political behaviours and politics within the organisation. To harness the true power in an organisation and work the politics of that organisation, a number of networks can be used (Ferris & Treadway, 2012). These include the:

▲ advice network, which reveals the people to whom others turn to get the work done;

▲ trust network, which tends to uncover who shares delicate information with whom; and

▲ communication network, which shows who talks to whom about work-related matters (Wood et al., 2012).

Language and power

Language is very powerful. It is the principal means by which reality is constructed and mediated; in other words, language creates meaning (Lei, 2006). It conjures up images and sends powerful messages about how things are positioned and where they sit in terms of power, status and prestige. To illustrate this, back in 2001 Britain re-introduced the term 'matron', to describe senior nurses whose role it was to oversee cleanliness and care standards across ward areas and whole hospitals (Duffin, 2001). Although some British nurses welcomed government moves to empower and increase the visibility of these nurses, the proposed title of 'matron' caused considerable and heated discussion. The term was said to be 'gender-oriented and specific to women', 'outdated', and to conjure up images of 'fearsome' women, 'housekeeper and surrogate mother' women, and women who lead through 'bullying and harassment' (Duffin,

2001, p. 7). Clearly these are not images nursing wishes to perpetuate and one can see that a nurse with a title such as nurse manager, nurse executive or director of nursing, could carry out the same activities, but without the connotations implicit in the word 'matron'. Thus it can be seen that the word, or the language, has created a set of understandings that may not have been intended, and which then created enormous controversy.

The ways that nurses use language has changed over the years; for example, changes in the ways nurses refer to patients at handover is noted in the literature (Smeulers, van Tellingen, Lucas, & Vermeulen, 2012; Wallis, 2010). The power of language is that it is not just a matter of matching objects with words, but it carries a moral and political dimension in the way that we use it. Nurses need to use language that accurately conveys meaning, but that is not denigrating and does not foster stereotypes or negativity about individuals or particular groups of people. The connotation or attitudes that people develop can be directly related to the language used to introduce or describe it. Take a look at the following 'lighthearted' list which uses very different language to describe the same phenomenon:

Table 3.1 How language can be used to manipulate meaning

Effective management label	Can be labelled as...
Fixing responsibility	Blaming others
Developing relationships	Kissing up
Demonstrating loyalty	Apple polishing
Delegating authority	Passing the buck
Documenting decisions	Covering your rear
Encouraging change/innovation	Creating conflict
Facilitating teamwork	Forming coalitions
Improving efficiency	Whistle blowing
Planning ahead	Scheming
Competent and capable	Overachieving
Career-minded	Ambitious
Astute	Opportunistic
Practical minded	Cunning
Confident	Arrogant
Attentive to detail	Perfectionistic

(Source: Krell, Mendenhall, & Sendry, 1987.)

It is clear from this listing that one's perception of the occurring behaviour is dependent on the situation in which the behaviour is manifest. Furthermore, description of the behaviour is also dependent on the situation.

Contributions to political behaviour

There are many factors that contribute to political behaviour. These can be described as those that are individual and those that are organisational (see Chapter 2 for further discussion of individual personality characteristics as they relate to leadership). Whether we choose to be political or not, and the degree to which we are political, depends on a number of factors. Within the individual domain, researchers have identified certain traits that will enhance one's political effectiveness. These include self-monitoring (Greenberg, 2010), locus of control (Robbins et al., 2008), the capacity to manipulate others (Buchanan & Badham, 2008), high self-esteem (Grossman & Valiga, 2013) and a variety of damage control techniques, all of which were comprehensively discussed in Chapter 2.

Organisational politics requires players to protect themselves, as well as promote their own interests. Behaving in a political manner requires reactive and protective 'defensive' behaviours to avoid action, avoid blame or avoid change. Extensive use of defensive behaviour will promote the political player's self-interest. In the longer term, however, it may become a liability. Defensive behaviour may become chronic, so that learned defensiveness becomes the only way one can behave. Eventually, this may lead to loss of support of peers, bosses and subordinates, who become aware of the limitations of this type of behaviour.

When used in moderation, defensive behaviour can be an effective device for surviving in organisations. However, frequent use tends to reduce effectiveness, delay decisions, increase interpersonal and intergroup tensions, reduce risk taking, make attributions and evaluations unreliable, and can restrict organisational change. If defensive behaviour is used often and for long periods of time, it can lead to organisational rigidity and stagnation, detachment from the organisational environment, and low employee morale (Buchanan, 2008; Wood et al., 2012).

Within the organisational domain, the individual who is highly adept politically will be well served by:

▲ an organisation in which there are finite resources and a win-lose approach to resource allocation;

▲ a culture of low trust and role ambiguity;

▲ an unclear performance evaluation system;

▲ 'supposed' democratic decision making that subverts the power of individuals;

▲ high performance pressures, where the greater the pressure, the more likely is the need to bend the rules; and

▲ a self-serving culture and politicking of seniors who role-model acceptability of 'playing politics' to those below them (Greenberg, 2010; Wood et al., 2012).

THE ETHICS OF BEHAVING POLITICALLY

Apart from personal and organisational contributions to political behaviour, there are a number of processes that can be used to enhance one's power in an organisation. Many people are not comfortable with talk of 'being political', and certainly are distinctly uncomfortable with behaving in political ways. Nurses are no exception. But politics is a fact of life in organisations; to avoid it is to reduce your own effectiveness and ability to pursue goals for change (Davies, 2004; McKenna, 2010). It is important that nurses can operate in ways that are politically astute because some degree of political savvy is expected in today's nurses (Daily, 2008; Kelly, 2010). On the other hand, some people enjoy the 'cut and thrust' of politics, while some are significantly more politically astute than others, regardless of their level in the organisation. The politically naive and inept tend to feel continually powerless to influence those decisions that most affect them. They look at actions around them and are perplexed when they are regularly shafted by colleagues, bosses and the so-called 'system'.

Powerful and political people can be very successful at justifying or explaining their own interests. They can, and often do, argue that unfair actions are really fair and just. When power and politics are not guided by moral behaviour, there are real dangers to organisations and individuals. Immoral people can justify almost any behaviour. They can be influential, articulate and persuasive, and sometimes get away with unethical practices because of these characteristics (Buchanan & Badham, 2008).

As Wood et al. (2012) suggest, survival in a highly political environment requires recognising political game playing, identifying power sources of key players and building alliances and connections, despite appearances of cooperation that may be demonstrated. Recognising that you need to behave politically, but also wanting to behave ethically, there are some guidelines that might be helpful. For example, you can use three types of criteria to judge the ethics of your proposed behaviour.

▲ The first is the criterion of utilitarian outcomes, which indicates that the behaviour should produce the greatest good for the greatest number of people. In this way, everyone inside the organisation and outside it would derive some satisfaction or value.

▲ The second is the criterion of individual rights, where the behaviour respects the basic rights of all affected parties, including the rights of free consent, free speech, freedom of conscience, privacy and due process.

▲ The third criterion is that of distributive justice, where the political behaviour respects the rules of justice and treats people equitably and fairly, not arbitrarily (Wood et al., 2012).

It is important to keep in mind that we may use rationalisations to justify unethical behaviour. For example, we might tell ourselves that some behaviour is not really illegal and thus could be moral, when by the judgement of others it is illegal (and immoral); or we might tell ourselves that the actions we have taken or are about to take are in the organisation's best interests, when a neutral judge might perceive otherwise; or we may convince ourselves that the behaviour/action is unlikely to be detected; or finally, we may convince ourselves that a particular action demonstrates loyalty to the boss or the organisation, and is thus justifiable.

CONCLUSION

It is clear that nursing and health care take place in dynamic and highly policitised environments. A strong understanding of political processes is essential to ensure that nurses' interests are brought to attention and that their voices are heard in key decision-making forums. Nurses have a well-established role as client/patient advocates, and it is essential that this advocacy role is maintained and expanded at all levels of political influence. It is also important to recognise the contribution that nurses make to political processes within organisations, even though this contribution may not be currently acknowledged or valued.

Gender remains an issue of key interest to nurses, both collectively and individually. Like other professions, evidence suggests that gender is a variable that can affect career development and progression in nursing. While there is still much to be done to redress gender-related advantage and disadvantage in nursing, the signs are that progress is being made (Knowledge@Australian School of Business, 2010). One of the tasks of nurse managers and leaders is to acknowledge the existence of gender issues in nursing, and to work towards equity in workplace practices (EOWWA, 2012).

As we move further into the twenty-first century it is crucial to acknowledge the complex nature of power and to appreciate that men and women may have totally different attitudes to, and understandings of, power. Misuse of power has the potential to impact strongly and negatively on the workplace and contribute to the oppression of nurses and nursing. It is essential that the use of power in nursing is accompanied by integrity and veracity, and that it reflects the values nurses espouse—values such as care, compassion and social justice. Collectively and individually, nurses have the potential to further develop the concept of professional autonomy. A full understanding of the nature of power can only help us to move ahead and improve nursing as a career choice, and further develop practice so as to better meet the needs of the communities we serve.

REFLECTIVE EXERCISE

There are some questions that you can ask yourself when you feel uncomfortable about political behaviour. These include:

1. Am I behaving in the best interests of myself or my organisation?
2. What about the other parties involved? What are their rights?
3. Does my behaviour and the behaviour of my colleagues conform to standards of equity and justice?

Working through these questions may be helpful in deciding how to behave.

Recommended Readings

Grossman, S., & Valiga, T. M. (2012). *The new leadership challenge: Creating the future of nursing.* Philadelphia: F.A. Davis Company.

Hughes, R. L., Ginnett, R. C., & Curphy, G. J. (2008). *Leadership: Enhancing the lessons of experience.* New York: McGraw-Hill.

Sinclair, A. (2007). *Disillusioned: Moving beyond myths and heroes to leading that liberates.* Crows Nest, NSW: Allen & Unwin.

Tannen, D. (2007). *You just don't understand: Women and men in conversation.* New York: Harper.

References

Alimo-Meltcalfe, B. (2010). An investigation of female and male constructs of leadership and empowerment. *Gender in Management: An International Journal, 25*(8), 640–648.

Allen, A. (2013). Feminist perspectives on power. In E. N. Zalta (Ed.), *The Stanford encyclopedia of philosophy.* Retrieved from <http://plato.stanford.edu/>.

Bal, V., Campbell, M., Steed, J., & Meddings, K. (2008). *The role of power in effective leadership.* Center for Creative Leadership. A CCL Research White Paper.

Blau, F. D., & DeVaro, J. (2007). New evidence on gender differences in promotion rates: An empirical analysis of a sample new hires. *Industrial Relations, 46*(3), 511–550.

Bruckmuller, S., & Branscombe, N. R. (2011). How women end up on the 'glass cliff'. *Harvard Business Review*, January.

Buchanan, D. A. (2008). You stab my back, I'll stab yours: Management experience and perceptions of organization political behavior. *British Journal of Management, 19*(1), 49–64.

Buchanan, D. A., & Badham, R. J. (2008). *Power, politics and organizational change: Winning the turf game* (2nd ed.). London: Sage.

Buerhaus, P. I. (2010). What is the harm in imposing mandatory hospital nurse staffing regulations? *Nurse Economics, 28*(2), 87–94.

Carter, N. M., & Silva, C. (2010). Women in management: Delusions of progress. *Harvard Business Review, March.* Retrieved from <http://hbr.org/2010/03/women-in-management-delusions-of-progress/ar/1>.

Chamorro-Premuzic, T. (2013). Why do so many incompetent men become leaders? *Harvard Business Review, August.* Retrieved from <http://blogs.hbr.org/2013/08/why-do-so-many-incompetent-men/>.

Choi, J. (2006). A motivational theory of charismatic leadership: Envisioning, empathy and empowerment. *Journal of Leadership and Organizational Studies, 13*(1), 24–43.

Committee for Economic Development of Australia. (2013). *Women in leadership: Understanding the gender gap.* Melbourne, Australia: CEDA.

Daily, M. A. (2008). Mastering the art of politics. *The Pennsylvania Nurse, 63*(3), 4–6.

Davies, C. (2004). Political leadership and the politics of nursing. *Journal of Nursing Management, 12*(4), 235–251.

Dewettinck, K., & Ameijde, M. V. (2011). Linking leadership empowerment behaviour to employee attitudes and behavioural intentions: Testing the mediating role of psychological empowerment. *Personnel Review, 40*(3), 284–305.

Duffin, C. (2001). Sexist, outdated...matron rejected for modern NHS. *Nursing Standard, 5*(3), 7.

Eagly, A. H., & Carli, L. L. (2007). Women and the labyrinth of leadership. *Harvard Business Review, September.* Retrieved from <http://hbr.org/2007/09/women-and-the-labyrinth-of-leadership/ar/1>.

Equal Opportunity for Women in the Workplace Agency (EOWW). (2012). *Australian census of women in leadership. Summary of key findings.* Research conducted by the UTS Centre for Corporate Governance. Australian Government.

Ernst, S. (2008). If the 'natural gender-arrangement falters': Ambivalent tensions and dynamics of power-interdependencies between the sexes. *International Seminar: Gender Difference and Democracy. Ideas, Experimentations and Routes.* March.

Evans, J. A. (2004a). Bodies matter: Men, masculinity and the gendered division of labour in nursing. *Journal of Occupational Science, 11*(1), 14–22. doi:10.1080./14427591.2004.9686527.

Evans, J. (2004b). Men nurses: A historical and feminist perspective. *Journal of Advanced Nursing, 47*(3), 321–328.

Feldt, G. (2012). *No excuses: Nine ways women can change how we think about power.* Berkeley, California: Seal Press.

Ferris, G. R. R., & Treadway, D. C. C. (2012). *Politics in organizations: Theory and research considerations.* New York: Taylor and Francis Group.

French, J. R. P., & Raven, B. (1959). The bases of social power. In D. Cartwright & A. F. Zander (Eds.), *Group dynamics: Research and theory.* New York: Harper and Row.

Goodall, J. (2013). Cracking the dress code. In J. Schultz (Ed.), *Griffith Review, 40, Women and Power.* Melbourne: Text Publishing Company.

Greenberg, J. (2010). *Behavior in organizations* (10th ed.). Upper Saddle River, New Jersey: Pearson Education/Prentice-Hall.

Grossman, S., & Valiga, T. M. (2013). *The new leadership challenge: Creating the future of nursing* (4th ed.). Philadelphia, PA: F.A. Davis Company.

Hakim, C. (2006). Women, careers and work-life preferences. *British Journal of Guidance and Counselling, 34*(3), 279–294.

Heilman, M. E., & Parks-Stamm, E. J. (2007). Gender stereotypes in the workplace: Obstacles to women's career progress. In S. Corell (Ed.), *Social psychology of gender: Advances in group processes.* Greenwick: JAI Press.

Hewlett, S. A., Peraino, K., Sherbin, L., & Sunberg, K. (2011). The sponsor effect: Breaking through the last glass ceiling. *HBR Research Materials,* January 2012.

Holmes, J. (2006). *Gendered talk at work: Constructing gender identity through workplace discourse*. Maiden, MA: Blackwell Publishing.

Hoss, M. A. K., Bobrowski, P., McDonagh, K. J., & Paris, N. M. (2011). How gender disparities drive imbalances in health care leadership. *Journal of Healthcare Leadership, 3*, 59–68.

Hughes, R., Ginnett, R. C., & Curphy, G. J. (2008). *Leadership: Enhancing the lessons of experience.* New York: McGraw-Hill International.

Husu, L., Hearn, J., Lamsa, A.-M., & Vanhala, S. (Eds.), (2010). *Leadership through the gender lens. Women and men in organisations. Hanlean School of Economics Research Reports, 71*. Helsinki, Finland.

Ibarra, H., Ely, R., & Kolb, D. (2013). Women rising: The unseen barriers. *Harvard Business Review, September.*

Inam, H. (2013). Why we're not sure we want to be #1. *InPower Women, October.* Retrieved from <http://www.theglasshammer.com/news/2013/04/03/why-were-not-sure-we-want-to-be-1/>.

Kelly, K. (2010). Women's leadership and the development of nursing. In K. O'Connor (Ed.), *Gender and women's leadership: A reference handbook.* Thousand Oaks, CA: Sage.

Knowledge@AustralianSchool of Business. (2010). *Gender mender: Are women getting even, at last?* Retrieved from <http://knowledge.asb.unsw.edua.au/article>.

Kowalski, C., Omnen, O., Driller, E., Ernstmann, N., Wirtz, M. A., Kohler, T., et al. (2010). Burnout in nurses—the relationship between social capital in hospitals and emotional exhaustion. *Journal of Clinical Nursing, 19*(11–12), 1654–1663.

Krell, T. C., Mendenhall, M. E., & Sendry, J. *Doing research in the conceptual morass of organizational politics.* Paper presented at the Western Academy of Management Conference, Hollywood, CA, April.

Lalanne, M., & Seabright, P. (2011). The old boy network: Gender differences in the impact of social networks on remuneration in top executive jobs. Toulouse School of Economics. *GREMAQ*, 1–51.

LaPierre, T. A., & Zimmerman, M. K. (2012). Career advancement and gender equity in health care management. *Gender in Management: An International Journal, 27*(2), 100–118.

Lei, X. (2006). Sexism in language. *Journal of Language and Linguistics, 5*(1), 87–94.

Linstead, S., Fulop, L., & Lilley, S. (2009). *Management and organization: A critical text* (2nd ed.). New York: Palgrave Macmillan.

Loughrey, M. (2008). Just how male are male nurses? *Journal of Clinical Nursing, 17*(10), 1327–1334.

Maher, J. M., Lindsay, J., Bardoel, A., & Advocat, J. (2008). *Flexibility and more? Nurses working and caring.* School of Political and Social Inquiry and the Australian Centre for Research in Employment and Work (ACREW). Monash University.

Martin, M. J. (2006). 'That's the way we do things around here': An overview of organizational culture. *Electronic Journal of Academic and Special Librarianship, 7*(1). Retrieved from <http://southernlibrarianship.icaap.org/content/v07n01/martin_m01.htm>.

Mason, D. J., Isaacs, S. L., & Colby, D. C. (2011). *The nursing profession: Development, challenges, opportunities.* San Francisco: Jossey Bass.

McClelland, D. C. (1975). *Power: The inner experience.* New York: Irvington.

McClelland, D. C., & Boyatzis, R. E. (1982). Leadership motive pattern and long-term success in management. *Journal of Applied Psychology, 67*(6), 737–743.

McKenna, H. (2010). Nurses and politics — laurels for the hardy. *International Journal of Nursing Studies, 47*(4), 397–398.

Ministry of Women's Affairs. (2013). *Realising the opportunity: Addressing New Zealand's leadership pipeline by attracting and retaining talented women.* Thorndon, Wellington: New Zealand Government.

O'Lynn, C., & Tranbarger, R. (2006). *Men in nursing: History, challenges and opportunities.* New York: Springer Publishing Company.

Painter-Morland, M. (2011). Systemic leadership, gender, organization. In P. Werhane & M. Painter-Morland (Eds.), *Leadership, gender, organization. Issues in Business Ethics, 27*. Netherlands: Springer.

Pfeffer, J. (2010). Women and the uneasy embrace of power. *Harvard Business Review, August.*

Pham, T. (2013). *Men in nursing. Minority Nurse.* Indiana Wesleyan University. Retrieved from <http://www.minoritynurse.com/article/men-nursing>.

Porter-O'Grady, T. (2011). Leadership at all levels. *Nursing Management, 42*(5), 32–37.

Powell, G. N. (2012). Six ways of seeing the elephant: The intersection of sex, gender and leadership. *Gender in Management: An International Journal, 27*(2), 119–141.

Raven, B. H. (1993). The bases of power: Origins and recent developments. *Journal of Social Issues, 49*(4), 227–252.

Raven, B. H. (2008). The bases of power and the power/interaction model of interpersonal influence. *Analyses of Social Issues and Public Policy, 8*(1), 1–22.

Robbins, S. P., & Coulter, M. (2013). *Management* (11th ed.). New Jersey: Prentice Hall.

Robbins, S. P., Judge, T. A., Millett, B., & Waters-Marsh, T. (2008). *Organisational behaviour* (5th ed.). Frenchs Forest, NSW: Pearson Education.

Ryan, M. K., & Haslam, S. A. (2007). The glass cliff: Exploring the dynamics surrounding the appointment of women to precarious leadership positions. *Academy of Management Review, 32*(2), 549–572.

Ryan, M. K., Haslam, S. A., & Kulich, C. (2010). Politics and the glass cliff: Evidence that women are preferentially selected to contest hard-to-win seats. *Psychology of Women Quarterly, 34*(1), 56–64.

Sabharwal, M. (2013). From glass ceiling to glass cliff: Women in senior executive service. *Journal of Public Administration Research and Theory.* Retrieved from <http://jpart.oxfordjournals.org>.

Sanford, K. D. (2012). Nurse advocates: Past, present and future. *OJIN: The Online Journal of Issues in Nursing, 17*(1), Overview and summary.

Simon, M. (2012). Nursing and political activism. *Queensland Nurse, 31*(3), 39.

Sinclair, A. (2005). *Doing leadership differently: Gender, power and sexuality in a changing business culture* (2nd ed.). Melbourne: Melbourne University Press.

Sinclair, A. (2007). *Leadership for the disillusioned: Moving beyond myths and heroes to leading that liberates.* Crows Nest, NSW: Allen & Unwin.

Smeulers, M., van Tellingen, I. C., Lucas, C., & Vermeulen, H. (2012). Effectiveness of different nursing handover styles for ensuring continuity of information in hospitalised patients. *Cochrane Summaries,* doi:10.1002/14651858.CD009979.

Snyder, K. A., & Green, A. I. (2008). Revisiting the glass escalator: The case of gender segregation in a female dominated occupation. *Social Problems, 55*(2), 271–299.

Tannen, D. (2007). *You just don't understand: Women and men in conversation.* New York: Harper.

Toegel, G., & Barsoux, J.-L. (2012). How to become a better leader. *MIT Sloan Management Review, 53*(3), March. Retrieved from <http://sloanreview.mit.edu/article/how-to-become-a-better-leader/>.

Wallis, S. (2010). *Nursing handover research project: How is nursing handover talked about in the literature?* Master of Nursing, Waikato Institute of Technology.

Waterford Technologies. (2013). *Story pitch: From email to scandal.* Retrieved from <www.waterfordtechnologies.com>.

Whitehead, D. K., Weiss, S. A., & Tappen, R. M. (2010). *Essentials of nursing leadership and management* (5th ed.). Philadelphia, PA: F.A. Davis Company.

Wolfenden, J. (2011). Men in nursing. *The Internet Journal of Allied Health Sciences and Practice, 9*(2), 1–6.

Wood, G., Fromholtz, M., Morrison, R., Seet, P.-S., Wiesneer, R., & Zeffane, R. M. (2012). *Organisational behaviour: Core concepts and applications.* Melbourne: John Wiley & Sons.

World Bank. (2012). *Gender differences in employment and why they matter.* Washington DC: World Bank. Retrieved from <http://econ.worldbank.org/>.

Yap, M. (2010). The intersection of gender and race: Effects on the incidence of promotions. *Canadian Journal of Career Development, 9*(2), 22–33.

Young, R. (2011). *Power dressing: First ladies, women politicians and fashion.* London: Merrell Publications.

CHAPTER FOUR

Leadership, ethics and nursing work environments

Debra Jackson & Marie Hutchinson

LEARNING OBJECTIVES

At the completion of this chapter, the reader will be able to:

▲ describe the role of ethics in leadership;

▲ elucidate leadership in the context of ethical behaviour;

▲ explain the influence of leadership ethics in shaping nursing work environments;

▲ clarify the role of moral courage in effective leadership;

▲ discuss the consequences of ethics failures in leadership;

▲ identify ways of recognising ethical and unethical leadership behaviours in the workplace; and

▲ demonstrate understanding of the need for ethical workplace behaviour in self and others.

KEY WORDS

Leadership, ethical behaviour, work environments, bullying, workplace incivility, whistleblowing

INTRODUCTION

In this chapter we consider the role of leaders in creating and maintaining ethical and principled working environments. It is widely accepted that leaders do have an essential role in shaping moral and just working environments, and for contributing to the creation of workplaces that reflect organisational missions and values (Lindy & Schaefer, 2010). However, there is a plethora of literature suggesting that all too often, espoused organisational values are not reflected in the work environment for nurses (Firtko & Jackson, 2005; Jackson, Cleary, & Mannix, 2013; Shirey, 2005). Indeed, there is a vast literature indicating quite the opposite—that for many nurses, the workplace is experienced as negative and even hostile, and characterised by inappropriate and disruptive behaviour (Hutchinson & Jackson, 2013a; McNamara, 2012; Vessey, DeMarco, & DiFazio, 2010).

Despite the extensive research and commentary on negative workplace behaviour, and notwithstanding some notable exceptions (such as Jackson, 2008a; Milton, 2009; Wong & Cummings, 2007) the place of ethical leaders' behaviours in creating or contributing to quality work environments for nurses has not, in our opinion, received adequate attention. In this chapter we draw broadly from the intersection of ethics and leadership literature to focus on issues such as moral courage in relation to the role that leaders have in shaping nursing work environments.

ETHICS IN LEADERSHIP

A strong adherence to ethical practice lies at the very heart of nursing. Ethical principles guide our actions with patients, and also the conduct of research and knowledge dissemination. In the patient-care, publication and research domains, any breach of ethical practice, or digression from accepted ethical norms, is viewed very seriously and carries considerable consequences, with swift action taken to restore ethically appropriate practice.

However, when considering behaviours within organisations and the collegial realm, the role of ethical leadership behaviour is rather less clear (Jackson, 2008a; Milton, 2009). Although there have been numerous policy and research reports that call for nursing leadership to address models of care, care outcomes and care environments (Cummings et al., 2010; The Joint Commission, 2009; Wong & Cummings, 2007), rarely has attention been given to whether the presence or absence of ethical leadership may influence care outcomes.

When faced with ethical dilemmas and challenges, individuals will look to those around them for guidance and make their decision according to what they perceive peers and leaders expect of them (Brown & Trevino, 2006). Leaders play an important role in creating and sustaining opportunities for ethical decision making and action in the workplace. The enactment of ethical leadership requires not only individual moral judgements and actions, but the ability to create and sustain work environments to enable others to make ethical judgements and resist pressures to behave in unacceptable or unethical ways. In order to have this effect and be perceived as an ethical leader by others, those in leadership roles must display behaviours and actions that make them stand out as an ethical figure.

So, what does it mean to enact ethics in leadership? Ethical leaders are those who commit to a moral and just form of leadership. This form of leadership has an explicit ethical dimension, and the values and behaviour of ethical leaders are guided by established ethical principles of respect for persons, justice, veracity, beneficence, non-maleficence and fidelity (Shirey, 2005). Some of the ways that ethical leaders might enact these ethical principles are shown in Table 4.1.

Table 4.1 Enacting ethical leadership

Ethical principle	Definition	Application to leadership
Respect for persons	An attitude towards others that perceives all persons are inherently worthy of respect	Acts to make others feel appreciated as a person
		Recognises, appreciates and communicates the important worth of other persons (this recognition is not rewards based)
		Confers responsibility, grants autonomy, considers others' needs
Justice	Ensuring fair treatment of all people	Treats others to be of equal worth
		Distribution of rewards according to merit
		Displays morality and fairness in decision making
		Promotes and rewards just conduct
Veracity	The principle of honesty in interactions	Listens and is attentive to others' concerns
		Transparent and engages in open communication and decision making
		Attention to integrity, true to themselves and others
		Upholds trust and confidentiality
		Role-models honesty, respect and sincerity
		Uncompromising and steadfast
		Do as they say, and follow-up and follow-through with regard to their principles
Beneficence	Acts with a commitment to the welfare of others	Displays appreciation of others and empowers others
		Displays authentic concern for others and demonstrates that they are individually valued
		Allows others to have a voice in decision making and listens to ideas and concerns
Non-maleficence	To prevent harm and promote wellbeing	Clear guidance on expectations and responsibilities
		Openly engages with discussion on the implications of actions
		Displays concern for the means used to achieve goals
		Is not primarily concerned with transactions and end results
Fidelity	Being loyal to others	Supports those facing adversity
		Develops inclusive processes and power sharing

Table content informed by: De Hoogh & Den Hartog, 2008; Jackson & Borbasi, 2000; Shirey, 2005; van Quaquebeke & Eckloff, 2010

In contemplating the nature of ethical leadership, Milton (2009) highlights 'fairness and honesty in being just and trusting human integrity' (p. 119) as important characteristics. Ethical leadership also encompasses moral courage (Hannah, Avolio, & Walumbwa, 2011). It is concerned not only with distinguishing what might be considered right or good in a given situation, but also with the commitment to act to do what is right or good—even in the face of considerable adversity. The crucial role of ethical and courageous leadership in achieving optimal standards of patient care has been reinforced by many public inquiries into poor standards of care (Alberti, 2009; Francis, 2010). It is also reflected in research into workplace problems and difficulties experienced by many nurses (Jackson, Hutchinson, Peters, Luck, & Saltman, 2013).

THE INFLUENCE OF LEADERSHIP AND LEADERSHIP ETHICS IN SHAPING NURSING WORK ENVIRONMENTS

In many workplaces, nurses and other health workers routinely experience pressures and tensions between acting in ways that uphold personal and professional principles of ethical conduct, and the expectation and pressure to attain other goals, such as cost efficiency, which may threaten ethical judgement and action (Judge & Piccolo, 2004; McGuire & Kennerly, 2006). In resource-pressured environments, bottom-line decision making can promote financial goals as the primary value considered in decision making. This type of transactional environment increases the likelihood of decisions and actions that are unethical and the erosion of the ethical climate (Zhu, Riggio, Avolio, & Sosik, 2011).

The prevailing perceptions about what is appropriate and inappropriate conduct within workplaces create an ethical climate within an organisation; this climate shapes the operation of formal and informal systems and processes and influences behaviour and action (Neubert, Carlson, Kacmar, Roberts, & Chonko, 2009). The ethical climate operates to signal and reinforce what is considered acceptable behaviour, and can operate to support either ethical or unethical conduct (Brown & Trevino, 2006). To influence the ethical climate and facilitate others in their ethical decision-making capacity, ethical leadership requires more than leaders simply making ethical decisions and treating others with dignity and respect; it requires that ethical values be made visible within the workplace.

Though many workplaces espouse certain workplace values and may even have conduct policies in place espousing 'zero-tolerance' for various negative workplace behaviours (Australian Nursing Foundation, 2002; NSW Health, 2003), these policies are only as effective as their implementation and administration (Jackson, Hutchinson et al., 2013). Indeed, it has been noted that bad behaviour in the workplace occurs because it is seen in others, and therefore considered to be acceptable, and because it so often remains unchallenged (McNamara, 2012). Repeated exposure to wrongdoing that is either actively or passively condoned can habituate individuals to its occurrence. Over time, repeated exposure can have a normative effect, shaping socialisation processes and dulling awareness through gradual desensitisation (Robinson & O'Leary-Kelly, 1998).

Shirey (2005) highlighted the importance of espoused workplace values and vision in shaping the climates or cultures of the workplace. Certainly, organisational values (such as equity, respect, etc.) should be translated into the day-to-day working environment (Shirey, 2005), and should be able to be reflected in the ways that personnel interact and engage with all stakeholders, including clients, patients and other personnel.

However, even the most cursory scan of the literature shows that there are many forms of aberrant conduct plaguing the nursing workplace, and these include behaviours that together comprise bullying and/or harassment, violence, abuse and also incivility (Hutchinson, Vickers, Jackson, & Wilkes, 2006a; Hutchinson, Vickers, Wilkes, & Jackson, 2010; Vessey et al., 2010). There are many terms used to describe these undesirable and damaging behaviours (Lindy & Schaefer, 2010; McNamara, 2012). The nature of the various terms and the images they conjure up are beyond the scope of this chapter; suffice to say they range from phrases such as 'nurses eating their young' and 'wrongdoing' (Milton, 2009, p. 117) through to 'horizontal violence' and 'abuse' (Vessey et al., 2010). However, notwithstanding the type of language used to describe this behaviour, the sheer volume of literature on this topic speaks for the extent of concern that surrounds it. It is also noteworthy that this literature comes from across the globe, suggesting that these problems are causing concern internationally (Lindy & Schaefer, 2010).

There are a number of explanations offered for the prevalence of inappropriate and damaging behaviours in the nursing workplace. These explanations include theorising about the effects of oppressed group behaviour (Corney, 2008; Roberts, Demarco, & Griffin, 2009), which leads to a cycle of enactment of damaging behaviours between nurses. An alternate interpretation positions wrongdoing and damaging behaviour as a feature of the operation of power within organisations, with these behaviours enabled through networked power relations and the use and misuse of formal and informal organisational position and process (Hutchinson, Vickers, Jackson, & Wilkes, 2010).

There is considerable evidence that the behaviour and responses of leaders to inappropriate behaviour in the workplace greatly influence both its prevalence and the willingness of nurses and others to report it (Jackson et al., 2010a; Keenan, 2002; Lindy & Schaefer, 2010). Lindy and Schaefer (2010) produce findings that indicate managers do view negative workplace behaviours as an issue they need to address in their roles as managers, but there is a clear subtext of ambivalence about how to actually go about this. The idea of turning a blind eye to inappropriate behaviour is visible as a clear subtext; for example, if the perpetrator of the bad behaviour was considered to be a 'good' clinician, then there seemed to be a view that they can 'get away with' inappropriate behaviour (Lindy & Schaefer, 2010, p. 289). Similarly, a study of nurses in the United States reported a very strong tendency towards peers overlooking wrongdoing when they positioned the wrongdoer as being a 'good' nurse (King & Scudder, 2013).

Minimising the complexity of the problem is another prevalent subtext, with a general framing of inappropriate behaviour as being associated with personality; reducing it to simply an interpersonal problem, and so the target personality is also scrutinised, and positioned as 'accommodating and passive' and willing to tolerate the behaviour (Lindy & Schaefer, 2010, p. 288). The notion that people are positioned as being either perpetrators or targets/victims is also problematic, and Milton (2009) cautions reflection on how the parties in these situations are positioned, urging leaders to avoid 'reducing and dehumanizing' (p. 119) the individuals involved, and instead focus on developing more innovative approaches to addressing the issues.

A secondary analysis of research into nurses' experiences of bullying and whistle-blowing revealed a strong undercurrent of avoidant leadership. In this context, avoidant leadership referred to those in leadership roles not responding appropriately when made aware of wrongdoing. Three ways of enacting avoidant responses were identified: these were through placating avoidance, equivocal avoidance and hostile avoidance (Jackson, Hutchinson et al., 2013). However, despite the clear differences in these responses, in all of these ways of avoiding addressing serious workplace issues, these leadership reactions reflect a lack of ethical and moral courage and highlight how avoidant responses in those with leadership roles can damage 'the ethical character of the workplace' (Jackson, Hutchinson et al., 2013, p. 6). To all intents and purposes, avoidant leadership is a leadership that is devoid of courage, and a leadership that contributes to the corruption of the workplace, thus posing a threat to the safety and wellbeing of those within it.

WHEN LEADERSHIP ETHICS FAIL

When considering the nursing workplace, it is also important to remember that this same space that is so often presented as hostile and characterised by inappropriate and undesirable behaviour is also, simultaneously, presented as a site of healing and therapeutic care for patients (Jackson & Daly, 2010). Indeed, some literature also highlights the damaging and deleterious effects of inappropriate behaviours to patients as well as to nursing and other health personnel (Cummings et al., 2008; Hutchinson, Jackson, Walter, & Cleary, 2013; Hutchinson, Jackson, Wilkes, & Vickers, 2008; Hutchinson et al., 2006a; Jackson, 2008a, 2008b; McNamara, 2012).

Although addressing the impact of wrongdoing and disruptive behaviours has been identified in policy documents emanating from the United States as a priority for healthcare leaders (The Joint Commission, 2008, 2009), the focus of these policies is upon leadership that addresses the behaviour of individuals, with sparse attention given to the nexus between ethical leadership and care failures, and the impact of these failures in corrupting the care environment. It is important to acknowledge that when the environment is corrupted, what is meant to be a healing and therapeutic environment is rendered devoid of care and can become toxic.

Evidence suggests that in healthcare institutions, leaders lie at the very heart of both the cause and solution to the corruption of care environments. Inquiries into large-scale care failures have repeatedly identified that most start with relatively small failures and indiscretions, that over time grow on a scale that is proportional to the failure in leadership (Francis, 2010; Garling, 2008). Figure 4.1 depicts the ways that ethically and morally weak leadership can influence patient outcomes, nursing morale

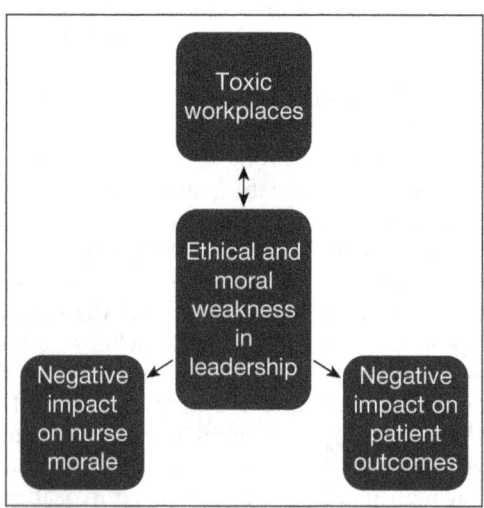

FIGURE 4.1
Leadership failure

and can corrupt the workplace to the point of rendering it toxic and potentially damaging to all those within it.

As depicted, the corruption of work and care environments impacts at a number of levels and can become widespread. At the level of patient care, deriving efficiencies that undermine care without due consideration of this impact or the likelihood of harm can undermine the ethical climate (Heggen & Wellard, 2004). In this context, the pursuit of targets and efficiencies, even when they impact the quality and standard of care, can be reframed as acceptable. To survive in this environment, nurses may disengage their moral compass and become indifferent or uncaring. This type of selective moral disengagement can lead to the further disregard of ethical standards (Bandura, 2002). Possible sequelae to organisations (Lindy & Schaefer, 2010) and nurses of toxic work environments are very well acknowledged in the literature and include a range of outcomes such as poor morale, disengagement and recruitment and retention issues (Jackson & Daly, 2010; Jackson et al., 2010b; McNamara, 2012; Peters et al., 2011; Spence Laschinger, Leiter, Day, & Gilin, 2009).

When a work environment becomes negative or toxic, bad behaviour can become normalised (Jackson, Hutchinson et al., 2013; Milton, 2009). At a workgroup level, repeated instances of silence on wrongdoing can reinforce a form of groupthink (Nielsen, 2003) that fosters continued moral silence (Clegg, 1997). Individuals are less likely to speak out about concerns or wrongdoing. The normalisation of withholding information or 'turning a blind eye' to transgressions or wrongdoing can have far-reaching consequences, including the erosion of patient safety.

Managers in the healthcare sector are under increasing pressure to perform (McMurray, Pullen, & Rhodes, 2011) and have been said to obscure information that may be considered detrimental to the organisation—including information about adverse events (Perra, 2001). Transactional leaders may be swayed to exploitation for organisational or personal gain (Trevino, Brown, & Hartman, 2003). This behaviour has a trickle-down effect across the workplace and can perpetuate silence and increase the likelihood of disruptive and unacceptable behaviours. One of the more powerful influences on voice perceptions in workgroups is the direct leader of the group, with negative leader behaviours negatively influencing perceptions about voice climate and increasing the likelihood of silence (Zohar & Luria, 2005).

Issues surrounding the ways that bullying or other wrongdoing can damage work teams and lead to behaviours that can negatively affect and even harm patients are still largely unacknowledged in the literature (Hutchinson & Jackson, 2013a). Indeed, and as we have stated earlier, all too often these difficulties are framed as interpersonal problems between staff, which minimises and greatly diminishes their potential damage to others, including potential harm to patients.

Notwithstanding the lack of general recognition, the evidence is clear. A recent case study report clearly revealed corruption of the work environment, through wrongdoing that was allowed to continue unabated, until the death of a patient brought the behaviour into the public realm (Hutchinson et al., 2013). This case highlights the need for scrutiny, and for a more critical stance on the nature of hostile and disruptive behaviours that can seriously impact the quality, safety, healing and therapeutic functions of the healthcare environment.

LEADERSHIP AND ETHICS IN THE WORK ENVIRONMENT

In their everyday work experiences, leaders will be confronted with myriad competing issues and perspectives (Aiken, Clarke, & Sloane, 2002). These multiple competing priorities and agendas create an ambiguous and difficult moral maze that must be navigated in decision making and action. So far in our discussion, we have positioned ethics as an obligation to respond to the other in just and moral ways (Ray, 2006). In considering multiple others, as leaders must in their decision making and actions, the notion of 'other' moves beyond dyadic relationships, to the competing demands of multiple individuals or groups and the systems and structures at play in organisations.

In considering multiple others in this way, ethical leadership is more complex, and the choices confronting leaders inevitably give rise to the play of politics in decision making (Weiskopf & Willmott, 2013). This requires that leaders give attention to the norms and ethical practices in organisations and critically locate themselves within this discourse (Clegg, Kornberger, & Rhodes, 2007). It is important that leaders recognise that power structures within institutions can facilitate ways of thinking and acting that become routine, and individuals within these environments may define their ethical position in relation to these everyday events (Prasad & Prasad, 1998). These shared understandings of organisational morality have a history and are reproduced over time through established practices and power dynamics, providing a way of interpreting, defining and dealing with issues.

Such ways of viewing the world are not power neutral; instead, they operate to reinforce certain worldviews and associated values, and these taken-for-granted worldviews can impede moral judgement and conduct (Hutchinson, Vickers, Jackson, & Wilkes, 2006b). Likewise, demands for loyalty and confidentiality (Jackson et al., 2010a; Jackson & Raftos, 1997) may work to silence dissent, and ensure agreement with the accepted order. In these situations, disagreement can be framed as undesirable or even disloyal, and those who challenge accepted values and frames of reference may be positioned as troubling dissenters.

In negotiating these complex dynamics, ethical leaders must build a bridge between power and politics in ethically managing competing demands (McMurray et al., 2011). This bridge involves making practical decisions about competing demands and decisions about which demands are a priority in the face of competing choices. In grappling with this complexity, there is a need to craft leadership practices that move beyond taken-for-granted rules and practices and create a leadership space that allows for different ways of acting and relating.

Ethical leadership in this context requires a critical stance, one which questions and problematises the ethics of accepted practices. In critically questioning what are otherwise taken for granted, ethical leaders can create 'ethical moments' (Weiskopf & Willmott, 2013, p. 475) that open up opportunities to question and challenge. Ethical leaders do not turn a 'blind eye' to ethical lapses (Trevino et al., 2003). This means they may need to take a stance against political or executive level decisions that erode the capacity to maintain standards. This requires that leaders have a high level of awareness of their own moral identity and awareness about their moral engagement and responsibility to others and its consequences.

CONCLUSION

We are not suggesting that leaders necessarily make deliberate decisions to neglect integrity, or that they are indifferent to ethics and integrity; instead, they may succumb to ways of thinking and acting that cumulatively erode their capacity for ethical behaviour. Insensitive or unaware unethical leaders may unintentionally lose sight of ethical issues and concerns with potentially devastating flow-on effects in the workplace.

While some leadership models, such as servant leadership, have an 'explicit moral component' (Jackson, 2008b, p. 28), many do not. In other models of leadership, ethical and moral conduct is implied, such as in transformational leadership (Hutchinson & Jackson, 2013b). Another concerning feature of many contemporary models of leadership is that ethical leadership is considered exceptional rather than the norm (Trevino et al., 2003). The idea that moral and ethical leadership is a taken-for-granted aspect of many leadership models is troubling and raises the need for self-monitoring and transparency in leadership. The place of ethical leaders' behaviours in creating or contributing to quality work environments for nurses has not received adequate attention, and emerging and current nurse leaders must turn their attention to making visible the nature and enactment of ethical leadership.

REFLECTIVE EXERCISE

1. Obtain and read the Mission or Value Statement from your workplace.
    a. Consider the nature of the workplace in relation to this Statement.
    b. What strategies can you identify that are in practice to uphold the Mission or Value Statement?
    c. Now reflect again on the issues raised in this chapter and consider the major personal qualities needed by leaders if they are to enhance the nursing workplace.
2. Obtain the relevant Code of Ethics governing nurses in your jurisdiction.
    a. Consider the nature of the workplace in relation to this Code.
    b. What strategies can you identify that are in practice to uphold the Code of Ethics?

Recommended Readings

Hutchinson, M., & Jackson, D. (2013). Transformational leadership in nursing: Towards a more critical interpretation. *Nursing Inquiry, 20*(1), 11–22.

Hutchinson, M., Jackson, D., Walter, G., & Cleary, M. (2013). Coercion and the corruption of care in mental health nursing: Lessons from a case study. *Issues in Mental Health Nursing, 34*(6), 476–480.

Jackson, D., Hutchinson, M., Peters, K., Luck, L., & Saltman, D. C. (2013). Understanding avoidant leadership in health care: Findings from a secondary analysis of two qualitative studies. *Journal of Nursing Management, 21*(3), 572–580.

Neubert, M. J., Carlson, D. S., Kacmar, K. M., Roberts, J. A., & Chonko, L. B. (2009). The virtuous influence of ethical leadership behavior: Evidence from the field. *Journal of Business Ethics, 90*, 157–170.

References

Aiken, L. H., Clarke, S. P., & Sloane, D. M. (2002). Hospital staffing, organization, and quality of care: Cross-national findings. *Nursing Outlook, 50*, 187–194.

Alberti, G. (2009). *Mid Staffordshire NHS foundation trust: A review of the procedures for emergency admission and treatment, and progress against the recommendation of the March Healthcare Commission Report*. The Health Care Commission. Retrieved from <http://www.midstaffspublicinquiry.com/key-documents>.

Australian Nursing Foundation. (2002). *Zero tolerance (occupational violence and aggression)*. Melbourne: Australian Nursing Foundation, Victorian Branch.

Bandura, A. (2002). Selective moral disengagement in the exercise of moral agency. *Journal of Moral Education, 31*(2), 101–119.

Brown, M. E., & Trevino, L. K. (2006). Ethical Leadership. *The Leadership Quarterly, 17*, 595–616.

Clegg, S. (1997). Foucault, power, social theory and the study of organisations. In C. O'Farrell (Ed.), *Foucault the legacy* (pp. 484–491). Brisbane, Australia: Queensland University of Technology.

Clegg, S. R., Kornberger, M., & Rhodes, C. (2007). Business ethics as practice. *British Journal of Management, 18*(2), 107–122.

Corney, B. (2008). Aggression in the workplace: A study of horizontal violence utilising Heideggerian hermeneutic phenomenolog. *Journal of Health Organisation and Management, 22*(2), 164–177.

Cummings, G., Lee, H., MacGregor, T., Davey, M., Wong, C., Paul, L., et al. (2008). Factors contributing to nursing leadership: A systematic review. *Journal of Health Services Research and Policy, 13*(4), 240–248.

Cummings, G. G., MacGregor, T., Davey, M., Leeab, H., Wong, C. A., Loab, E., et al. (2010). Leadership styles and outcome patterns for the nursing workforce and work environment: A systematic review. *International Journal of Nursing Studies, 47*(3), 363–385.

De Hoogh, A. H. B., & Den Hartog, D. N. (2008). Ethical and despotic leadership, relationships with leader's social responsibility, top management team effectiveness and subordinates' optimism: A multi-method study. *The Leadership Quarterly, 19*, 297–311.

Firtko, A., & Jackson, D. (2005). Do the ends justify the means? Nursing and the dilemma of whistleblowing. *Australian Journal of Advanced Nursing, 23*(1), 51–57.

Francis, R. (2010). *Independent inquiry into care provided by Mid Staffordshire NHS Foundations*. Healthcare Commission. Retrieved from <http://www.midstaffspublicinquiry.com/report>.

Garling, P. (2008). *Final report of the special commission of inquiry. Acute care services in NSW public hospitals*. Special Commission of Inquiry, New South Wales Government, Sydney. Retrieved from <http://www.dpc.nsw.gov.au/__data/assets/pdf_file/0003/34194/Overview_-_Special_Commission_Of_Inquiry_Into_Acute_Care_Services_In_New_South_Wales_Public_Hospitals>.

Hannah, S. T., Avolio, B. J., & Walumbwa, F. O. (2011). Relationships between authentic leadership, moral courage, and ethical pro-social behaviors. *Business Ethics Quarterly, 21*(4), 555–578.

Heggen, K., & Wellard, S. (2004). Increased unintended patient harm in nursing practise as a consequence of the dominance of economic discourses. *International Journal of Nursing Studies, 41*(3), 293–298.

Hutchinson, M., & Jackson, D. (2013a). Hostile clinician behaviours in the nursing work environment and implications for patient care: A mixed-methods systematic review. *BMC Nursing, 12*(25), doi:10.1186/1472-6955-1112-1125

Hutchinson, M., & Jackson, D. (2013b). Transformational leadership in nursing: Towards a more critical interpretation. *Nursing Inquiry, 20*(1), 11–22.

Hutchinson, M., Jackson, D., Walter, G., & Cleary, M. (2013). Coercion and the corruption of care in mental health nursing: Lessons from a case study. *Issues in Mental Health Nursing, 34*(6), 476–480.

Hutchinson, M., Jackson, D., Wilkes, L., & Vickers, M. (2008). A new model of bullying in the nursing workplace: Organizational characteristics as critical antecedents. *Advances in Nursing Science, 31*(2), E60–E71.

Hutchinson, M., Vickers, M. H., Jackson, D., & Wilkes, L. (2006a). 'They stand you in a corner; you are not to speak': Nurses tell of abusive indoctrination in work teams dominated by bullies. *Contemporary Nurse, 21*(2), 228–238.

Hutchinson, M., Vickers, M. H., Jackson, D., & Wilkes, L. (2006b). Workplace bullying in nursing: Towards a more critical organisational perspective. *Nursing Inquiry, 13*(2), 118–126.

Hutchinson, M., Vickers, M. H., Jackson, D., & Wilkes, L. (2010). Bullying as circuits of power: An Australian perspective. *Administrative Theory & Praxis, 32*(1), 25–47.

Hutchinson, M., Vickers, M., Wilkes, L., & Jackson, D. (2010). A typology of bullying behaviours: The experiences of Australian nurses. *Journal of Clinical Nursing, 19*, 2319–2328.

Jackson, D. (2008a). Collegial trust: Crucial to safe and harmonious workplaces. *Journal of Clinical Nursing, 17*(12), 1541–1542.

Jackson, D. (2008b). Servant leadership in nursing: A framework for developing sustainable research capacity in nursing. *Collegian (Royal College of Nursing, Australia), 15*(1), 27–33.

Jackson, D., & Borbasi, S. A. (2000). The caring conundrum: Potential and perils for nursing. In J. Daly, S. Speedy, & D. Jackson (Eds.), *Contexts of nursing: An introduction* (pp. 65–74). Sydney: MacLennan and Petty.

Jackson, D., Cleary, M., & Mannix, J. (2013). Ethical sensitivity: Shaping the everyday work environment. *Contemporary Nurse, 44*(1), 2–4.

Jackson, D., & Daly, J. (2010). Improving the workplace: The pivotal role of nurse leaders. *Contemporary Nurse, 36*(1–2), 82–85.

Jackson, D., Hutchinson, M., Peters, K., Luck, L., & Saltman, D. C. (2013). Understanding avoidant leadership in health care: Findings from a secondary analysis of two qualitative studies. *Journal of Nursing Management, 21*(3), 572–580.

Jackson, D., Peters, K., Andrew, S., Edenborough, M., Halcomb, E., Luck, L., et al. (2010a). Trial and retribution: A qualitative study of whistleblowing and workplace relationships in nursing. *Contemporary Nurse, 36*(1), 34–44.

Jackson, D., Peters, K., Andrew, S., Edenborough, M., Halcomb, E., Luck, L., et al. (2010b). Understanding whistleblowing: Qualitative insights from nurse whistleblowers. *Journal of Advanced Nursing, 66*(10), 2194–2201.

Jackson, D., & Raftos, M. (1997). In uncharted waters: Confronting the culture of silence in residential care institutions. *International Journal of Nursing Practice, 3*(1), 34–39.

Judge, T., & Piccolo, R. F. (2004). Transformational and transactional leadership: A meta-analytic test of their relative validity. *Journal of Applied Psychology, 89*(5), 755–768.

Keenan, J. P. (2002). Whistleblowing: A study of managerial differences. *Employee Rights and Responsibilities Journal, 14*(1), 17–24.

King, G., & Scudder, J. M. (2013). Reasons registered nurses report serious wrongdoings in a public teaching hospital. *Psychological Reports, 112*(2), 626–636.

Lindy, C., & Schaefer, F. (2010). Negative workplace behaviours: an ethical dilemma for nurse managers. *Journal of Nursing Management, 18*, 285–292.

McGuire, E., & Kennerly, S. M. (2006). Nurse managers as transformational and transactional leaders. *Nursing Economics, 24*(4), 179–185.

McMurray, R., Pullen, A., & Rhodes, C. (2011). Ethical subjectivity and politics in organisations: A case of health care tendering. *Organization, 18*(4), 541–561.

McNamara, S. (2012). Incivility in nursing: Unsafe nurse, unsafe patients. *AORN Journal, 95*(4), 535–540.

Milton, C. L. (2009). Leadership and ethics in nurse-nurse relationships. *Nursing Science Quarterly, 22*, 116–119.

Neubert, M. J., Carlson, D. S., Kacmar, K. M., Roberts, J. A., & Chonko, L. B. (2009). The virtuous influence of ethical leadership behavior: Evidence from the field. *Journal of Business Ethics, 90*, 157–170.

Nielsen, R. P. (2003). Corruption networks and implications for ethical corruption reform. *Journal of Business Ethics, 42*(2), 125.

NSW Health. (2003). Zero tolerance: Response to violence in the NSW Health Workplace, policy and framework guidelines. Retrieved from <www.wslhd.health.nsw.gov.au/>.

Perra, B. M. (2001). Managing clinical outcomes. *Journal of Nursing Care Quality, 15*(2), 68–73.

Peters, K., Luck, L., Hutchinson, M., Wilkes, L., Andrew, S., & Jackson, D. (2011). The emotional sequelae of whistleblowing: Findings from a qualitative study. *Journal of Clinical Nursing, 20*(19–20), 2907–2914.

Prasad, A., & Prasad, P. (1998). Everyday struggles at the workplace: The nature and implications of routine resistance in contemporary organisations. In P. A. Bamburger & W. J. Sonnestohl (Eds.), *Research in the sociology of organisations: Deviance in and of organisations* (pp. 225–255). Stamford, Connecticut: JAI Press.

Ray, S. (2006). Whistleblowing and organisational ethics. *Nursing Ethics, 13*(4), 438–455.

Roberts, S. J., Demarco, R., & Griffin, M. (2009). The effect of oppressed group behaviour on the culture of the nursing workplace: A review of the evidence and interventions for change. *Journal of Nursing Management, 17*, 288–293.

Robinson, S. L., & O'Leary-Kelly, A. M. (1998). Monkey see, monkey do: The influence of work groups on the antisocial behavior of employees. *Academy of Management Journal, 41*(6), 658–671.

Shirey, M. (2005). Ethical climate in nursing practice: The leader's role. *JONA's Healthcare Law, Ethics, and Regulation, 7*(2), 59–67.

Spence Laschinger, H. K., Leiter, M., Day, A., & Gilin, D. (2009). Workplace empowerment, incivility, and burnout: Impact on staff nurse recruitment and retention outcomes. *Journal of Nursing Management, 17*, 302–311.

The Joint Commission. (2008). Behaviors that undermine a culture of safety (Vol. Sentinel Event Alert #40). Retrieved from <http://www.jointcommission.org/SentinelEvents/SentinelEventAlert/sea_40.htm>.

The Joint Commission. (2009). Leadership committed to safety. *Sentinel Event Alert #43*: The Joint Commission on Accreditation of Healthcare Organisations.

Trevino, L. K., Brown, M., & Hartman, L. P. (2003). A qualitative investigation of perceived executive ethical leadership: Perceptions from inside and outside the executive suite. *Human Relations, 56*(1), 5–37.

van Quaquebeke, N., & Eckloff, T. (2010). Defining respectful leadership: What it is, how it can be measured, and another glimpse at what it is related to. *Journal of Business Ethics, 91*(3), 343–358.

Vessey, J. A., DeMarco, R., & DiFazio, R. (Eds.). (2010). Bullying, harassment, and horizontal violence in the nursing workforce: The state of the science. *Annual Review of Nursing Research, 28*, 133–157.

Weiskopf, R., & Willmott, H. (2013). Ethics as critical practice: The 'Pentagon Papers', deciding responsibility, truth-telling, and the unsettling of organisational morality. *Organization Studies, 34*(4).

Wong, C., & Cummings, G. (2007). The relationship between nursing leadership and patient outcomes: A systematic review. *Journal of Nursing Management, 15*(5), 508–521.

Zhu, W., Riggio, R. E., Avolio, J. B., & Sosik, J. J. (2011). The effect of leadership on follower moral identity: Does transformational/transactional style make a difference. *Journal of Leadership & Organizational Studies, 18*, 150.

Zohar, D., & Luria, G. (2005). A multilevel model of safety climate: Cross-level relationships between organisation and group-level climates. *Journal of Applied Psychology, 90*, 587–596.

CHAPTER FIVE

Organisation violations: Implications for leadership

Sandra Speedy

LEARNING OBJECTIVES

At the completion of this chapter, the reader will be able to:
▲ understand the nature of organisation violations and the purposes they serve;
▲ consider the causes of organisation violations from a range of perspectives;
▲ develop a deeper understanding of the consequences of organisation violations;
▲ discuss the problem and consequences of trust violation in organisations; and
▲ insightfully identify ways of reducing organisation violations in the workplace.

KEY WORDS

Organisation violations, resistance, whistleblowing, horizontal violence, bullying, sexual harassment

INTRODUCTION

While organisations are created for a diverse range of purposes, they are recognised as having a 'dark side' (Slattery, 2009). This dark side has been identified as behaviours that are unacceptable to management because they disturb the goals of the organisation (generally profit-seeking) and may significantly disrupt its functioning. A number of scholars have historically given a range of descriptors to such 'unacceptable behaviours' including 'oppositional practices' (Collinson & Ackroyd, 2005), 'organisational retaliatory' or 'anti-citizenship' behaviours, including those labelled 'deviant', 'dysfunctional' and 'antisocial' (Barnes & Taska, 2012; Furnham & Siegel, 2012; Greenberg, 2010; Grieve, Palmer, & Pozner, 2010; Kets de Vries, 2006); and 'recalcitrant', demonstrated by sabotage, absenteeism, disobedience and decreased productivity (Bryman, Collinson, Grint, Jackson, & Uhl-Bien, 2011; Collinson & Ackroyd, 2005). Other researchers have used the term 'counterproductive work behaviours' to include aggression, violence and theft (Furnham & Siegel, 2012; Hershcovis, 2011); sexual harassment (Sinclair, 2005), and incivility (Kelloway, Francis, Prosser, & Cameron, 2010; Porath & Pearson, 2013); and horizontal violence and bullying, which has specifically been used in the nursing context (Demir & Rodwell, 2012; Hutchinson, Vickers, Jackson, & Wilkes, 2010; Hutchinson, Vickers, Wilkes, & Jackson, 2010; Poilpot-Rocaboy, 2006).

In 2001, Hearn and Parkin produced insightful work that conceptualised the above types of behaviour as 'organisation violations' in order to provide an inclusive framework that takes into account the structure of the organisation, its culture, its enactment of authority and its organisational processes; in other words, the context in which such behaviours occur. They stated that the 'ordinary and extraordinary tactics perpetuating oppressions—bullying, isolation, exclusion, harassment, physical violence, emotional assault, demeaning actions, along with cultural ideological and symbolic violences—need to be named as violations' (p. 87). Failure to recognise and deal with organisation violations results in poor standards of healthcare and ultimately high-level governmental inquiries, such as the Francis Report (Francis, 2013), the Garling Report (Garling, 2008), otherwise known as the Final Report of the Special Commission of Inquiry Acute Care Services in New South Wales Public Hospitals, and the Douglas Inquiry (Department of Health, Government of Western Australia, 2005).

This chapter, therefore, considers the contexts of organisation violations and examines the range of violations that can occur. It then addresses some of the causes of organisation violation, using a range of examples to demonstrate how workplace abuse is manifest, particularly from the perspective of the employee. Some of the consequences of organisation violations will be examined to see how this knowledge can be used by those in leadership positions to enhance organisational environments. Leaders of organisations need a high level of understanding of organisation violations and destructive leadership if they wish to be part of the reform process within such organisations (Gundmundsson & Southey, 2011).

CONTEXTS OF ORGANISATION VIOLATIONS

Organisation violations occur in any organisation. Healthcare organisations are no exception. In fact, there may be more potential for abuse of workers due to the unique characteristics of healthcare organisations. While all organisations seek efficiencies, productivity and cost containment in order to maximise profits, healthcare organisations have complexities of function and structures that are not generally characteristic of profit-making organisations. Their goals are often more abstract, authority is more diffuse and there are fewer performance indicators than 'for profit' organisations. Because of their mandate to meet socially recognised public health needs, healthcare organisations emphasise health rather than organisational issues, making them accountable in a range of ways that do not apply to private sector organisations. Typically, healthcare organisations are funded by the 'public purse', although increasingly there is a private funding imperative at work.

The major difference between healthcare organisations and 'for profit' organisations is the division between the 'professional' capacity for control over the 'bureaucratic' function of organisations. Specifically, professionals have the capacity to determine power relationships between the medical, nursing and administrative groups, which results in a political process that is entirely about the control that is exercised. Nevertheless, healthcare organisations do conform to the generic form of organisations, and hence, organisation violations are likely to occur.

'Unacceptable behaviours' of employees in the workplace, or 'organisation violations' are identified and interpreted by those who have power over those whose behaviour is being judged. Sometimes such behaviours have been labelled 'dysfunctional' or 'pathological'. This label is provided from the perspective of those who are in a position to sanction such behaviours, as their supervisory roles are being made more difficult. Collinson and Ackroyd (2005) insightfully analyse 'organisational misbehaviour', suggesting that the 'sociology of opposing interests' would be a useful lens with which to examine organisations. Rather than viewing persistent 'troublemakers' as having a personal pathology, they suggest that many misbehaviours are underpinned by informal workgroup norms, and that the organisation has a degree of dependency on them. This dependency is created by the organisation's structural imbalances of power (Collinson & Ackroyd, 2005). The organisation context, both internal and external, can be critical in determining the level of abuse that occurs; however, it is also clear that certain individuals are psychologically predisposed to using brutality to achieve their goals. An important contribution to this literature was made in 1995 by Gherardi, who asserted that authoritarian, highly centralised leadership often sets the scene for tyrannical behaviour of managers.

Power inequalities are embedded in organisational structures and contain the antecedents of organisation violations. It cannot be assumed that managers will responsibly wield their power to achieve organisational objectives; managers are certainly capable of misbehaviour (Richards, 2008). As demonstrated in the cited research, they do not always wield their power responsibly, despite attempts to downplay their abuses of power and discredit those who resist or react against it.

Misbehaviour is defined very broadly to be anything done at work that one is not supposed to do. In 1998 Ashforth and Mael explored the concept of 'acts of resistance', defined as attempts to assert power over those who have legitimate authoritative and organisational power. They suggested that the power of resistance is 'partly in its potential to contest meaning' (p. 92), because employees negotiated their 'work selves' with the organisation. Whether employees are regarded as behaving constructively or destructively is dependent on from whose perspective dysfunctionality is assessed. What is adaptive and functional for an individual (or a workgroup) may not be adaptive and functional for the organisation, such as whistleblowing behaviour, which may be negative from a management perspective, but positive from the public's perspective. There are many examples of behaviours that are counterproductive to management, but which assist individuals in adapting to situations that become intolerable (Kelloway et al., 2010). For example, employee theft or aggression may be a response to perceptions of gross injustice, such as being passed over for promotion.

Counterproductive work behaviours are often an emotional response to what the employee perceives as organisational work stressors, or any other perceived organisational injustice (Levine, 2010; Spector et al., 2006). This raises the issue of workplace abuse as a stress agent (Barling & Cooper, 2008), to be examined later in this chapter. Some employees may be treated unfairly and then seek justice through the use of retaliatory behaviours, which is not an individually neurotic event* (Folger, Cropanzano, & Goldman, 2005). There may be considerable justification for what has been labelled dysfunctional, deviant and antisocial behaviour (Elias, 2013).

This chapter takes the focus of employees' organisation violations, rather than violations more likely to be committed by senior management, including, for example, fraud, corporate crime and destructive leadership (Einarsen, Aasland, & Skogstad, 2007; Krasikova, Green, & LeBreton, 2013). Managers will be examined in so far as they define, interpret and sanction organisation violations of their workforce, and are, in fact, complicit in their management of 'misbehaviour' (Hearn & Parkin, 2001). This is particularly the case for sexual harassment and bullying, but has also been identified in 'the ordinary enactment of managerial "policy"' (Hearn & Parkin, 2001, p. 149). Managers can, for example, be actively involved in violations, ignore them, or collude with practices that lead to 'cultures of intimidation' (p. 150). Additionally, managers may be rewarded for bullying behaviours and thus continue to behave in this way. Observers are likely to emulate such abuses if they are viewed as acceptable in the work setting. Specifically, therefore, they may be the sexual harasser, or treat the harassed individual as 'imagining' the event, or allow the creation of opportunities within the organisation for violation to occur.

THE ROLE OF CULTURE

The culture of an organisation is significant when examining organisation violations because understanding culture is critical for effective leadership (Dalglish & Miller, 2010). Graetz, Rimmer, Smith, and Lawrence (2011) suggested that organisational culture comprised beliefs, values, norms, expectations and subsequent behaviours of a particular group of people, and, in this case, employees. If an organisation has particular values it may well socialise employees to engage in violations.

Other research demonstrates that highly ethical cultural environments encourage and facilitate organisational behaviours that are ethical and honest (Linstead, Fulop, & Lilley, 2009). However, in an organisational culture that is focused on self-interest, employees may lie in order to achieve rewards; conversely, if the lying is to protect a workmate, it may be viewed as justifiable if the culture values relationships.

Senior managements have been known to manipulate the culture of an organisation in order to create a 'strong culture' that will acquire the commitment and dedication of employees. Cultural values reflect the workgroup's shared understanding and subsequent behaviour, and, depending on those values, a trusting or distrusting environment can be created. Highly centralised, formalised and hierarchical organisations, whose focus is on efficiency, will not generate managerial trustworthiness (Choo & Ringquist, 2011) or employee empowerment (Rao, 2012). Conversely, organisations can encourage trustworthy managerial behaviours when interpersonal values of inclusiveness, open, honest communication, concern and valuing of colleagues are the norm. Managers who engender trust are more likely themselves to be trusting, inviting and to expect reciprocity of trust.

Managerial subcultures within organisations are also significant to organisation violations. Sinclair (2005) documents a study suggesting that managerial subcultures are built around masculinities, expressed in a variety of ways. These include traditional authoritarianism, advanced through bullying and fear; protective paternalism (otherwise known as 'the gentleman's club'); entrepreneurialism, expressed as task-focused, excessive commitment to work; and informalism, demonstrated by a boyish,

*This is a classic victim blaming strategy which places all responsibility on the targeted individual.

larrikin-like culture. Such subcultures, Sinclair (2005) asserts, require organisational women to exhibit a higher level of personal sacrifice and greater emotional toughness, and leaves them vulnerable to sexual harassment, aggression and bullying.

THE ROLE OF THE INDIVIDUAL

An individual's perception and interpretation of the work situation impacts on whether or not workplace abuse is recognised or acknowledged. Jones and Skarlicki (2013) assert that the psychological effect of a situation depends on how a person interprets the situation, and that these interpretations will depend on individual differences. Furthermore, they suggested that unfair treatment would not affect everyone subjected to it in the same way. They noted that some individuals had greater sensitivity to environments that had negative effects on them, suggesting that responses to such situations involved personality characteristics, perceptions of fairness, and also the person's perception of common practice. Of course, the relative power of the person abused, and their avenues of support within the organisation, can also impact on how the individual will deal with organisation violation (Shao, Rupp, Skarlicki, & Jones, 2013).

Resistance within an organisation can be rationalised by the individual if it is in that individual's best interests. For example, nurses who subject others to horizontal violence may justify such behaviours as being necessary to point out the 'shortcomings' of the target victim. The target victim, on the other hand, may try to resist this by behaving in unprofessional ways (that can be justified) with patients—a psychological mechanism known as displacement.

Individual attributes and emotions can influence organisational behaviour (Morgan, 2007; Shahzad, 2012). Shahzad suggests, for example, that aggression, greed, hate, fear and sexual desire, while having no official status, often break through, and may be rapidly punished or rationalised. However, any retaliation does not necessarily have a long-standing effect. Irrationality is banished, as it is feared as 'dangerous' and in need of controlling. Rationality, on the other hand, is designed to enhance our security. However, it will not necessarily result in understanding the impact of our actions on the organisation: hence the metaphor Morgan (2007) uses to describe the organisation as a 'psychic prison', in which all are imprisoned. This does highlight the importance of recognising the role that emotions and emotionality play in organisational life.

There is extensive literature taking the perspective that misbehaviour is due to psychological and biological causes (Langan-Fox, Cooper, & Klimoski, 2007). Bodankin and Tziner (2009) and Kets de Vries (2006) relate personality to organisational sabotage. Kets de Vries (2006) suggests that individuals use their defences to protect themselves against stressful work events, and that in most circumstances such defences are not pathological. Defences become pathological when they are overused or overdeveloped. However, psychological defences do tend to restrict the individual's perceptions, range and appropriateness of behavioural responses, particularly in emotion-laden situations. Other individual factors identified include locus of control, attributions and emotional stability (Spector & Fox, 2005). Psychological causes of misbehaviour have been framed as individuals having counterproductive workplace behaviours or 'dark-side' traits, which include argumentativeness, interpersonal insensitivity, narcissism, perfectionism, impulsivity and fear of failure.

There is now some recent more critical literature that suggests that previous research has not been able to elucidate the value (or otherwise) of counterproductive workplace behaviours. This research suggests, for example, that 'dark-side' traits may be useful for work success and productivity (Bolino, Klotz, Turnley, & Harvey, 2013; Furnham, Trickey, & Hyde, 2012; Judge, Piccolo, & Kosalka, 2009; Krischer, Penney, & Hunter, 2010; Spector, 2012; Spitzmuller & Van Dyne, 2013), which frames this behaviour in a more positive way.

CAUSES OF ORGANISATION VIOLATION

As previously established, behaviours that have a direct and visible negative effect on the organisation or members of the organisation can be caused by a range of factors and will, if unchecked, have a corruptive influence on organisational climate. Counterproductive work behaviours have the potential to decrease organisational productivity and damage the wellbeing of individuals. Note that self-destructive behaviours, such as drug or alcohol abuse, suppression of negative emotions, consistently working overtime, the expression of fake positive emotions (known as emotional labour), and even suicide are all possible responses to an abusive workplace.

As noted above, organisational cultures, structures and processes play a determining role in deeming what is unacceptable workplace behaviour. It is also clear that particular circumstances can be instrumental in encouraging 'misbehaviour'. In a now classic work, Ackroyd and Thompson (1999) suggested that 'misbehaviour' can take four directions (pp. 25–27). The first direction was disagreement over the appropriation of work, with conflict taking the possible form of destructiveness or sabotage. The second is the appropriation of materials used in work, and, in this case, conflict can result in pilferage, sometimes referred to as 'stock shrinkage' or 'unplanned overheads', also known as 'fiddling' (Linstead et al., 2009). The third direction is the amount of time spent on the work, and where conflict occurs, employees may engage in a range of behaviours, including time-wasting (often known as 'being absent at work', where toilets are often the place of refuge), or simply leaving the organisation altogether. The final direction is the extent to which employees identify with their work and their employer (known as the appropriation of identity), and where this does not occur, the behaviours can range from joking rituals based on horseplay and banter, to subjecting each other to existing subcultural rituals, which may involve initiations that are humiliating to newcomers.

ABUSIVE LEADERS AND ABUSIVE WORK SETTINGS

Employees who suffer 'work stress' are often operating under abusive work climates that organisations either refuse to acknowledge or take responsibility for (Barling, Kelloway, & Frone, 2005). These individuals may then be labelled as 'disgruntled' or 'troublemakers', therefore denying the role that organisations can play in creating an unnecessarily conflictual or unsupportive environment. This is another 'blame the victim' strategy that does not account for the often-sanctioned violence that occurs.

Inequality, oppression, toxic leadership and the abuse of power are fundamental to organisation violations (Babiak, Newmann, & Hare, 2010; Barnard, 2008; Hearn & Parkin, 2001; Itzen & Newman, 1995; Pelletier, 2010; Walton, 2007). Hearn and Parkin (2001) consider that 'gendered, sexualed power provides the material and ideological backcloth' (p. 85) to these violations, while Itzen and Newman (1995) acknowledge the damaging effects on both employer and employee. Such oppressiveness effectively silences or excludes employees, resulting in increased denial of violations, since these are not acknowledged. Hearn and Parkin (2001) also note that management takes an explicit and complicit role in violations, particularly those of sexual harassment and bullying, but point out that the ordinary enactment of managerial policy can have the same effect (p. 149).

Historically, there are a range of studies that seek to determine the characteristics, attributes and behaviours of abusive bosses, and, in some cases, why these occur. These include the following behaviours:

▲ sarcastic, verbally abusive, dishonest, intimidatory, harassing and cruel, due to poor interpersonal skill development, low self-esteem, and inadequate competencies (Sheehan, 1996);

▲ abusive due to lack of personal power (Jacques, 1995; Wyatt & Hare, 1997);

▲ argumentative, interpersonally insensitive, narcissistic, impulsive, perfectionist and having a fear of failure (Harms, Spain, & Hannah, 2011; Hughes, Ginnett, & Curphy, 2008; Northouse, 2013);

▲ abusive due to severe anxiety, thus justifying the need to 'strike first', citing 'lex talionis', the law of retaliation, commonly described as 'an eye for an eye, a tooth for a tooth' (Kets de Vries, 2006);

▲ petty, tyrannical behaviour (Ashforth, 1994; Bies & Tripp, 2005; Leonard, Lewis, Freedman, & Passmore, 2013). Variously described as the 'intolerable boss', the 'psycho boss from hell' or the 'brutal boss', the abusive boss primarily seeks to control others, and for various reasons;

▲ micro-manages, while demonstrating 'mercurial' mood swings, denigrates employees, exercises raw power for personal gain, coercive in corrupting employees (Bies & Tripp, 2005; Gilbert, Carr-Ruffino, Ivancevich, & Konopaske, 2012). This socially toxic behaviour has a poisonous effect on professional and personal lives (p. 210);

▲ bossy, abusive, ruthless, authoritarian, manipulative, dishonest, coercive (Buchanan & Badham, 2008);

▲ sense of entitlement, lacking in conscience, aggressive, narcissistic, disloyal, lacking in empathy, emotionally impoverished (Babiak & Hare, 2006; Barnard, 2008);

▲ snooping, excessive surveillance, no respect for privacy (Hasan & Subhani, 2012).

A well-recognised form of abuse resulting from power inequities is bullying, a distinct form of aggressive behaviour, which has been the focus of much recent study (e.g. Bies & Tripp, 2005; Bryman et al., 2011; Furnham & Siegel, 2012; Hutchinson, Vickers, Jackson et al., 2010; Hutchinson, Vickers, Wilkes et al., 2010; Yildirim, 2009). Bullying has various grades of intensity, ranging from physical actions to slander and individual isolation. Whether behaviour is bullying or not is dependent on the perception of the individual, but it always involves unwanted behaviour that is intimidating, humiliating, offensive and embarrassing conducted in public or private.

Bullying also has a component that is known as 'mobbing' (Einarsen, Hoel, Zapf, & Cooper, 2011; Zapf & Einarsen, 2005). This refers to situations where the bully uses power and influence to incite others to be part of the bullying process, to marginalise and persecute the target, either knowingly or unknowingly, which is common in healthcare and other organisations. Mobbing can be successful due to a mechanism known as 'identifying with the aggressor' (Sinclair, 2005), which involves building alliances with the abuser in order to be in the 'winning camp' (Kets de Vries, 2006). This serves to legitimise scapegoating the 'losers', resulting in the 'victim' developing power over another, while becoming the oppressor.

There are a number of elements in bullying: the desire to hurt; the perpetuation of hurtful behaviour by a more powerful person; unjustified and repeated actions enjoyed by the perpetrator, and which the target feels oppressed by (Dellasega, 2009;

Hutchinson, Vickers, Wilkes et al., 2010; Johnson, 2009; Johnston, Phanhtharath, & Jackson, 2009; Liefooghe & Davey, 2010; Oade, 2009; Rigby, 2012). Researchers have identified an extensive range of interpersonal bullying behaviours including scapegoating, aggressive teasing and joking at another's expense, trading of insults (Hearn & Parkin, 2001), as well as aggressive behaviour directly targeting the organisation, including vandalism, theft and sabotage (Ackroyd & Thompson, 1999).

Hearn and Parkin (2001) and Jordon (2002) cite a range of studies indicating that bullying and lateral violence is very common by line managers and those in authority over subordinates, particularly when it is used as a method of disciplining the workforce (Cleary, Hunt, & Horsfall, 2010; Croft & Cash, 2012). Typically, bullying can last for many years, having a debilitating effect on the individual and the organisation.

There can be enormous organisational costs associated with unchecked bullying, including counter-aggression towards others, withdrawal of services, increased absenteeism, reduction in productivity and 'citizenship' behaviours, increased turnover, incivility (Pearson, Andersson, & Porath, 2005; Porath & Pearson, 2013), demotivation (Kupers, 2009) and a range of stress reactions that can have major physical and psychological impacts on employees. In such situations, an increasingly likely option for employees is litigation against the organisation. A study by Greenberg (2010) found that workplace aggression and violence was common when there was job insecurity, unfair justice procedures and excessive surveillance of employees.

A major form of disruption occurs when there is violation of trust in organisations. Systematic research relating to trust in organisations has been carried out for more than 40 years (Bligh & Kohles, 2013). Organisations in which violations are prevalent will not have a trusting climate or culture (Covey, 2009). Ackroyd and Thompson (1999) noted that there are low trust and high trust managerial regimes, the former characterised by suspicion of employees, and increased regulation of activities and surveillance, 'bureaucratized, rule bound, introspective and a slave to its history' (p. 89). Employees are typically loath to cooperate with such managements, and may then be defined by them as 'recalcitrant'.

Breaches of trust can create vengeful and destructive attitudes among employees, jeopardising organisational processes. Folger et al. (2005), Hearn and Parkin (2001), and Restubog, Hornsey, Bordia, and Eposo (2008), note that perceptions of injustice will determine whether employees will indulge in counterproductive work behaviours, such as theft, aggression and withdrawal. Employees who for any reason feel betrayed by an employer will have little reason to trust in the future, creating a climate of suspicion and vigilance against wrongdoing. Violations of trust include supervisor behaviours such as coercive or threatening behaviour, withholding of promised support, favouritism, improper dismissal, blaming employees for their own mistakes, misuse of private information, stealing of ideas, lying and sexual harassment.

One classic example of trust violations occurs when psychological contracts are not honoured. The psychological contract refers to the tacit understanding between an employer and an employee concerning the mutual and reciprocal obligations of both and is subject to individual perception and interpretation (Restubog et al., 2008). When psychological contracts are violated, distrust, anger, betrayal, dissatisfaction and strong hostile reactions can occur, which results in a decline in loyalty and productivity. In extreme cases where employees feel violated and betrayed, they may engage in revenge and retaliatory behaviour such as sabotage, theft or aggression, or may initiate expensive legal proceedings.

The issue of sexual harassment and sexuality in organisations is an important one to briefly address in the context of organisation violations. Sexual harassment usually involves 'unwanted sexual advances, requests for sexual favors (quid pro quo), and any verbal or physical sexualized conduct resulting in a situation where cooperation is used to determine employment-related decisions or unreasonably interfere with a person's performance including the creation of a hostile work environment' (Stockdale & Nadler, 2012, pp. 149–150).

Sexual harassment can have a serious impact on women (and men), ranging from feelings of shame and humiliation, loss of confidence, psychological and/or physical illnesses, absenteeism from work to exiting the workplace. This is particularly the case when the dominant discourse is 'that of the isolated harasser harassing the isolated victim' (Hearn & Parkin, 2001, p. 51; Willness, Steel, & Lee, 2007). It is also recognised that such harassment is a problem in workplaces because of gendered power relations. Sexual harassment is an abuse of power (Itzen & Newman, 1995; Lunenburg, 2010), which is damaging to those who are on the receiving end, and to those who are dominant.

Sexual harassment demands attention, but this should not be at the expense of sexuality. Sexualisation of the workplace is becoming increasingly recognised as vital to organisational functioning, particularly when sexual behaviour is categorised as misbehaviour, disrupting the social and industrial order, thus posing difficulties for employers. It is obvious that the sexuality of employees is not and cannot be 'parked at the door' for the period of working time, then assumed as one leaves the workplace. This is particularly relevant to a workplace where one gender dominates, such as occurs in nursing, which creates its own vulnerabilities and complexities.

Sinclair (2005) points out that our sexualities affect social relations, influencing the effectiveness of employee and employer behaviour. It becomes the business of organisations because it impacts on their dynamics and culture. Sexuality is not simply about sexual harassment or sexual affairs that the organisation seeks to suppress or outlaw, or make marginal (Sinclair, 2005).

Ackroyd and Thompson (1999) note that the 'declining male control of sexuality inside and outside of work' has resulted in increased anger and violence towards women, often manifest in workplaces that are traditionally male dominated (pp. 132–133). This lays the foundation for sexual abuse. The most common forms are joking rituals, sexual banter, pranks, flirting and various forms of 'horseplay', and what Ackroyd and Thompson call 'shop-floor resistance' (p. 136). It has been noted that when there is a breakdown in the authority of the employer, one solution to sexual misbehaviour is to ensure that 'women ... got the bullet' (Ackroyd & Thompson, 1999, p. 138).

Sexuality may be related to the occurrence of gendered violence in organisations, since the operation of sexuality within organisations (including sexual harassment, sexual dominance and power relations) is now recognised as impacting on organisations (McMillan, 2007). A more subtle form of workplace abuse is subjecting the target to silence and exclusion, which can be very powerful (Robinson, O'Reilly, & Wang, 2013). Nurses may practise this by targeting their colleagues (Estes, 2013). Patients may also be a target. Nurses who are not available to patients in the full context of a caring environment may be regarded as 'silent'. This could be interpreted as a form of violating patient rights. When employees fail to be heard, they are effectively silenced (Beheshtifar, Borhani, & Moghadam, 2012). While men can and are silenced, it is more likely to be a problem for women, who are not only silenced by the structure of organisations, but also through interactional processes. In general, men dominate in meetings, interrupt and talk over women, silence women with subtle put-downs, ignore contributions made by women and even attribute them to men (Tannen, 2007). The opposite to 'organisational silence' is 'organisational voice' (Greenberg & Edwards, 2009; Harlos, 2010). This refers to employees communicating concerns to employers and conceivably reducing levels of discontent, distress and dissatisfaction. Alternatively, disgruntled employees may choose to voice their issue through what are considered more negative channels, as they have other options denied them.

RESISTANCE TO ORGANISATION VIOLATION

This chapter has identified a range of resistance behaviours, as evident in the literature. Resistance is demonstrated when there is, usually, subordinate defiance and opposition to another's power. Acts of resistance are either positive or negative, depending on the perspective taken. If viewed from an employer's perspective they are negative; from the employee's perspective they may be positive and justifiable.

Researchers propose that resistance serves a range of purposes. For example, Ashforth and Mael (1998) suggest that it seeks to contest meaning, which defines the role and identity of the individual in the workplace. Organisations seeking to colonise the emotionality of their workers, or to define how they should feel about their work, may find resistance from employees who endeavour to assert their 'valued sense of identity independent of—or antagonistic to—the organization's definition' (p. 113). Because this impacts on the employee's sense and definition of self, the workplace becomes an invasive and threatening place, to be resisted. Such workplaces may make excessive demands on employees, and have been described as 'greedy organizations' (Burchielli, Bartram, & Thanacoody, 2008; McCarthy, 2010).

Collinson and Ackroyd (2005) propose that resistance can occur either through distancing or persistence mechanisms. Resistance through distance occurs when employees try to escape or avoid the demands of employers. This strategy, however, reinforces the legitimacy of hierarchical control, fails to challenge management practices, and increases the employees' vulnerability to discipline. An example of resistance through distance is provided by Martin and Myerson (1998), whose study of female executives found that their resistance mechanism to tyrannical and aggressive male behaviour was to not take abuse personally. Further research in this area might consider whether these are gendered responses, or whether they are more generalised.

Resistance through persistence contrasts with this, as employees demand greater involvement in the organisation by challenging decision-making processes for example, or by attempting to make management more accountable (Collinson & Ackroyd, 2005). It is a more proactive means of behaviour because it involves gaining information and knowledge that will assist employees to critically analyse organisational practices. Nevertheless, current organisational practices of control and discipline derive from a perspective that treats resistance as a form of deviance, aberrant and unjustifiable. Resisters may be called hysterical reactionaries (Ashforth & Mael, 1998) by employers, but they can play a valuable role in the organisation. First, they challenge it in various ways to check the validity of arguments for change, and second, they provide an understanding of subversive tactics that can be evaluated for positive value.

Power and resistance questions are central to a gendered analysis of organisations, and the violations occurring therein (Broadbridge & Hearn, 2008; Hearn & Parkin, 2001). However, one of the problems of gendered resistance is that it is rarely organised, thus rendering it less effective. This uncoordinated reaction by women is called 'disorganised coaction', and is relatively futile as a resistance and change mechanism. There are many forms of resistance, including sabotage, avoiding tasks, withholding labour or 'working to rule', insubordination, violence and whistleblowing.

Whistleblowing is an interesting example of organisational dissenting action that directly challenges managerial authority and power. Whistleblowing is concerned with disclosing illegal, unethical or harmful practices in the workplace so that rectifying action can be taken (Davis, 2013). Whistleblowers usually believe that the organisation's mission is being undermined or that harm is being done to the public good; their principles are being violated and their position usually has an ethical foundation (Lewis, 2011; Lipman, 2011). For many it is a struggle for dignity and integrity that cannot be suppressed by threats or reprisals from the organisation. This is particularly the case when whistleblowers are nurses who take a patient advocate role (Jackson et al., 2013; Jackson et al., 2010; Jones, 2005; Wilkes, Peters, Weaver, & Jackson, 2011).

The literature shows us that responses to whistleblowers are often swift and vindictive. They have destroyed the tranquillity of the workplace and created problems for management that might have been known but ignored. Whistleblowers are usually discredited in a range of ways, being regarded as being mentally unbalanced, disaffected, liars and a variety of other negative adjectives (Delk, 2013). This we can recognise as a 'blame the victim' strategy and it can have a severe, incapacitating psychological impact, sometimes resulting in resignation from the organisation. Hearn and Parkin (2001) believe that '[u]ntil whistleblowing is seen as contributing to a violation-free environment, violations will continue to be denied, silenced and confined to the subtext of worker grievances' (p. 155). This is an issue of great importance in the workplace and readers are urged to explore it further (Bahl & Dadhich, 2011; Brown, 2008).

One of the difficulties that can occur in organisations is that management sometimes makes concessions towards accepting a certain level of 'misbehaviour'. Turning a blind eye to petty theft, various perks of office, or tyrannical behaviour does implicate management and makes them complicit. In fact, managers themselves may be 'misbehaving' when they are the ones who are expected to be 'responsible for defining and policing the formal and informal rules governing acceptable behaviour' (Ackroyd & Thompson, 1999, p. 80). Thus, misbehaviour cannot become too visible, and managers must not be seen to bend the rules too far. Hearn and Parkin (2001) note the complicit and explicit role of management in organisation violations, as they are known to be actively involved in harassment, bullying, intimidation and ignoring known perpetrators of violations. Managements who impose unreasonable work demands and policies that disadvantage their workers are included in the violator category (Burchielli et al., 2008; McCarthy, 2010). The protection and rewarding of these perpetrators adds significantly to the extent of, and difficulties in resolving, the problem of organisation violations.

CONCLUSION

Organisation violations produce workplace traumas that brutalise their employees. Given our knowledge and understanding of such behaviours, it is important to break the conspiracy of silence. Given the complexity of organisational cultures, power structures and the idiosyncratic nature of humankind, is it ever going to be possible to eradicate violations, given the purposes these serve? Employees are innovative in finding alternative and possibly more subtle ways to meet their needs. From the perspective of the employer, misbehaviour is to be dealt with; from the perspective of the employee, misbehaviour is normal, as it is an appropriate reaction to the situation. The workplace thus becomes a contested terrain in which conflict is inevitable because of the competing nature of outcomes in organisations. An examination of organisation violations has exposed complex structures and individual features that require a level of consciousness-raising that is unlikely to occur because of the threat to existing power bases. While it may be claimed that organisational processes are transparent, it is apparent that most organisations have a 'dark side' that is only informally acknowledged (and often only in tea rooms and corridors).

Workplaces should aim to develop and maintain a caring, empathetic environment, career-enriching opportunities, job security, enhanced conflict management, trust, interpersonal cooperation, empowerment and incentives for ethical behaviour. Finally, an important contribution to organisation violation reduction is the focus that has been developed among a body of researchers who explicitly and relentlessly expose, politicise and critique contemporary organisational life.

REFLECTIVE EXERCISE

1. Consider your current workplace, or a former workplace.
    a. In your experience, do/did organisation violations occur?
    b. What form do/did these take?
    c. Can you identify how such abuses impact on the morale, behaviours and motivation of those who are subject to this abuse?
    d. Are you aware of any legitimation or rewarding of abusive behaviours by supervisors of staff?
2. This chapter has addressed organisation violations and suggested ways to reduce abuses. Do any of these suggestions seem valid to you? Or are they well meaning, but unlikely to be successful?
3. If you think they are unlikely to be successful, what reasons can you give for this?
4. What are you now going to do about abusive behaviour in your workplace?

Recommended Readings

Barnes, A., & Taska, L. (2012). *Rethinking misbehavior and resistance in organizations*. Bingley, UK: Emerald Publishing Group.

Broadbridge, A., & Hearn, J. (2008). Gender and management: New directions in research and continuing patterns in practice. *British Journal of Management, 19*(Suppl. s1), S38–S49.

Elias, S. M. (Ed.), (2013). *Deviant and criminal behavior in the workplace*. New York: New York University Press.

Hearn, J., & Parkin, W. (2001). *Gender, sexuality and violence in organizations*. London: Sage.

References

Ackroyd, S., & Thompson, P. (1999). *Organizational misbehaviour*. London: Sage.

Ashforth, B. E. (1994). Petty tyranny in organizations. *Human Relations, 47*(7), 755–788.

Ashforth, B. E., & Mael, F. (1998). The power of resistance: Sustaining valued identities. In R. M. Kramer & M. A. Neale (Eds.), *Power and influence in organizations*. Thousand Oaks, California: Sage.

Babiak, P., & Hare, R. D. (2006). *Snakes in suits: When psychopaths go to work*. New York: Regan Books.

Babiak, P., Newmann, C. S., & Hare, R. D. (2010). Corporate psychopathy: Talking the walk. *Behavioral Sciences and the Law, 28*(2), 174–193.

Bahl, K. T., & Dadhich, A. (2011). Impact of ethical leadership and leader-member exchange on whistleblowing: The moderating impact of the moral intensity of the issue. *Journal of Business Ethics, 103,* 485–496.

Barling, J., & Cooper, C. L. (Eds.), (2008). *The SAGE handbook of organizational behavior. Volume 1: Micro Perspectives*. London: Sage.

Barling, J., Kelloway, E. K., & Frone, M. R. (2005). *Handbook of work stress*. London: Sage.

Barnard, J. W. (2008). Narcissism, over-optimism, fear, anger and depression: The interior lives of corporate leaders. *University of Cincinnati Law Review*, William & Mary Law School Research Paper No 08-10.

Barnes, A., & Taska, L. (Eds.), (2012). *Rethinking misbehaviour and resistance in organizations*. Bingley, UK: Emerald Publishing Group.

Beheshtifar, M., Borhani, H., & Moghadam, M. N. (2012). Destructive role of employee silence in organizational success. *International Journal of Academic Research in Business and Social Sciences, 2*(11), 275–282.

Bies, R. J., & Tripp, T. M. (2005). The study of revenge in the workplace: Conceptual, ideological and empirical issues. In S. Fox & E. Spector (Eds.), *Counterproductive work behavior: Investigations of actors and targets* (pp. 65–81). Washington DC: American Psychological Association.

Bligh, M. C., & Kohles, J. C. (2013). Do I trust you to lead the way? Exploring trust and mis-trust in leader-follower relations. In H. S. Leonard, R. Lewis, A. M. Freedman, & J. Passmore (Eds.), *The Wiley-Blackwell handbook of the psychology of leadership, change and organizational development*. Oxford: John Wiley & Sons.

Bodankin, M., & Tziner, A. (2009). Constructive deviance, destructive deviance and personality: How do they interrelate? *Economic Interferences, XI*(26), 549–564.

Bolino, M. C., Klotz, A. C., Turnley, W. H., & Harvey, J. (2013). Exploring the dark side of organizational citizenship. *Journal of Organizational Behavior, 34*(4), 542–559.

Broadbridge, A., & Hearn, J. (2008). Gender and management: New directions in research and continuing patterns in practice. *British Journal of Management, 19*(Suppl. s1), S38–S49.

Brown, A. J. (Ed.), (2008). *Whistleblowing in the Australian public sector: Enhancing the theory and practice of internal witness management in public sector organisations*. Canberra: Australian National University Press.

Bryman, A., Collinson, D., Grint, K., Jackson, B., & Uhl-Bien, M. (Eds.), (2011). *The SAGE handbook of leadership*. London: Sage.

Buchanan, D., & Badham, R. (2008). *Power, politics and organizational change: Winning the turf game* (2nd ed.). London: Sage.

Burchielli, R., Bartram, T., & Thanacoody, R. (2008). Work-family balance or greedy organizations? *Industrial Relations, 63*(1), 108–133.

Choo, Y. J., & Ringquist, E. J. (2011). Managerial trustworthiness and organizational outcomes. *Journal of Public Administration, Research and Theory, 21*(1), 53–86.

Cleary, M., Hunt, G. E., & Horsfall, J. (2010). Identifying and addressing bullying in nursing. *Issues in Mental Health Nursing, 31*(5), 331–335.

Collinson, D., & Ackroyd, S. (2005). Resistance, misbehavior and dissent. In S. Ackroyd, R. Batt, P. Thompson, & P. S. Tolbert (Eds.), *The Oxford handbook of work and organization*. New York: Oxford University Press.

Covey, S. M. R. (2009). How the best leaders build trust. *Leadership now: Building a community of leaders*. Retrieved from <http://www.LeadershipNow.com/>.

Croft, R. K., & Cash, P. A. (2012). Deconstructing contributing factors to bullying and lateral violence in nursing using a postcolonial feminist lens. *Contemporary Nurse, 42*(2), 226–242.

Dalglish, C., & Miller, P. (2010). *Leadership: Understanding its global impact.* Victoria: Tilde University Press.

Davis, M. (2013). *Whistleblowing. The International Encyclopedia of Ethics.* Chichester: John Wiley & Sons.

Delk, K. L. (2013). Whistleblowing—is it really worth the consequences? *Workplace Health and Safety, 61*(6), 61–64.

Dellasega, C. A. (2009). Bullying among nurses. *American Journal of Nursing, 109*(1), 52–58.

Demir, D., & Rodwell, J. (2012). Psychological antecedents and consequences of workplace aggression for hospital nurses. *Journal of Nursing Scholarship, 44*(4), 376–384.

Department of Health, Government of Western Australia. (2005). *Implementation of the Douglas Inquiry Recommendations.* King Edward Memorial Hospital. Review Final Report.

Einarsen, S., Aasland, M. S., & Skogstad, A. (2007). Destructive leadership behaviour: A definition and conceptual model. *Leadership Quarterly, 18*(3), 207–216.

Einarsen, S., Hoel, H., Zapf, D., & Cooper, C. (Eds.), (2011). *Bullying and harassment in the workplace: Developments in Theory, Research and Practice* (2nd ed.). Boca Raton, Florida: Taylor and Francis Group.

Elias, S. M. (Ed.), (2013). *Deviant and criminal behavior in the workplace.* New York: New York University Press.

Estes, B. C. (2013). Abusive supervision and nursing performance. *Nursing Forum, 48*(1), 3–16.

Folger, R., Cropanzano, R., & Goldman, E. C. (2005). What is the relationship between justice and morality? In J. Greenberg & J. A. Colquitt (Eds.), *A handbook of organizational justice.* New Jersey: Lawrence Erlbaum Associates.

Francis, R. (2013). *The Mid-Staffordshire NHS Foundation Trust. Report of the Public Inquiry.* London: Skipton House.

Furnham, A., & Siegel, E. M. (2012). Reactions to organizational injustice: Counter work behaviours and the insider threat. In E. Kals & J. Maes (Eds.), *Justice and conflicts.* Berlin: Springer-Verlag.

Furnham, A., Trickey, G., & Hyde, G. (2012). Bright aspects to dark side traits: Dark side traits associated with work success. *Personality and Individual Differences, 52*(8), 908–913.

Garling, P. (2008). *Final Report of the Special Commission of Inquiry.* Acute Care Services in NSW Public Hospitals.

Gherardi, S. (1995). *Gender, symbolism and organizational cultures.* London: Sage.

Gilbert, J. A., Carr-Ruffino, N., Ivancevich, J. M., & Konopaske, R. (2012). Toxic versus cooperative behaviours at work: The role of organizational culture and leadership in creating community-centered organizations. *International Journal of Leadership Studies, 7*(1), 29–47.

Graetz, F., Rimmer, M., Smith, A., & Lawrence, A. (2011). *Managing organisational change* (3rd ed.). Brisbane: John Wiley & Sons.

Greenberg, J. (Ed.), (2010). *Insidious workplace behavior.* New York: Taylor & Francis Group.

Greenberg, J., & Edwards, M. S. (2009). *Voice and silence in organizations.* Bigley, U.K.: Emerald Group Publishing Ltd.

Grieve, H. R., Palmer, D., & Pozner, J. E. (2010). Organizations gone wild: The causes, processes and consequences of organizational misconduct. *The Academy of Management Annals, 4*(1), 53–107.

Gudmundsson, A., & Southey, G. (2011). Leadership and the rise of the corporate psychopath: What can business schools do about the 'snakes inside'? *e-Journal of Social and Behavioural Research in Business, 2*(2), 18–27.

Harlos, K. (2010). If you build a remedial voice mechanism, will they come? Determinants of voicing interpersonal mistreatment at work. *Human Relations, 63*(3), 311–329.

Harms, P. D., Spain, S. M., & Hannah, S. T. (2011). *Leader development and the dark side of leadership*. University of Nebraskan-Lincoln: Management Department Faculty Publications. Paper 82.

Hasan, S. A., & Subhani, M. I. (2012). Top management's snooping: Is sneaking over employees productivity and job commitment a wise approach? *MPRA Paper No. 35691*, January.

Hearn, J., & Parkin, W. (2001). *Gender, sexuality and violence in organizations*. London: Sage.

Hershcovis, S. M. (2011). 'Incivility, social undermining, bullying...oh my!': A call to reconcile constructs within workplace aggression research. *Journal of Organizational Behavior, 32*(3), 499–519.

Hughes, R., Ginnett, R. C., & Curphy, G. J. (2008). *Leadership: Enhancing the lessons of experience*. New York: McGraw-Hill International.

Hutchinson, M., Vickers, M. H., Jackson, D., & Wilkes, L. (2010). Bullying as circuits of power: An Australian nursing perspective. *Administrative Theory and Praxis, 32*(11), 25–47.

Hutchinson, M., Vickers, M. H., Wilkes, L., & Jackson, D. (2010). A typology of bullying behaviours: The experiences of Australian nurses. *Journal of Clinical Nursing, 19*, 2319–2327.

Itzen, C., & Newman, J. (1995). *Gender, culture and organizational change*. London: Routledge. doi:10.1108/17465641011042017

Jackson, D., Hutchinson, M., Peters, K., Luck, L., & Saltman, D. (2013). Understanding avoidant leadership in health care: findings from a secondary analysis of two qualitative studies. *Journal of Nursing Management, 21*(3), 572–589.

Jackson, D., Peters, K., Andrew, S., Edenborough, M., Halcomb, E., Luck, L., et al. (2010). Understanding whistleblowing: Qualitative insights from nurse whistleblowers. *Journal of Advanced Nursing, 66*(10), 2194–2201.

Jacques, E. (1995). Why the psychoanalytical approach to understanding organizations is dysfunctional. *Human Relations, 48*(4), 343–350.

Johnson, S. L. (2009). International perspectives on workplace bullying among nurses: A review. *International Nursing Review, 56*(1), 34–40.

Johnston, M., Phanhtharath, P., & Jackson, B. S. (2009). The bullying aspect of workplace violence in nursing. *Critical Care Nursing Quarterly, 32*(4), 287–295.

Jones, D. A., & Skarlicki, D. P. (2013). How perceptions of fairness can change: A dynamic model of organizational justice. *Organizational Psychology Review, 3*(2), 138–160.

Jones, J. (2005). 'I had to act': A conversation with a whistleblower. *Australian Journal of Advanced Nursing, 23*(1), 4–6.

Jordon, P. (2002). *Uncontrolled emotions in organizations: Coercion and bullying in the workplace*. Paper presented at the Third Conference on Emotions and Organizational Life, Bond University, Gold Coast.

Judge, T. A., Piccolo, R. F., & Kosalka, T. (2009). The bright and dark sides of leader traits: A review and theoretical extension of the leader trait paradigm. *Leadership Quarterly, 20*(6), 855–875.

Kelloway, E. K., Francis, L., Prosser, M., & Cameron, J. E. (2010). Counterproductive work behavior as protest. *Resource Management Review, 20*, 18–25.

Kets de Vries, M. (2006). *The leader on the couch: A clinical approach to changing people and organizations*. Chichester: John Wiley.

Krasikova, D. V., Green, S. G., & LeBreton, J. M. (2013). Destructive leadership: A theoretical review, integration and future research agenda. *Journal of Management, 39*(5), 1308–1338.

Krischer, M. M., Penney, L. M., & Hunter, E. M. (2010). Can counterproductive work behaviors be productive? CWB as emotion-focused coping. *Journal of Occupational Health Psychology, 15*(2), 154–166.

Kupers, W. (2009). Embodied and emotional dimensions of demotivation in organisations. *International Journal of Behaviour, 14*(1), 41–53.

Langan-Fox, J., Cooper, C. L., & Klimoski, R. J. (Eds.), (2007). *Research companion to the dysfunctional workplace: Management challenges and symptoms*. Cheltenham, UK: Edward Elgar Publishing Ltd.

Leonard, H. S., Lewis, R., Freedman, A. M., & Passmore, J. (2013). When leaders are bullies: Concepts, antecedents and consequences. In S. Einarsen, A. Skogstad, & L. Glaso (Eds.), *The Wiley-Blackwell handbook of the psychology of leadership, change and organizational development*. Oxford: John Wiley & Sons.

Levine, E. L. (2010). Emotion and power (as social influence): Their impact on organizational citizenship and counterproductive individual and organizational behavior. *Human Resource Management Review, 20*(1), 4–17.

Lewis, D. (2011). Whistleblowing in a changing legal climate: Is it time to revisit our approach to trust and loyalty in the workplace? *Business Ethics: A European Review, 20*(1), 71–87.

Liefooghe, A., & Davey, M. K. (2010). The language and organization of bullying at work. *Administrative Theory and Praxis, 32*(1), 71–95.

Linstead, S., Fulop, L., & Lilley, S. (2009). *Management and organization: A critical text* (2nd ed.). New York: Palgrave Macmillan.

Lipman, F. D. (2011). Establishing a robust whistleblower system. In *Whistleblowers: Incentives, disincentives and protection strategies*. New Jersey: John Wiley & Sons Inc.

Lunenburg, F. C. (2010). Sexual harassment: An abuse of power. *International Journal of Management, Business and Administration, 13*(1), 1–7.

Martin, J., & Myerson, D. (1998). Women and power: Conformity, resistance and disorganized coaction. In R. Kramer & M. Neale (Eds.), *Power, Politics and Influence*. Newbery Park, CA: Sage.

McCarthy, S. (2010). Thought leader: Greedy organisations will suffer most. *New Zealand Management Magazine, February*, 25.

McMillan, L. (2007). *Feminists organising against gendered violence*. New York: Palgrave MacMillan.

Morgan, G. (2007). *Images of organization* (updated ed.). London: Sage.

Northouse, P. G. (2013). *Leadership: Theory and practice* (6th ed.). Thousand Oaks, California: Sage.

Oade, A. (2009). *Managing workplace bullying*. Hampshire, UK: Palgrave Macmillan.

Pearson, C. M., Andersson, L. M., & Porath, C. L. (2005). Workplace incivility. In S. Fox & P. E. Spector (Eds.), *Counterproductive work behavior: Investigations of actors and targets*. Washington, D.C.: American Psychological Association.

Pelletier, K. L. (2010). Leader toxicity: An empirical investigation of toxic behavior and rhetoric. *Leadership, 6*(4), 373–389.

Poilpot-Rocaboy, G. (2006). Bullying in the workplace: A proposed model for understanding the psychological harassment process. *Research and Practice in Human Research Management, 14*(2), 1–17.

Porath, C., & Pearson, C. (2013). The price of incivility: Lack of respect hurts morale and the bottom line. *Harvard Business Review, January-February*, 115–121.

Rao, A. (2012). The contemporary construction of nurse empowerment. *Journal of Nursing Scholarship, 44*(4), 396–402.

Restubog, S. L. D., Hornsey, M. J., Bordia, P., & Eposo, S. R. (2008). Effects of psychological contract breach on organizational citizenship behavior: Insights from the group value model. *Journal of Management Studies, 45*(8), 1377–1400.

Richards, J. (2008). The many approaches to organisational misbehaviour: A review, map and research agenda. *Employee Relations, 30*(6), 653–678.

Rigby, K. (2012). Bullying in schools: Addressing desires, not only behaviours. *Educational Psychology Review, 24*(2), 339–348.

Robinson, S. L., O'Reilly, J., & Wang, W. (2013). Invisible at work: An integrated model of workplace ostracism. *Journal of Management, 39*(1), 203–231.

Shahzad, K. (2012). Vision or psychic prison. *Business Intelligence Journal, 5*(2), 207–213.

Shao, R., Rupp, D. E., Skarlicki, D. P., & Jones, K. S. (2013). Employee justice across cultures: A meta-analytic review. *Journal of Management, 39*(1), 263–301.

Sheehan, M. (1996). Case studies in organisational restructuring. In P. McCarthy, M. Sheehan, & W. Wilkie (Eds.), *Bullying: From backyard to boardroom*. Alexandria, NSW: Millenium Books.

Sinclair, A. (2005). *Doing leadership differently: Gender, power and sexuality in a changing business culture* (2nd ed.). Melbourne: Melbourne University Press.

Slattery, C. (2009). *The dark side of leadership: Troubling times at the top*. Sydney: Seemann & Slattery.

Spector, P. E. (2012). *Industrial/organizational psychology. Research and practice* (6th ed.). Hoboken, New Jersey: John Wiley & Sons.

Spector, P. E., & Fox, S. (2005). The stressor-emotion model of counterproductive work behavior. In S. Fox & P. E. Spector (Eds.), *Counterproductive work behaviour* (pp. 151–174). Washington, DC: American Psychological Association.

Spector, P. E., Fox, S., Penney, L. M., Bruurema, K., Goh, A., & Kessler, S. (2006). The dimensionality of counterproductivity: Are all counterproductive behaviors created equal? *Journal of Vocational Behavior, 68*(3), 446–460.

Spitzmuller, M., & van Dyne, L. (2013). Proactive and reactive helping: Contrasting the positive consequences of different forms of helping. *Journal of Organizational Behavior, 34*(4), 560–580.

Stockdale, M. S., & Nadler, J. T. (2012). Situating sexual harassment in the broader context of interpersonal violence: Research, theory and policy implications. *Social Issues and Policy Review, 6*(1), 148–176.

Tannen, D. (2007). *You just don't understand: Women and men in conversation*. New York: Harper.

Walton, M. (2007). Leadership toxicity—An inevitable affliction of organizations? *Organisations and People, 14*(1), 19–27.

Wilkes, L. M., Peters, K., Weaver, R., & Jackson, D. (2011). Nurses involved in whistleblowing incidents: Sequelae for their families. *Collegian (Royal College of Nursing, Australia), 18*(3), 101–106.

Willness, C. R., Steel, P., & Lee, K. (2007). A meta-analysis of the antecedents and consequences of workplace sexual harassment. *Personnel Psychology, 60*(1), 127–162.

Wyatt, J., & Hare, C. (1997). *Work abuse: How to recognize and survive it*. Rochester, Vermont: Schenkman Books.

Yildirim, D. (2009). Bullying among nurses and its effects. *International Nursing Review, 56*, 504–511.

Zapf, D., & Einarsen, S. (2005). Mobbing at work: Escalated conflicts in organizations. In S. Fox & P. E. Spector (Eds.), *Counterproductive work behaviour* (pp. 237–270). Washington, DC: American Psychological Association.

CHAPTER SIX

Leadership and healthcare change management

John Daly, Martha N. Hill
& Debra Jackson

*All courses of action are risky, so prudence is not in avoiding danger (it's impossible),
but calculating risk and acting decisively. Make mistakes of ambition and not
mistakes of sloth. Develop the strength to do bold things, not the strength to suffer.*

— Niccolò Machiavelli

LEARNING OBJECTIVES

At the completion of this chapter, the reader will be able to:

▲ identify drivers of healthcare change management;
▲ analyse current issues in facilitating change in nursing;
▲ describe and discuss critical change management competencies;
▲ assess effectiveness of change management;
▲ implement strategies for facilitating change management.

KEY WORDS

Change process, leading change, management principles, planning, evaluation

INTRODUCTION

Change has become an almost permanent feature of leadership and management in the corporate, public and health sectors internationally. Launching and completing change is said to be one of the most difficult, challenging and potentially disastrous undertakings a leader is required to engage in. However, risky as it can be for a leader, there are high expectations for nursing internationally to participate in health system improvement, including leading change to maximise quality of care and health outcomes. These expectations recognise that 'because nurses make a major contribution to healthcare provision and to the experiences of those using health services they need to be equipped and enabled to take a lead role in developing services' (Hewitt-Taylor, 2013, p. 38).

In this chapter we explore some of the key issues in change management, to inform nursing leadership about how to bring about change in healthcare environments. The concepts we present may apply at all levels of the healthcare system but the complexity of a change initiative may increase exponentially as the scale and scope of the target entity grows. In doing so, we will identify drivers of healthcare change management; scrutinise current issues in facilitating change in nursing; describe and discuss critical change management competencies; and consider efficacy and implementation strategies for successfully facilitating change management in healthcare.

DRIVERS OF HEALTHCARE CHANGE MANAGEMENT

Transformation efforts are under way in many healthcare systems and change management has become embedded in system development, redesign, service evaluation and sustainability initiatives. Improvement science has become a new interdisciplinary applied field. To compete and survive, healthcare organisations must 'embrace continuous, emergent change' (Iles & Sutherland, 2001, p. 14) and accept that it cannot be avoided despite the fact that change in healthcare organisations is often highly complex and intentionally disruptive for a range of reasons. The emerging field of improvement science focuses on methods to transform healthcare by promoting the integration of research findings and evidence into healthcare practice and policy. Implementing innovations through such changes may require intentional disruption, a process that can be carefully managed (Christensen, 1997). The goal of improvement science is to improve quality of care based on evidence of best practices (Shojania & Grimshaw, 2005). In efforts to accelerate the rate at which new therapies and cures are delivered to patients, traditional methods of care must be intentionally changed, transforming processes and policies (Vijayaraghaven & O'Donnell, 2011). Many national and local healthcare institutions now have online resource-rich repositories which clinicians can readily access for information on many facets of leadership including leading change management, preparing business plans, analysing administrative data sets and implementing and evaluating change processes.

Basic quality, economic and political factors are driving change in healthcare availability and delivery. In addition, rapid advancement of technology, effectiveness research showing improved processes and outcomes and increasing demand for cost containment are major drivers of change. There is perhaps inevitable tension between healthcare practitioners who have been trained to give the best possible care to all, and health administrators who have been trained to run businesses, some of which are for profit. Thus, basic management skills are needed by health leaders, to enable the formation of teams with shared goals and the commitment to manage changes that will facilitate the achievement of organisational goals. In 2003 Leatt and Porter noted that:

In the last decade healthcare throughout the world has experienced broad strategic management strategies, such as restructuring, regionalisation, downsizing of personnel, reduced bed capacity, and decreased funding. At the same time consumers are expecting higher quality services, more information about treatment options, as well as more accountability. At the service delivery level, health professionals are burnt out, feel undervalued and under rewarded, have lost trust in their employers and governments, and appear dissatisfied. Health service workers appear more resistant to change, and less open to creativity and to innovation (Leatt & Porter, 2003, p. 22).

This quote would undoubtedly resonate with many healthcare professionals across the world over a decade later. In many settings little progress has been made in implementing constructive and meaningful change to improve care and outcomes, and maximise quality, while containing costs. The issues confronting many governments and healthcare organisations are common across national and international borders: the growing burden of chronic disease, ageing populations, fluctuations in human resources for health, quality and safety, clinical education challenges as a consequence of system redesign, the struggle to promote evidence-based practice, and tribalism among the health professional team, which can block innovation (particularly the introduction of new models of care, which require authentic teamwork, genuine collaboration, power sharing and shared governance).

Of central concern to many clinicians is the need to ensure that patients and communities continue to have access to responsive and high-quality health services, even in the context of rapid, imposed structural and organisational change and diminished resources. Unfortunately it is the case that in the desire to implement change, particularly change driven by economic, political or other resource pressures, there have been some disastrous flow-on effects that have negatively influenced patient care and have become the focus of various inquiries into organisational failure in the health sector (for example, Francis, 2013). Herein lies the challenge for healthcare leaders—to design, implement and effect change to promote fiscal and resource containment, while continuing to provide responsive and high-quality services for end-users. Furthermore, despite the extent of the challenges, there is the need, and the opportunity to create, implement and evaluate sustainable, accessible and affordable healthcare across the world.

ISSUES IN FACILITATING CHANGE IN NURSING

Calls for building nursing capacity for change leadership have recently been made by a number of important health policy organisations across the world. In 2010 the US Institute of Medicine (IOM), in collaboration with the Robert Wood Johnson Foundation (RWJF), released the report *The Future of Nursing: Leading Change, Advancing Health* (2010). The report states: 'the nursing profession has the potential capacity to implement wide-reaching changes in the health system' (IOM, 2010, p. 1) and it asserts that professional nurses need to be prepared to participate in healthcare from the bedside to the boardroom (IOM, 2010). Moreover, the IOM/RWJF Report made the following four major recommendations:

▲ Nurses should practise to the full extent of their education and training.

▲ Nurses should achieve higher levels of education and training through an improved education system that promotes seamless academic progression.

▲ Nurses should be full partners, with physicians and other healthcare professionals, in redesigning healthcare in the United States.

▲   Effective workforce planning and policy making require better data collection and information infrastructure (IOM, 2010).

Effective management of the changes that will be necessary for these recommendations to be implemented, within health systems, as well as within nursing education, practice and policy, will be required. The following quote, while drawn from the IOM report and made in relation to the situation in the United States is applicable worldwide.

The United States has the opportunity to transform its health care system, and nurses can and should play a fundamental role in this transformation. However, the power to improve the current regulatory, business, and organizational conditions does not rest solely with nurses; government, businesses, health care organizations, professional associations, and the insurance industry all must play a role. Working together, these many diverse parties can help ensure that the health care system provides seamless, affordable, quality care that is accessible to all and leads to improved health outcomes (IOM, 2010).

The importance of nursing as a profession and its capacity to contribute with strength in healthcare reforms and systems level change have also been noted in both developed and developing countries (Munjanja, Kibuka, & Dovlo, 2005; Stokowski, 2010; Tomajan, 2012). Indeed, the World Health Organization (WHO) has a strategic plan for strengthening nursing and midwifery globally to assist in making healthcare systems more accessible and robust (WHO, 2011). However, it is important to remember that while nursing does have great transformative potential, nursing does not practise alone. Nursing cannot bring about healthcare change or manage healthcare change alone. Thus, in order to effect meaningful change it is crucial that nurses effectively engage with other key health stakeholders. Leaders in nursing therefore need well-developed competencies in high-level communication and negotiation, as well as in leading change; not just as providers of 'vision' for required changes, but as active and effective leading agents in implementing and evaluating organisational change initiatives (Shirley, 2011).

COMPETENCIES FOR HEALTHCARE CHANGE MANAGEMENT

The highly politicised and dynamic nature of healthcare means that health leaders are regularly challenged to adjust and recalibrate organisational aspirations and objectives. This need for fairly continuous revising of organisational priorities may be approached by taking account of a range of drivers in both internal and external environments, to maximise performance in increasingly competitive and complex environments. Numerous competencies for leading change can be identified. Successful leadership in this context requires assiduous commitment to understanding organisational challenges within a given context, taking account of organisational climate and cultural issues (Shipton, Armstrong, West, & Dawson, 2008), the ability to plan strategically for effective change, high-level skills in communication, negotiation and dispute resolution, the capacity to influence stakeholders and gain commitment to objectives and the drive to deliver on related action plans (Shirley, 2011).

Trevelyan (2001, p. 42) noted two critical roles of leaders as change agents. The first of these highlights the role of leaders in generating change through the identification and articulation of new objectives, goals and visions for the future. The other critical role of the leader in relation to change is to be able to inspire constituents to follow and commit to contributing to and achieving the new vision. Thus, to be effective change agents, leaders must be able to not only develop and articulate a vision for the future, that vision must be able to be expressed and presented in ways that constituents can firstly engage with, and secondly want to become a part of. Similarly, in 2008 Shipton and colleagues observed that:

> *the leadership literature reveals that leaders are responsible for creating a vision of where the organization is going and implementing initiatives to achieve the vision. They generate enthusiasm for goal achievement and communicate employees' roles in contributing to the organization's strategy. Furthermore, effective leaders engage with the external environment, building collaborative relationships within the wider community in order to promote the necessary change orientation*
> *(Shipton et al., 2008, p. 440).*

In the United Kingdom, the National Health Service (NHS) advises that to be effective as agents of change, there is a need to focus on five competency clusters. These are:

▲ clarity in specifying goals/adapting to changing goals;

▲ adapting to different roles: teambuilding abilities, networking, tolerance of ambiguity;

▲ communication: interpersonal skills, self and other motivation;

▲ negotiation: selling the vision and negotiating in a political environment;

▲ managing up: demonstrating political awareness, influencing and taking a helicopter perspective (NHS, 2009).

Each of these complementary clusters subsumes numerous skills and competencies. These include gathering the key stakeholders, eliciting critical incentives, setting and resetting priorities and excellent communication and negotiation skills. Additionally, it is important to anticipate, recognise and meet the challenges associated with resistance, constituent anxiety in times of uncertainty, and the presence of any competing agendas that could sabotage the desired change process.

Very few individuals have the breadth and depth of necessary competency and skill to effectively design, implement and manage change initiatives that can improve healthcare and health service delivery. Thus, to effect change, there is a basic need to ensure a strong team with complementary and diverse skill sets. This means that effective team building becomes a crucial skill set that is needed very early in the change process. Finally, another crucial competency is that of efficacious evaluation of change initiatives. Knowing the value and process of evaluation and how it can be integrated throughout the life of the change process (and beyond) is important. Nothing justifies change better than valid and legitimate evidence, detailing changes that have been implemented, and being able to clearly demonstrate the positive differences the changes have made to a variety of stakeholders, such as providers, administrators, clinicians, communities and patients and their families.

EFFECTIVENESS OF HEALTHCARE CHANGE MANAGEMENT

The scientific literature on leadership and change management poses limitations with regard to the evidence base, particularly in relation to healthcare and nursing. In a high-quality review of the literature conducted for the NHS in the United Kingdom more than a decade ago, it was noted that there were a number of challenges associated with the change management literature. In addition to some of the usual difficulties associated with aggregating a large body of literature; for example, differences in methodologies, definitional issues and so forth, some specific challenging issues were identified. These challenges were framed as six key difficulties as listed below:

1. It contains contributions from several different academic disciplines including psychology, sociology, business policy, social policy and others.

2. Its boundaries can be set differently, according to the definition of change management employed.

3. Valuable contributions to the literature have been made in all of the past five decades, with the later not necessarily superseding the earlier.

4. It contains evidence, examples and illustrations generated in a wide variety of organisations and from a diverse range of methodologies with varying degrees of rigour.

5. Some material is not readily accessible to non-specialists and does not readily lend itself to cumulative review.

6. The concepts included within it range in scale from whole academic schools, through methodologies to single tools (Iles & Sutherland, 2001, p. 12).

What was clear from this authoritative review was that the science underpinning approaches leading change in nursing and healthcare is in an early stage of development. However, despite the embryonic state of the evidence in 2001, Iles and Sutherland were able to state that 'An important (arguably the central) message of recent high-quality management of change literature is that organisation level change is not fixed or linear in nature but contains an important emergent element' (Iles & Sutherland, 2001, p. 14). More recently, it has been noted that the evidence regarding change leadership in nursing and healthcare remains rather tenuous (NHS, 2009). Indeed, while there is considerable research examining issues around organisational change processes, there is a lack of longitudinal studies that can show meaningful and sustained changes over time. Furthermore, the contextual nature of work in the area and the difficulty in controlling variables also presents challenges in trying to establish a clear evidence base.

Numerous accounts of leadership and change management endeavours can be found in the nursing and health literature (see, for example, Kassean & Jagoo, 2005; McMurray, Chaboyer, Wallis, & Fetherston, 2010; Rosen et al., 2006). In nursing, the majority are small-scale context-bound studies, some of which are focused on changing aspects of nursing practice within defined areas, and others are concerned with translational science designed to build the evidence base for practice (Hewitt-Taylor, 2013). Although meta-analysis was attempted with a high number of high-quality systematic reviews of nursing leadership and impact, the wide diversity of outcomes, samples and settings precluded meta-analysis procedures and limited the consolidation of findings (Pearson et al., 2007; Wong & Cummings, 2007).

STRATEGIES FOR LEADING CHANGE

Managing change is very similar to managing nursing care. One must be able to analyse a situation, plan appropriate interventions, intervene and evaluate outcomes. The nursing process provides a parallel process involving: assessment, planning, implementing and evaluation in an iterative process. Like the nursing process, the change management process requires robust concurrent formative and summative evaluation.

Assess need for change

Recognise need for change. It is critical to take the time to clarify the fundamental problem that needs to be changed and to whom positive outcomes matter. Focus on the vision that supports the change and the mission that guides the organisation. Identify what changes will be brought about, how the proposed change is to be measured and how its success is to be defined. This analysis will benefit from objective data. Identify and interview key stakeholders to develop consensus about the basic problem(s) and need for change. Analyse existing administrative data sets. Gather external data to benchmark one's own situation against peer organisations. Have an outside person(s) gather and review data. Share these findings in a case to build support for moving forward. This will take time but will save time in the end.

It is not uncommon to hear someone say that they want to implement a change when they have drawn a conclusion and identified a preferred solution without accurately defining the problem that needs to be addressed. This is a recipe for ineffective leadership, unsuccessful change management processes, wasted resources and harmed reputations. Such a situation is particularly likely to occur when an individual, or a group of individuals, are identified as the target that has to be changed by being removed from their positions, transferred to other positions, leaving the organisation and/or eliminating the positions. While people can become so enmeshed in their positions and their own needs, attitudes and skills that the 'goodness of fit' is a reasonable concern, it is critical for human resource, ethical and legal reasons to objectively analyse dysfunctional (and potentially dysfunctional) situations carefully. There is a tendency for many to begin with an assumption that if an organisational structure or a part of it is changed, improvement performance and outcomes will follow.

Plan for change

The planning process should be as transparent as possible. Key stakeholders should be involved and regular communications should be sent to more distant stakeholders. Town meetings, question and answer postings and other methods keep people informed and encourage exchange, input and involvement. The only thing lost by including all key and distant stakeholders is time, hence the importance of effective planning and time management strategies.

Clarify desired outcomes. Consider the organisational mission. Use it as the guiding set of principles that defines the common overall goals and objectives of the organisation. Work back from that and ask 'What do we want to do?' 'What will it take?' Identify necessary resources including human capital and competencies. Think through the what, why, when, how, who and 'so what' elements of the change initiative. Develop a business plan and a communication plan.

Decide and make clear who is in charge and who has specific responsibilities for planning, implementing and evaluating change. It is critical that the importance of evaluation is appreciated from the outset and that evidence is gathered to support leaders' effectiveness in managing change. Consider planning for sustainability as well as the initial achievement of goals. Planning for allocation of resources is important from the beginning of the change process. Include evaluation as well as initial implementation costs and plan for sustainability costs. Ask 'Are resources allocated to optimise use of available data and data that needs to be collected during planning and implementation phases?' Incentives may need to be identified and reconciled with policies. Resources will need to be provided. Many a change initiative has failed because it was under-financed and under-staffed.

Consider unintended consequences. Assess risks and benefits. The literature is full of tools and strategies, including the use of consultants and facilitators. Identify teams of leaders within the organisation who have change management as a major part of their duties.

Prepare people and the environment for change. Communicate. Communicate. Communicate. Assess readiness for change. Help prepare people. Include them. Welcome their ideas and suggestions. Anticipate resistance from some.

Implement change

As the planning phase moves towards closure and implementation a preliminary phase may be required to train staff for the 'roll out' phase. Staff who will implement change on the front line, the leaders of the troops, may need training before beginning to implement, and coaching throughout, the process. Organisational leaders, the champions and faces of change, may need media training to optimise their communication. The importance of ongoing evaluation and regular communication cannot be overestimated.

Evaluate change

Collect qualitative as well as quantitative data throughout the process. Provide feedback on progress towards goals on an announced schedule (i.e. weekly, monthly, quarterly) and keep this commitment. At every stage avoid drawing conclusions by objectively analysing quantitative and qualitative data. Take corrective action as soon as data indicates that deadlines are not being met, results are sub-optimal or not on time.

Celebrate success

The desired outcomes are difficult to achieve and to sustain. When major outcomes are achieved, communicate the good news and recognise the contributions of people at all levels who contributed to the success.

CONCLUSION

Change is inevitable. An effective leader must anticipate the need for change and be proactive to survive and to thrive. The IOM's *Roundtable on Value & Science-Driven Health Care* has summarised their deliberations in *Making a Difference ... Roundtable strategy, tactics, impact* (IOM, 2013). Their vision of a continuously learning health system speeds progress by mapping strategies, clarifying concepts and opportunities, stewarding action, informing policy, spreading the word, engaging broadly and linking leaders. Their synthesis complements and reinforces this chapter's emphasis on planning and implementing change to improve outcomes.

The challenges to leading change management are many. Effective change requires risk taking and courage. That must be balanced with careful analysis, planning, focused interventions and aligned evaluation. This chapter describes a process with which the change process can be conceptualised and implemented. Change management can be exciting and impactful. Effective leaders welcome change, anticipate it and manage it decisively. They either manage it or find it has managed them.

REFLECTIVE EXERCISE

Answer the following questions in relation to the last formal change process in your workplace.

1. What was the nature of the change?
2. Who led the development and implementation of the change plan?
3. What key strategies were used to garner support in the workplace?
4. How much time elapsed between the rollout of the change plan and the change being adopted?
5. Do you consider the change process was successful or unsuccessful?
6. What would you do differently if you had to lead a similar change process in the future?
7. Try to think of three additional strategies you could implement that would enhance the outcomes of this change process.

Recommended Readings

Best, A., Greenhalgh, T., Lewis, S., Saul, J. E., Carroll, S., & Bitz, J. (2012). Large-system transformation in health care: A realist review. *Milbank Quarterly, 90*, 421–456.

Corazzini, K., Twersky, J., White, H. K., Buhr, G. T., McConnell, E. S., Weiner, M., et al. (2014). Implementing culture change in nursing homes: An adaptive leadership framework. *The Gerontologist*, doi:10.1093/geront/gnt170.

Martin, G. P., Sutton, E., Willars, J., & Dixon-Woods, M. (2013). Frameworks for change in healthcare organisations: A formative evaluation of the NHS Change Model. *Health Services Management, 26*(2–3), 65–75.

Schyve, P. M. (2009). *Leadership in healthcare organisations: A guide to joint commission leadership standards.* San Diego: Governance Institute. Retrieved from <www.governanceinstitute.com>.

Shipton, H., Armstrong, C., West, M., & Dawson, J. (2008). The impact of leadership and quality climate on hospital performance. *International Journal for Quality in Health Care, 20*(6), 439–445.

References

Christensen, C. (1997). *The innovator's dilemma: When new technologies cause great firms to fail.* Boston: Harvard Business School Press.

Francis, R. (2013). *Report of the Mid Staffordshire NHS Foundation Trust Public Inquiry.* London: The Stationery Office.

Hewitt-Taylor, J. (2013). Planning successful change incorporating processes and people. *Nursing Standard, 27*(38), 35–40.

Iles, V., & Sutherland, K. (2001). *Managing change in the NHS-organizational change: A review for health care managers, professionals and researchers.* London: NCCSDO.

Institute of Medicine (IOM). (2010). *The future of nursing: Leading change, advancing health.* Retrieved from <http://www.iom.edu/Reports/2010/The-future-of-nursing-leading-change-advancing-health.aspx>.

Institute of Medicine (IOM). (2013). *Roundtable on Value & Science-Driven Healthcare*. Retrieved from <http://iom.edu/vsrt>.

Kassean, H. K., & Jagoo, Z. B. (2005). Managing change in the nursing handover from traditional to bedside handover—a case study from Mauritius. *BMC Nursing, 4*(1), Retrieved from <http://www.biomedcentral.com.ezproxy.lib.uts.edu.au/1472-6955/4/1>.

Leatt, P., & Porter, J. (2003). Where are the healthcare leaders? The need for investment in leadership development. *Health Care Papers, 4*(1), 14–31.

McMurray, A., Chaboyer, W., Wallis, M., & Fetherston, C. (2010). Implementing bedside handover: Strategies for change management. *Journal of Clinical Nursing, 19*, 2580–2589.

Munjanja, O. K., Kibuka, S., & Dovlo, D. (2005). *The nursing workforce in sub-Saharan Africa*. The Global Nursing Review Initiative, International Council of Nurses. Retrieved on 9 March 2014 from <http://www.ghdonline.org/uploads/The_nursing_workforce_in_sub-Saharan _Africa.pdf>.

National Health System (NHS). (2009). *What is change?* Retrieved from <http://webarchive .nationalarchives.gov.uk/+/www.dh.gov.uk/en/publicationsandstatistics>.

Pearson, A., Laschinger, H., Porritt, K., Jordan, Z., Tucker, D., & Long, L. (2007). Comprehensive systematic review on developing and sustaining nursing leadership that fosters a healthy work environment in healthcare. *International Journal of Evidence Based Healthcare, 5*, 208–253.

Rosen, J., Mittal, V., Degenholtz, H., Castle, N., Mulsant, B. H., Hulland, S., et al. (2006). Ability, incentives, and management feedback: Organizational change to reduce pressure ulcers in a nursing home. *Journal of the American Medical Directors Association, 7*(3), 141–146.

Shipton, H., Armstrong, C., West, M., & Dawson, J. (2008). The impact of leadership and quality climate on hospital performance. *International Journal for Quality in Health Care, 20*(6), 439–445.

Shirley, M. R. (2011). Addressing strategy execution challenges to lead sustainable change. *Journal of Nursing Administration, 1*, 1–4.

Shojania, K. G., & Grimshaw, J. M. (2005). Evidence-based quality improvement: The state of the science. *Health Affairs, 24*(1), 138–150.

Stokowski, L. A. (2010). *Healthcare reform and nurses: Challenges and opportunities*. Retrieved from <http://www.medscape.com/viewarticle/721049>.

Tomajan, K. (2012). Advocating for Nurses and Nursing. *OJIN: The Online Journal of Issues in Nursing, 17*(1), 4.

Trevelyan, R. (2001). *Unit 11 Organisational transformation in managing people and organisations, Part B, (11-1,11-48)*. Sydney: Australian Graduate School of Management.

Vijayaraaghaven, V., & O'Donnell, R. (2011). *Sentara healthcare: A case series on disruptive innovations within integrated health systems*. San Mateo, CA: Innosight Institute.

Wong, C. A., & Cummings, G. G. (2007). The relationship between nursing leadership and patient outcomes: A systematic review. *Journal of Nursing Management, 15*, 508–521.

World Health Organization (2011). *Strategic directions for strengthening nursing and midwifery services, 2011–2015*. Geneva: WHO.

CHAPTER SEVEN

Leading research to enhance nursing practice

Hugh McKenna

LEARNING OBJECTIVES

At the completion of this chapter, the reader will be able to:

▲ understand the role of a good leader in developing a research culture;

▲ describe the steps to be followed in establishing a research culture;

▲ understand how high-quality research can underpin evidence-based practice.

KEY WORDS

Leadership, vision, evidence-based practice, research culture

INTRODUCTION

By the time you have reached this chapter in a book on Leadership and Nursing you will have been provided with several definitions of leadership and management. To set the scene for my contribution I too want to clarify these terms. By now you will have seen that leadership is about an individual influencing members of a group towards achieving some agreed goals. To do so, this individual needs the group members to recognise some legitimacy in this endeavour. A leader sets a new direction or vision for a group that they follow. In contrast, a manager controls or directs people/resources in a group according to principles or values that have been established (Myers, 2013). Similarly, it has been asserted that the style of a leader influences the performance and morale of a team (Crookes et al., 2010).

There are probably as many definitions of research as there are definitions of leadership. The one I favour is that used by the OECD (2002). It is perceived as creative work undertaken on a systematic basis in order to increase the stock of knowledge, including knowledge of man (sic), culture and society, and the use of this stock of knowledge to devise new applications. Therefore, the aim of nursing research is to investigate in a rigorous and systematic manner so as to increase our body of knowledge in order to improve nursing practice. This is strongly linked to evidence-based practice. Appleby, Walshe, and Ham (1995) maintained that evidence-based practice was 'A shift in the culture of health care provision away from basing decisions on opinion, past practice and precedent toward making more use of research evidence to guide clinical decision making' (p. 1). It should be mentioned at this stage that evidence might also be based on patient reports and clinician observations or clinician intuition. However, for the purposes of this chapter let us assume that the best type of evidence to underpin practice has its basis in systematic and rigorous research.

Such research does not happen accidentally; it has to be planned, funded, undertaken and reported. In other words someone must lead the research and the research team. Without a leader, the research will not happen and there is little hope of enhancing nursing practice. Therefore, I want to address the title of this chapter by focusing on leadership that is centred on leading high-quality nursing research.

LEADING HIGH-QUALITY RESEARCH

You will have gathered that research leadership is about having a clear vision and inspiring, enthusing and motivating others to pursue that vision. This means it is about being focused. This is best explained in the following two case studies.

CASE STUDY 7.1

The Clinical Medicine Unit (CMU) in Waddington Regional Hospital was opened in the mid-1980s. It has 38 beds of which half are for female patients. The Unit is almost always full to capacity. The patients range in age from 25 to 82 years and are hospitalised for a range of medical conditions. The average length of stay is two weeks. There are 32 nursing staff covering all shifts including night duty. There is one ward manager, 20 staff nurses, and 11 healthcare assistants. At any one time there are five student nurses from the local university School of Nursing. The CMU has three medical consultants who each have more junior physicians reporting to them. In the morning shift there are 10 nurses on duty, which decreases to seven in the afternoon and evening. There are two nurses and two healthcare assistants on night duty. Miss Jane Wright, the ward manager, is 54 years old and has many years' experience in medical nursing. She prides herself on being able to manage a complex clinical setting. She has seen fads come and go such as the nursing process, primary nursing, nursing models and feels that evidence-based practice is the latest craze embraced by the profession. In fact, she often reminisces on the good old days where there were no highfalutin' degree courses and nursing was a vocation. She sees the core business of the CMU to be caring for patients and not undertaking research; that is what university academics do and in her opinion it has little impact on patient care. She never wished to undertake a degree course and feels that her original nurse training amply prepared her for her current role. The nursing workload is quite heavy and the nurses have little time to consider research ideas. Anyway, they are not encouraged to think about what they could or should research. There are some small funding sources but no nurse in the CMU has ever applied for such grants. Some of the physicians carry out research in the Unit but none of this is multidisciplinary in nature. There are also very little research collaborations or partnerships with colleagues within and outside the CMU.

Readers will note that at Waddington Regional Hospital the CMU is really a traditional medical setting. The clinical practice that is being undertaken there is not likely to be based on the best research findings. It could be argued that Miss Wright is a good manager and runs a 'tight ship'. There may also be good leadership from Miss Wright but it is focused on the day-to-day running of the CMU rather than on leading a research-active unit. Compare this scenario with that of another clinical facility.

CASE STUDY 7.2

Keystone Hospital opened its General Medical Department (GMD) in 1987. It is a mixed gender clinical setting with 40 beds. The Unit is always full to capacity. The patients range in age from mid-twenties to mid-eighties and the two consultants in charge of the GMD specialise in a range of medical conditions. The average length of stay is two weeks. There are 30 nursing staff covering all shifts including night duty. This includes one ward manager, 18 staff nurses, and 11 clinical support workers. The local university School of Nursing sends six students to the GMD for their medical placement. The department has four shifts, morning, afternoon, evening and night. In the morning shift there are 10 nurses on duty, which decreases to seven in the afternoon and evening. There are three nurses and one healthcare assistant on night duty. Miss Mary Wilkes is the nurse manager and is 52 years old. She has worked in medical settings for over 30 years and has been the clinical nurse manager in the GMD for four years. She undertook a degree course part time in the 1990s and followed this with a master's degree in nursing. Her interest in research started during her primary degree and she undertook a research project as part of her master's dissertation. Since then she has collaborated with medical and social work colleagues in the GMD and obtained small amounts of funding for clinical projects. Prior to Miss Wilkes taking up her current role, there was very little research being undertaken by nurses within the GMD. Research was an afterthought in the minds of most staff. Shortly after her appointment she let it be known that she expected the majority of the staff to be research active and to ensure that their research is informed by their practice and that their research findings are returned to inform practice. She realised many years ago that the GMD research activities can not be of any quality by trying to do everything. Rather it was important to focus on a small number of research topics with which to concentrate scarce resources and efforts. She held numerous brainstorming events with her staff. This led to the identification of four research areas where they could reasonably attract research funding and undertake investigations that would produce findings that would enhance nursing practice. The staff were allocated to four research groupings, each with a Research Group Leader. These were: Care of Stroke Patients; Personalised Care for Chronic Obstructive Airways Disease; Diabetes Research Group; and Cardiac Research Group. These groups were multidisciplinary and soon developed links with other researchers. While there were external funding sources for these research topics, Miss Wilkes managed to get the hospital to provide some matching funds to support staff to attend and speak at conferences and to visit centres of excellence. She also encouraged the nurses to publish their work. There were strong links with the local university and several of the staff there had joint appointments in the hospital. A number of the GMD staff was asked to give lectures and in time the GMD established a reputation for its focused areas of research. Over time it was perceived as a centre of excellence and other nurse managers and researchers saw this as a clinical setting that they must visit.

Readers should be able to see the difference in both case studies. I can assure you that there are more clinical settings in the world similar to the first case study than to the second. I also assure you that these are real-life case studies of two clinical medical units with which I am familiar. But let me tease out for you what contributed to the success of the General Medical Department at Keystone Hospital. In a word it was the leadership of Mary Wilkes. She knew exactly what had to be done if she was to change the culture of the department to being a setting where knowledge and skills are generated, challenged and tested as well as being practised.

I am going to go into greater detail of how Mary Wilkes set the direction for the GMD and encouraged and motivated the staff to sign up to her vision. This was relatively easy for most of the staff because they all wished to be part of a research-oriented facility where evidence-informed practice was the norm and that had a high profile and produced research that enhanced nursing care.

The vision and its targets

When she became the nurse manager for the GMD, Mary Wilkes knew that what was required was a more clearly articulated research strategy. The following 16 elements were part of that strategy and fed into the vision that she had for the department.

1.   Emphasis on capacity building and sustainability

One of her targets was to grow the capacity of her staff to undertake clinical research. This was done through mentoring existing staff with colleagues who were research active in other disciplines or from the local university's School of Nursing. During her four years in the job she also hired some new nursing staff who had expertise in the clinical topics that the GMD wished to focus upon and who had some experience in doing research as part of their degree. Her mantra was to recruit and retain the very best nurses who were interested in using and testing the very best evidence for excellence in patient care. An important aspect of her vision was to ensure that newly qualified nurses were supported. They were given some 'seed money' and mentored by more experienced colleagues. She knew that the emphasis on supporting young nurses to get involved in research was an important aspect of future proofing the department's research profile. In addition, the research esteem of the staff was a priority. They were encouraged to write articles, sit on the boards of journals, on funding bodies, on health service research governance panels, on policy-making committees and to attend conferences. They were also encouraged to attend classes in the university on appraising research evidence and implementing research findings. Two were asked to sit on the hospital's research ethics committee. This was part of a strategy to build close mutually beneficial relationships with other more research-oriented disciplines, with researchers in the university's School of Nursing and with funders, policy makers and health service managers.

2.   Research linked to national and international priorities

Mary Wilkes realised that for the GMD to raise its research profile it had to focus on research themes that were priority areas for the government and were perceived as important international health problems. This meant a move away from studies that were of interest to individual staff to studies that were addressing national and international strategic priorities. After a small number of meetings with her staff these themes emerged. No one could argue that stroke, chronic obstructive airways disease, diabetes and heart disease were not high on the World Health Organization's list of global problems. However, Mary Wilkes did not want the department to be doing medical research or nurses acting as research assistants for doctors. Therefore, the emphasis across the four themes was enhancing the care and wellbeing of patients and their families. While research grant proposals were often sent to medical research funders, the emphasis was always on care rather than cure.

3.   Modern and high-quality infrastructure

To attract and retain the best staff it was important that the environment was conducive. One large store room was transformed into an area where staff had the opportunity to discuss research ideas in a comfortable work area. There were numerous whiteboards where impromptu brainstorming could take place. The tea, coffee, refreshment areas were close by and this meant that staff from different research groups and disciplines would 'bump' into each other several times each day. Mary Wilkes knew that the day was long gone where a researcher could do serious research on their own. The four topics that were the focus of their research lent themselves well to multidisciplinary studies. In other parts of the hospital there were small meeting rooms where multidisciplinary teams would discuss research ideas and where research proposals could be drafted. Sandpits were often held in these meeting rooms. This is where a research question regarding one of the research topics was identified and researchers from a range of different health professions would 'play' with this, bringing their own expertise to the problem. One of these involved post-stroke mobilisation. Nurses, doctors, occupational therapists, physiotherapists and social workers were just some of the disciplines that took part in that sandpit. It was facilitated by a nursing professor from the local university. The objective was to design at least one research proposal that would be sent to a funding body. Furthermore, regular research days were organised for nursing staff to share their research with other hospital staff and external colleagues from the university and from the local diabetes and chest, heart and stroke charities.

4.   Competitive peer-review funding sources

It has been said already but it merits repeating. There is no point in having enthusiastic nurses keen on doing research and having a good research environment if no one wants to fund the studies. Therefore, the identification of the four themes was crucial. Not only was there funding regionally for these areas but there were also national and international funding bodies who wished to see such research being carried out. Initially, some internal seed funding was made available. This was mainly to conduct some pilot studies so that larger funding sources could be pursued. Mary Wilkes referred to this as using a 'sprat to catch a mackerel'. Such internal research funding showed commitment but it had to be allocated strategically and fairly. There were also staff development courses on how to capture peer-reviewed grants. Here, successful and unsuccessful research proposals were shared and analysed. Junior staff were mentored by more experienced colleagues and in many cases taken onto a research proposal team to get experience in grant writing. These strategies resulted in 5–10-year program grants replacing 1–3-year project grants.

5.   Appropriate and productive links with partners in the university

The relationship between clinical staff and university staff grew stronger. The main reason for this was that the university staff needed access to patients to do their research and the clinical staff needed access to university staff to help them write grant applications. Such mutually beneficial relationships led to many collaborative research projects. An important aspect of Mary Wilkes' vision was to involve academic nurses in the research not as advisors but as partners, from design right through to dissemination. She formed strategic links with COPD, diabetes, stroke and cardiac researchers in the university and in relevant charities. This meant that from day one, there were discussions about the impact of the research on changing practice or enhancing nursing care. She also encouraged the development of joint appointment positions where a researcher worked part time in the GMD and part time in the university's School of Nursing. There were four of these and one was fully funded by the university. The university staff knew that such joint appointment posts would lend them clinical credibility while the clinical staff knew that such joint appointments would provide them with the opportunity to form partnerships with high-profile researchers.

6.   Appropriate and well-developed collaborative research partnerships

In the early days of her appointment as the department's nurse manager, Mary Wilkes was able to get several computers installed in the clinical setting. Here staff searched the internet and the nursing journals to identify best evidence and research recommendations within their themed areas. They were also able to identify other hospitals where similar research was being undertaken. Mary Wilkes lost no time in contacting the directors of those centres and arranging visits for her staff. This resulted in fruitful collaborative partnerships between her department and similar departments and units in the USA, Canada, South Africa, Australia and in several European countries. Mary Wilkes also had an idea to approach clinical researchers in these countries and ask them to be a member of a GMD International Advisory Board (IAB). This meets every six months using the hospital's videoconferencing technology. They share success stories and also problem areas where joint research could be undertaken.

7.   Rigorous methodologies and theoretical sophistication

Mary Wilkes did not want the GDM to be associated with poor-quality research. It had taken a few years to build up a reputation and she knew that this could be lost if the department was associated with any shoddy investigations. It was a given from the emergence of the research groupings that quality was the watchword for all research emanating from the GDM. Staff worked with experts from the university to ensure that methodologies were designed that withstood the scrutiny of the most high-profile peer reviewers. Similarly, the theoretical underpinnings for the research studies had to add to the nursing knowledge base.

8.   A better balance between practice and research

Mary Wilkes knew from experience that in a busy clinical setting research could be perceived as a luxury. She also knew that the most important role that the nurses had was caring expertly for the patients. Therefore, the research activities undertaken in the department had to focus on making that care better through generating or testing new knowledge and skills. If the research did not enhance practice she saw it as a waste of valuable staff time. It was crucial that the quality of clinical care did not suffer and that patients and their families were happy that their care was of the highest standard. It was also important to ensure that patients were not 'over researched' or did not suffer survey fatigue. Full and ongoing informed consent was always a high priority and the Hospital Research Ethics Committee was involved in monitoring the department's research activity. Mary Wilkes and four of her senior staff nurses undertook a 'root and branch' review of all the clinical procedures in the department. Most were high quality but in the early days of her appointment she also noted that there were routines and rituals that were not based on any research and while they probably did not do the patients any harm, they also did not do them any good. Several procedures were no longer fit for purpose. The result of the review was that all the procedures in the department were based on the best available evidence. Where the best evidence was not available, this formed the basis for research projects.

9. PhD students

In the past, potential PhD students tended to approach staff in the local School of Nursing with their own research ideas and invariably the staff member agreed to supervise them, even though they did not have relevant expertise in the topics. Most of the students were part time and in their mid-thirties. While they brought a great deal of experience to the project, it was Mary Wilkes' vision that clinical staff would partner with School of Nursing staff and would only supervise students who wished to undertake a PhD in one of the four research themes. If not, the student was informed that they may wish to go to another university to get the relevant supervision or that they could undertake their research training in one of the four research groups but on a related topic. Furthermore, Mary Wilkes ensured that clinical researchers and research students presented to the final year undergraduate students and masters students so as to encourage them to consider undertaking postgraduate clinical research.

10. Evidence of research impact

Research for the sake of research is not an option; research findings must have an impact. For Mary Wilkes, it was not enough for staff to claim that their research had impact; they had to have evidence to show this. Therefore, staff began to collect the evidence as it happened. So if clinical practice was changed as a result of findings from a research study, the views of patients, senior managers and other disciplines were collected to identify what and how practice had changed and the effect this had on staff and patients. Similarly, if a government minister or civil servant changed policy as a result of research findings, this was noted and filed. This meant that when the staff claimed that their research had benefit they could show the evidence for this.

11. Knowledge transfer—strategic links with industry

For nursing research the impact could be on enhanced nursing practice or improved quality of life; it can also be of benefit to society and to business. For example, Mary Wilkes saw that research on stroke care could have a very powerful impact on a local community or on society. Similarly, she saw that nursing research could also lead to new products and health-related smart phone applications that would be of commercial interest to business and industry. Staff established links with a local seating company that was interested in developing seating products for people with stroke and with a company that was developing oxygen masks for patients with COPD. Another staff member is working with a university spin-out company on a smart phone app for foot care in diabetes. Some of these have led to companies helping to fund the research and PhD scholarships.

12.   A research publicity strategy

The research often provided stories for the local media. This further enhanced the reputation of the department. However, Mary Wilkes knew that a publicity strategy was required for the department's research activities. It was not enough to publish them in professional or academic journals; they had to show the local population that they were undertaking research in the department that was making a positive difference to patients. Fortunately, the topics of COPD, diabetes, heart disease and stroke were newsworthy. The department built strong relationships with local journalists and this meant that some of the work was referred to on local radio or in local newspapers. This also engendered a sense of community pride in the hospital.

13.   Establish an institutional repository

An institutional repository is a virtual storehouse of research publications and reports. Taking into account the embargoes by publishers, Mary Wilkes made sure that when a paper was published it was put onto the online institutional repository. This meant that it was accessible online to anyone in the world whether academic, clinician or patient. One of the benefits of this was that research papers were available as soon as possible after publication. This was in line with the open access publication policy of many funding bodies. It also meant that the number of citations for the research increased considerably.

14.   High-quality research publications

Researchers are mainly judged by the quality of their publications. Mary Wilkes was initially concerned that some staff concentrated on the quantity of publications rather than the quality of publications. This trend was soon reversed. She introduced a system where senior staff undertook a voluntary internal review of young researchers' draft publications. They were asked to always stress in their papers the international implications of the research. This was part of the mentoring strategy for early career researchers. Staff were also encouraged to publish in those journals that were included in the SCOPUS and web of science databases as this meant they were more likely to be cited. However, to get the attention of other clinicians, staff were also encouraged to publish a more sanitised version of their research in professional journals and health service newsletters. Increasingly, more of the researchers began to keep a record of their H and G indices to show that their work was being cited nationally and internationally. They began to consistently publish in the top 25% of journals in their discipline or (in the case of books) with highly selective publishers. Senior staff were also encouraged to be on the editorial boards of peer-reviewed journals while more junior staff were encouraged to review manuscripts for prestigious journals.

15.   Celebrate a success

One key element of Mary Wilkes' leadership was that success has to be celebrated. Therefore, when a staff member was successful with a grant proposal a small party was organised. The same or similar celebrations occurred when an article was accepted for publication, when a staff member was asked to do a presentation at a conference, when policy or practice changed as a result of research findings, when a PhD student was awarded a doctorate, or when a staff member was appointed to a high-profile committee or board. Often, colleagues in the university and in external patient pressure groups were invited to the celebrations. This became part of the culture within the department, a culture constructed by Mary Wilkes.

16.   Enhancing nursing practice

The best quality research can be carried out and the findings disseminated and yet practice may not be enhanced. We know that researchers tend to publish in journals read by other researchers and speak at conferences attended by other like-minded researchers. So I would argue that there are two leadership positions—one to lead the research like Mary Wilkes and one to lead the change in practice as a result of that research. They may or may not be the same individual and in the majority of instances they are not. However, I would argue that both these types of leaders need to have the vision, energy and enthusiasm to create change. Both need to build the capacity and skills of their team, both need to partner with each other, both need a conducive environmental culture to enthuse their staff, both require resources, both have the enhancement of patient care as their goal, both need to see impact in their work and both need to celebrate success. In the case of the GMD, Mary Wilkes held both these roles.

Therefore, whether a person is leading research to enhance nursing practice or leading a clinical team to embrace evidence-based practice the same leadership skills are required. Such leaders are focused on the future, they are interested in changing things, they are focused on a culture based on shared values and they seek the highest possible standards of care.

There is the danger that once leaders like Mary Wilkes leave or retire, the research activities will stop and the environmental culture will disappear. This was addressed in the GMD by effective mentoring of future leaders and ensuring that the four research-themed areas were each led by a senior staff nurse. This helps to future proof the department and ensure that the reputation for discovery, dissemination and development continues.

There follows one example from many of a research project that was undertaken in the GMD that had global impact. Tricia Reid, a staff nurse, noticed that compared with the GMD an adjacent medical ward had longer lengths of patient stay. In the GMD there was a consistently shorter length of stay than in the other ward. What puzzled Tricia was that they were both medical assessment units that were admitting similar types of patients. Furthermore, they employed the same two medical consultants. In fact, the only difference that she could see between both settings was that the GMD had open visiting and the other ward did not. She was intrigued by this phenomenon and sought confirmation of her perceptions with colleagues. When it was brought to their attention, they too noticed this and found it strange.

Tricia decided to investigate the phenomenon further and research it as part of her master's degree dissertation. She started by searching the literature and did not come up with any published papers or reports on open visiting being linked to shorter lengths of stay. She then used a retrospective quantitative design to check for a statistical significant difference in discharge rates over the previous five years across both wards. She took into account demographic and other variables of patients. These included gender, age, diagnosis and consultant. She also used observation to check the number and types of visitors (family, friends, work colleagues, etc.) on both units. The data collected supported her hunch that this is an interesting and important phenomenon to study.

In this example, the 'Length of Stay' research emerged from practice. Tricia and her supervisor decided to publish her research in a medical journal. As a result of the publication, a nurse researcher in Australia decided to carry out a study to see if the findings can be verified or refuted when applied to patients in medical wards in Sydney.

CONCLUSION

This chapter was about leading research in order to enhance nursing practice. You were informed at the outset that leadership is where an individual influences group members towards achieving some agreed goals. In contrast, a manager controls or directs people/resources in a group according to principles or values that have been established (Myers, 2013). Two real-life case studies were presented. In the first one it was obvious that a culture of research or evidence-based practice did not exist to any extent. While the quality of management was high there did not appear to be anyone leading a vision for knowledge generation and the production of evidence that could change practice. It could be argued that Miss Jane Wright was a manager rather than a leader. In the second case study, readers could see how the vision and tenacity of a leader could bring a general medical department from being a place where there were several rituals and routines with little evidence to inform practice, to become a place where care was based on the best available evidence and where research was undertaken with the sole aim of enhancing practice. I can state without fear of contradiction that it was due entirely to the leadership of Mary Wilkes. She had a vision for where the department could be and she also knew how to achieve it. The best clinical nursing departments in the world made it there because of similar leadership and most have also introduced the 16 approaches used at Keystone Hospital by Mary Wilkes.

REFLECTIVE EXERCISE

1. When it comes to encouraging a culture of research, what is the difference between leadership and management in a busy clinical setting?
2. Is good leadership a trait one is born with or one can learn?
3. A transformational research leader is a great asset in a clinical setting but can represent a single point of failure. How would you ensure succession planning?
4. Think about your current workplace. Name three things that could enhance its research profile.
5. What strategies would you introduce to enable good-quality multidisciplinary research to take place?
6. How would you support early career researchers in the clinical setting?
7. Next time you are in practice, listen to the handover between shifts. Do the nurses refer to research studies or evidence-informed practices?
8. Imagine you are a new clinical manager or ward sister. How would you assess the clinical setting for a research culture? What would you look for?

Recommended Readings

Borbasi, S., & Jackson, D. (Eds.), (2008). *Navigating the maze of research: Enhancing nursing and midwifery practice* (2nd ed.). Sydney: Elsevier.

Gifford, W. A., Davies, B., Edwards, N., & Graham, I. D. (2006). Leadership strategies to influence the use of clinical practice guidelines. *Nursing Leadership, 19*(4), 72–88.

Gifford, W. A., Davies, B., Edwards, N., Griffin, P., & Lybanon, V. (2007). Managerial leadership for nurses' use of research evidence: An integrative review of the literature. *Worldviews on Evidence-based Nursing, 4*(3), 126–145.

Sandstrom, B., Borglin, G., Nilsson, R., & Willman, A. (2011). Promoting the implementation of evidence-based practice: A literature review focusing on the role of nursing leadership. *Worldviews on Evidence-based Nursing, 8*(4), 212–223.

Wong, C. A., & Cummings, G. G. (2007). The relationship between nursing leadership and patient outcomes: A systematic review. *Journal of Nursing Management, 15*(5), 508–521.

References

Appleby, J., Walshe, K., & Ham, C. (1995). *Acting on the evidence*. Research Paper. NAHAT.

Crookes, P., Griffiths, R., & Brown, A. (2010). Becoming part of a multidisciplinary healthcare team. In J. Daly, S. Speedy, & D. Jackson (Eds.), *Contexts of nursing: An introduction*. Sydney: Elsevier.

Myers, S. (2013). *Differences between leadership and management*. <http://www.teamtechnology.co.uk/leadership/management/definitions-of-leadership-and-management/>.

OECD (2002). *Frascati Manual: Proposed standard practice for surveys on research and experimental development* (6th ed.). Retrieved 27 May 2012 from <www.oecd.org/sti/frascatimanual>.

CHAPTER EIGHT

Leadership in health informatics: A pathway to twenty-first century patient care

Jen Bichel-Findlay & Cathy Doran

LEARNING OBJECTIVES

At the completion of this chapter, the reader should be able to:

- ▲ describe the articulation between health information technology and quality and safety of healthcare delivery;
- ▲ define health informatics, nursing informatics, ehealth and big data analytics;
- ▲ recognise nursing's unique position to lead health informatics at a local and national level;
- ▲ justify the value of a chief nursing informatics officer position within the healthcare environment;
- ▲ discuss the educational opportunities that will provide a skilled informatics workforce;
- ▲ describe the skills that a nurse leader requires to contribute to successful health information technology implementations;
- ▲ discuss the potential that health information technology has to transform practice and improve evidence-based decision making.

KEY WORDS

Health informatics, nursing informatics, health information technology, HIT, data analytics, Chief Nursing Informatics Officer, CNIO

INTRODUCTION

The Future of Nursing: Leading Change, Advancing Health report, released by the Institute of Medicine (IOM), highlighted the need to transform and remodel many aspects of the health system in order to provide seamless, affordable, accessible, evidence-based and patient-centric quality care (IOM, 2011). The authors recommended that the largest sector of the healthcare workforce, nurses, address four areas—scope of practice, education, leadership and equal partners in health opportunities, and data collection for workforce planning and policy making (IOM, 2011). As the report points out, nurses' consistent and close proximity to patients and their scientific understanding of care processes across the continuum of care places them in a unique position to both lead and contribute to the improvement and redesign of the healthcare system across all practice environments so that high-quality and safe care is delivered to every patient (IOM, 2011).

Numerous international reports and publications in the last two decades, including some released by the IOM (Amarasingham, Plantinga, Diener-West, Gaskin, & Powe, 2009; Committee on Quality of Health Care in America, 2001; Hillestad, Bigelow, & Bower, 2005; Holroyd-Leduc, Lorenzetti, Straus, Sykes, & Quan, 2011; IOM, 2012; Jha & Classen, 2011; Kohn, Corrigan, & Donaldson, 1999; Ortiz & Clancy, 2003; RAND Health, 2005), have identified health information technology (HIT) as a vehicle that can make substantial improvements to healthcare costs, quality and safety. All aspects of current care delivery are becoming increasingly digital, with the adoption of HIT expected to increase efficiency and effectiveness of clinician interactions, reduce the human potential for error and create a better work environment (Sensmeier, 2011). Unfortunately, the availability of technology does not guarantee that it will be used correctly or that it improves patient outcomes and maximises clinician effort. Current critics of health information technology highlight that systems often impede clinical processes and activities and detract from patient care, and call for the health informatics community to ensure that new systems follow workflow rather than the data-collection procedures (Bowens, Frye, & Jones, 2010; Carayon, Karsh, & Cartmill, 2010; Cusack, 2008; Lorenzi, Kouroubali, Detmer, & Bloomrosen, 2009).

In the current era of personalised and value-based healthcare, both nursing and health informatics are in need of strong leadership in order to progress a vision of what healthcare should deliver to patients. Leadership in health informatics by nurses is crucial, given nursing's large footprint in the delivery of care through its sizable population, its coverage of every healthcare setting and its direct contact with patients. Nurses have the ability to ensure a clear connection between people, process and technology so that the technology supports the workflow and provides for better patient outcomes and clinician effort. Leading health informatics will involve four key areas—education, scope of practice, policy participation and innovative vision.

BACKGROUND

Ever since the release of the findings of both the Harvard Medical Practice Study (Brennan et al., 1991; Leape et al., 1991) and the Quality in Australian Health Care Study (Wilson, Runciman, & Gibberd, 1995) and the publication of *To Err is Human: Building a Safer Health System* (Kohn et al., 1999), healthcare environments in most countries have been attempting to reduce adverse events and improve the safety and quality of care through a range of reform measures. These have included clinical redesign, innovative models of care, implementation of root cause analysis, application of efficiency theories such as lean thinking and six sigma, and so on. Yet, it seems that despite all these best efforts, the prevalence of harm to patients has not improved substantially and the delivery of highly variable and often unsuitable care remains an issue (Runciman et al., 2012). It is now increasingly clear that healthcare is unlikely to see any transformation without successful implementation of advanced technologies and the presence of a culture that accepts information technology as part of providing care. Just as electronic means of information exchange pervade our personal lives, healthcare needs to leverage technology to improve decision making, reduce the time it takes to diagnose and treat illness, eliminate redundancy, personalise care activities to the specific needs of the individual and improve the overall accuracy of healthcare activity. It is also hoped that digitised information will not only facilitate targeted information for treating patients but also allow healthcare organisations to conduct population analytics and deliver more personalised healthcare to the community.

Under-investment in information technology in healthcare is a common issue in most countries, and this is compounded by information technology resulting in improved clinical quality not playing the same role it does in other industries (Bates, 2002). The potential for information technology in healthcare is enormous, and includes improving communication between clinicians and patients and between clinicians, providing easier access to critical information, monitoring variation, delivering clinical decision support at the point of care, encouraging delivery of evidence-based healthcare, and reducing errors and near-miss adverse events through alerts and forced functions. Recent changes in information technology make rapid adoption of this technology attractive, such as the declining cost of computer processing, widespread availability of the internet and web-based platforms, availability of a plethora of software for a wide variety of activities, and the increased accessibility of handheld devices and applications (Bates, 2002). It certainly has the potential to reduce errors attributed to communication failures and those resulting from insufficient information. Nursing informatics leaders will play a vital role in transforming patient care into new models of clinical practice with the assistance of HIT (Health Information and Management Systems Society (HIMSS), 2011).

HEALTH INFORMATICS AND NURSING INFORMATICS

The discipline of health informatics evolved from medical informatics, gaining prominence in the 1980s (Bichel-Findlay & Doran, 2014). Health informatics refers to the science and practice around information in health that results in informed and assisted healthcare, where 'informed' means the right information about the consumer, patient or population together with pertinent health knowledge available at the right time in a usable form, and 'assisted' means the actions of the clinician are made safer and easier and the health consumer is supported in their decisions and activities (Health Informatics Society of Australia (HISA), 2013). Nursing informatics, despite dating back to Florence Nightingale, also evolved from medical informatics, and was defined by Graves and Corcoran in 1989 as the combination of computer, information and nursing science to support the management and processing of nursing data, information and knowledge to sustain the practice of nursing and the delivery of nursing care (Graves & Corcoran, 1989). In 2009, the Nursing Informatics Special Interest Group of the International Medical Informatics Association (IMIA-NI SIG) updated the definition to highlight that the science and practice of nursing informatics incorporates nursing, its information and knowledge, and how it manages the use of information and communication technologies in order to promote the health of people, families and communities worldwide (IMIA-NI SIG, 2013).

Two other common terms are used in the health sector when discussing technology—ehealth and big data analytics. Firstly, ehealth refers to the transfer of health resources and healthcare by electronic means, comprising three areas—the delivery of health information, for health providers and health consumers, through the internet and telecommunications, using the capacity of information technology and ecommerce to improve public health services, and the use of ecommerce and ebusiness practices in health systems management (World Health Organization, 2013). Lastly, big data analytics describes the ability to capture, store, manage and analyse the deluge of data we are generating in the current 'digital datafied world'. It is quite astounding to realise that the data generated from the dawn of civilisation to 2003 (five exabytes) is now what we produce every two days (Schmidt, 2010, cited by Woodill, 2012). Big data is also changing our perception of an expert from someone who possesses a range of information to someone who knows where to locate the latest and best information needed to solve a specific problem (Woodill, 2012). Due to this significant conceptual shift, we have to alter our learning approaches so that staff not only know how to access the most appropriate information for their current needs, but also how to critically judge that information and how to convey it to others who require that information to complete an activity or make a business case (Woodill, 2012). Big data has enormous potential for the healthcare sector, which is often described as data-rich and information-poor, as it will provide credible and relevant information to support evidenced-based healthcare practice.

LEADERSHIP IN HEALTH INFORMATICS

The world of health informatics is quite broad and encompasses the daily lives of all clinicians; however, nurses are often the greatest users of technology in most healthcare settings in part due to their direct contact with the patient (IOM, 2011). It is important, therefore, to foster a united voice for health informatics and increase the awareness of the health informatics community. Nursing is well placed to lead this voice and awareness, as they are the largest single clinical group in the workforce and deliver direct care to patients in virtually all healthcare environments. Clear paths need to be established for a national health informatics leader presence, particularly focusing on developing and promoting talented and upcoming leaders in the field of health informatics. Healthcare needs to provide a single point of connection between health informatics individuals and groups and the broader nursing and healthcare community, and the position of Chief Nursing Informatics Officer (CNIO) at the local level can guide the implementation and optimisation of information technology systems within the health environment and provide the vital link between the technical staff and the clinicians. The nurse in this position does not imply that they are responsible for nursing only but rather the person occupying this position is a nurse prepared as an informatician (Swindle & Bradley, 2010).

The role of the CNIO within healthcare organisations has gained recognition in the United States and the focus in the United Kingdom is on the creation of Chief Clinical Information Officers (Department of Health, 2012); however, this role has not gained any traction in Australia. Murphy (2010b) perceives this leader position as having both a strategic and operational role, as well as educative responsibilities in both roles. The CNIO must be able to explain what is possible with the deployment of HIT, and how the interaction with people and process changes must be addressed to realise the full benefits of this deployment (Murphy, 2010b). Strategic leader role examples include guiding the system selection process, defining the governance process, advising on the sequencing of module implementations, consulting on methodology for implementation, engaging senior management in culture and practice changes required during implementation, and assisting in identifying appropriate value proposition and key performance indicators for system implementations

(Murphy, 2010b). Examples of the operational leader role includes overseeing system design and implementation, designing implementation and key performance indicator metrics, establishing an enhancement request system and corresponding prioritisation process, and supervising ongoing process improvement initiatives (Murphy, 2010b). Tupper and Alexander (2012) view the future CNIO role as also being involved with data warehousing (central repositories that integrate data from one or more disparate sources which is then used for reporting and analysis), particularly in relation to clinical data being appropriately tagged and organised against industry standards.

EDUCATION

Clinicians are currently experiencing a catch-22 situation—the importance of clinician input into decisions about HIT infrastructure and deployment is acknowledged throughout the world yet the majority lack a basic understanding of informatics and how HIT can be effectively utilised in day-to-day practice. This often leads to implementation failure or a protracted implementation that is costly to the healthcare organisation and demoralising to the clinicians. Utilising informatics is a core competency required of all healthcare professions (IOM, 2011), and as the healthcare environment moves towards the widespread adoption of HIT, particularly the electronic medical record, nursing must transform itself as a profession if it is to enjoy all the benefits that this is purported to provide towards patient outcomes. Nursing curricula in many countries do not currently address health informatics, so it will be necessary to reform nursing education so that nurses embrace the rapidly changing technology environment.

In 2005, the Technology Informatics Guiding Educational Reform (TIGER) initiative was formed in the United States, and a summit was held in 2006 to address how practising nurses and students of nursing could become more engaged in the evolving digital era (DuLong & Ball, 2010; Skiba et al., 2010). It not only highlighted the need for core competencies for all clinicians, but identified three competency areas—basic computer skills, information literacy, and information management (Nahm & Wilson, 2011). It has since brought together over 1500 nurses to fill the healthcare quality chasm with information technology, through identifying information/knowledge best practices and effective technology capabilities for nurses and developing a shared vision and expected outcomes that will improve nursing practice, education and the delivery of patient care through the use of health information technology (TIGER, 2013).

Europe has taken a different approach to health informatics competencies and has developed the European Computer Driving Licence (ECDL) that defines the skills and competencies required to be proficient in the use of computers and computer applications. Specialised modules of the ECDL have been developed that address health informatics system users. A modified version of the ECDL known as the International Computer Drivers Licence (ICDL) has been adopted by Great Britain to ensure that all nurses have basic computer skills (Gugerty & Sensmeier, 2010).

Achieving a level of competency in clinical information technology is a crucial foundational tool for the leadership practice of nurse managers and leaders and will become even more important in the future as more sophisticated information technology is available (Nickitas & Kerfoot, 2010). It is also important that nurse leaders expand their understanding of information technology concepts and issues such as system interoperability (ability of different information technology systems and software applications to communicate and exchange data) and health data exchanges (electronic movement of clinical information among healthcare organisations which maintains the meaning of the information being exchanged) (Nickitas & Kerfoot, 2010). Exposure to clinical information systems for decision making and error mitigation, the use of the internet to improve access to information for themselves and their patients, and the ability to use email to communicate and coordinate with colleagues and patients are minimum skills in which clinicians should be proficient (Greiner & Knebel, 2003).

A range of educational paths should be available for nurses to become health informaticians. Not only should undergraduate health degrees provide content on health informatics, postgraduate programs addressing health informatics and health information management ought to be available, both at a graduate diploma and masters level. The availability of these programs will ensure that nurses are prepared to improve patient care by embracing HIT. Credentialling is a mechanism that many countries are pursuing to overcome the lack of formal recognition for health informatics skills, comprising agreed core competencies being tested, and the Health Informatics Society of Australia (HISA), in collaboration with the Australasian College of Health Informatics (ACHI) and the Health Information Association of Australia (HIMAA), recently launched the Certified Health Informatician Australasia certification program. Many other similar programs exist, such as those offered by the American Medical Informatics Association (AMIA), the International Medical Informatics Association (IMIA), the Health Information and Management Systems Society (HIMSS) and the Canadian Health Informatics Association (COACH). The American Nurses Credentialing Center has also been offering certification for informatics nurses since 1995, and there are over 500 nurses who have successfully completed the examination, which addresses system analysis, design, implementation, support, testing and evaluation, as well as human factors, computer technology, information management and professional practice trends and issues (Murphy, 2010a). Nursing leaders need to strongly support the three areas identified in the TIGER initiative in order to raise awareness of informatics—developing a nursing workforce capable of using HIT to improve the delivery of healthcare, securing more nurses in the development of a national healthcare information technology infrastructure, and fast-tracking the adoption of smart, standards-based, interoperable technology that will make care delivery safer, more efficient, timely, accessible and patient-focused (TIGER Initiative Advisory Council, 2009).

HealthWorkforce Australia (2013) has acknowledged that the capture, storage and use of electronic health data has grown and increased in complexity, and this reliance on HIT has driven demand for a specialised workforce of health informaticians. They are in the final stages of overseeing an analysis of this much-needed workforce, which will estimate shortfall between supply and demand, and recommend a range of possible education and training solutions (HealthWorkforce Australia, 2013). This skilled informatics workforce will be needed in the next decade, given the substantial government investment (both state and federal) in electronic health information systems in Australia, as well as private healthcare service corporations.

In 2011, HIMSS developed a position statement recommending that nursing informatics leaders transform nursing education to include informatics competencies at all levels of academic preparation and promote the continuing education of all levels of nursing, particularly in the areas of electronic health data and HIT (HIMSS, 2011). Nursing informatics leaders need to take heed of the HIMSS recommendations and ensure that we are developing a nursing workforce that is prepared to embrace and use HIT to improve patient care.

SCOPE OF PRACTICE

Nurse leaders (executives) need to be involved in all HIT activities, including the development of any infrastructure, system selection and evaluation, data entry and information retrieval procedures, through the extent of embedding clinical decision support, practice guidelines, protocols and pathways, and political partnerships. Various studies have demonstrated that involving nurses in the design, planning and implementation of technology systems leads to fewer problems during implementation (Hunt, Sproat, & Kitzmiller, 2004).

In order to support the delivery of clinical care, nurse leaders will need to develop a new set of skills and knowledge that encompasses information tools and technology (Nagle, 2012). Nurse leaders need to be strategically involved in the selection process of HIT to ensure that the HIT supports the organisation's mission and goals in the same way they would be involved in any strategic activities (Sensmeier, 2010; Simpson, 2011). Nurse leaders need to ensure that the HIT integrates with existing systems such as rostering and finance and that the HIT will provide information to support the delivery of patient care. Other considerations include the incorporation of data standards and establishing the flow of information to external systems such as national electronic health records (EHRs). In order to achieve this, nurse leaders will need to establish partnerships with the CNIO or the nursing informatics specialists within their organisation.

Nurse leaders will also need to advocate that the HIT solution is nursing centric (Simpson, 2006) and that it supports the acquisition of nursing knowledge and evidence-based nursing practice. The transition of data into information and knowledge into the application of wisdom is the cornerstone of nursing practice and enables nurses to practise patient-centric care in the twenty-first century. The transition of wisdom from data, information and knowledge cannot be achieved in isolation, requiring changes to current clinical practice and the redesign of clinical processes in order to realise a successful HIT implementation.

Workflow redesign is an integral aspect of health informatics and nurses are pivotal in the process analysis and redesign activities associated with the implementation of HIT (Hammel-Jones, 2012). Process analysis and redesign is a critical component of all HIT implementations, ensuring that information technology supports safe patient care (Hammel-Jones, 2012). The redesign of processes is the first step in change management activities that must be clearly articulated and led by the nurse executive. The impact of change and the change management associated with the introduction of HIT is often neglected and downplayed by nursing executive and clinical staff alike (Hammel-Jones, 2012). Change management in any HIT implementation requires clear communication, support and planning and should be championed by nurse leaders. An essential component of any change management activity for a successful HIT implementation and adoption requires the nurse leader to partner with nursing informatics specialists and the workforce to ensure organisational readiness and development. This involves incorporating the redesign of clinical processes, change management and ensuring that these activities are included in end-user education and training on the HIT.

POLICY PARTICIPATION

Nurse leaders need to hold positions in multidisciplinary health informatics organisations and to encourage the nursing population to become actively involved in these organisations in order to garner support for policy changes that will benefit nursing practice. Traditionally, nurses have not demonstrated a strong voice in the development of healthcare public policy (Hebda & Czar, 2013). It has now become critical for nurses to influence public policy as it is the only way that HIT will address the needs of nurses and their patients. A number of organisations exist that attempt to progress the needs of health informaticians and ensure that relevant standards related to HIT and electronic communication are developed and adhered to. Examples of these organisations are the American Medical Informatics Association, the Alliance for Nursing Informatics, the Health Information Management Systems Society, the European Federation for Medical Informatics in Europe, Health Informatics New Zealand, the Health Informatics Society of Australia, Nursing Informatics Australia and the Australasian College of Health Informatics. It is useful that health informatics is represented by a unified voice when policy and advocacy issues are raised, as well as ensuring human factors concepts are incorporated into the HIT so that care delivery truly is transformed. Nursing should have a strong presence at these organisations, and representatives of these organisations should, in turn, educate more generic health organisations about health informatics, such as the American Nurses Association, the American Organization of Nurse Executives, the American Academy of Nursing, the Australian College of Nursing and the College of Nurses Aotearoa to name a few.

At a state and national level, data metrics, standards of care and the documentation of patient care delivery processes are shaped by public policy (Walker, 2011). Nurse leaders are in a unique position to influence public policy. HIMSS (2011) advocates that nursing informatics leaders need to be active participants in the development of HIT policy and engage in all areas of strategy-setting committees and initiatives. In order to do this nursing informatics leaders need to ensure that they are up to date in HIT initiatives and must be able to articulate the needs of nursing to public policy decision makers (HIMSS, 2011). In order to influence public policy, nurse leaders need to develop skills in strategy, leadership and communication and ensure the engagement of stakeholders within their own organisations and government agencies (Walker, 2011). Nurse leaders influencing public policy in the areas of healthcare reform and the adoption of HIT will give patients a voice and ultimately result in new improved models of patient care (Padavano & Morton, 2011).

One of the pillars of *The TIGER Summit Report Evidence and Informatics Transforming Nursing: 3-Year Action Steps Towards a 10-Year Vision* was aimed at addressing public policy (TIGER Initiative 2007 cited in Hebda & Czar, 2013). The TIGER Initiative calls for nurses to take an active role in shaping the United States HIT in the areas of infrastructure and leadership in order to implement the changes required to improve healthcare (Hebda & Czar, 2013). Although the TIGER Initiative is focused on the United States healthcare environment, this initiative represents a call to action and should be adopted globally so that nurse leaders take the lead and embrace the need to transform healthcare by influencing public policy.

INNOVATIVE VISION

Innovative vision is required in order to transform the nursing care of the twenty-first century into high-quality care that is patient centric, delivered safely and efficiently (Murphy & Alexander, 2011), and nursing leaders have to recognise this need to transform practice and develop creative solutions and new models of care. As HIT has the capability to support and innovate patient care (Murphy & Alexander, 2011), nursing leaders need to embrace HIT, communicate, sustain the vision, and champion and support their staff in order to optimise evolving care delivery models.

As far back as Florence Nightingale, nurses have been using data as evidence to improve nursing care. Data, information, knowledge and wisdom are the cornerstone of the nursing care improvement process. Data alone has little meaning as it is an aggregation of alphanumeric or numeric code (character facts or numbers) captured for possible use at a later date and time thereby becoming information (Hebda & Czar, 2013). From a nursing perspective, data is usually captured at the point of care, for example vital signs, and plotted in order to compare against normal values and to identify trends and patterns in the measurement (Hebda & Czar, 2013). Knowledge applies analysis, synthesis and validation to information from multiple sources in order to form a single concept or idea and provides an order to thoughts and ideas that can be used again (Hebda & Czar, 2013). Wisdom is the application of knowledge and experience to solve and manage problems (Hebda & Czar, 2013). This is the basis of evidenced-based practice, which in turn is the foundation of nursing practice and knowledge.

It is evidence-based practice that assists nurses to improve care delivery and outcomes using the best available research (Hebda & Czar, 2013). It is a process based on the use of the best available research evidence combined with clinical expertise and the references of the patient (University of Minnesota cited in Simpson, 2006). The five steps involved in evidence-based practice include identifying a problem or issue, undertaking a literature search for the problem or issue, evaluating evidence, changing nursing practice and evaluating the effect of the change on nursing practice and patient care (Hebda & Czar, 2013).

Although evidence-based practice is pivotal in the innovation of nursing care, many nurses do not have the skills, knowledge or time to search for the best available evidence (Hanson, 2011). It must be remembered that data collection has only become a clinical responsibility in the last decade, whereas it was previously an administrative activity (Grain, 2005). HIT has the ability to support and progress evidence-based practice by embedding evidence into HIT systems in the form of clinical practice guidelines, clinical decision support tools and evidence-based clinical pathways (Hanson, 2011). As HIT becomes more accepted with a wider spread the power of the data captured within these systems will drive evidence-based practice to a new level. The term 'big data' is becoming commonplace and refers to very large data sets that cannot be processed in the conventional way, necessitating new cost-effective and reliable methods to extract value from all this data (Minelli, Chambers, & Dhiraj, 2013). This new data analytics methodology will process the data quickly and efficiently to drive informed decisions. Various authors (Murphy, Wilson, & Newhouse, 2013; Tupper & Alexander, 2012) believe that data analytics will be the next evolution in healthcare as it generates opportunities for business intelligence and provides and supports informed decision making at a facility, state and national level. Nurse leaders need to drive this process and push for data standards in order to be able to benchmark against like facilities and improve patient-centred care.

CONCLUSION

Outside of the health environment, the community is learning to use the numerous types of technology as part of their daily lives, whereas health has lagged behind in the use of information technology. There is a need for strong health informatics leadership in the areas of education, scope of practice, policy participation and innovative vision in order to progress a vision of what healthcare should deliver to patients in the twenty-first century. It is vital that nursing informatics leaders play a significant role in transforming patient care into new models of clinical practice with the assistance of HIT. The role of a CNIO can assist nursing executives to leverage HIT in order to guide improvements in clinical practice. Achieving a level of competency in HIT is a crucial foundational tool for the leadership practice of nursing managers and leaders, and postgraduate programs should be available for nurses who wish to specialise in this area. Nurse leaders will need to expand their scope of practice to include all aspects of HIT so that successful implementation of these systems that follow the clinical workflow can be realised. They also need to hold positions in multidisciplinary health informatics organisations so they can influence public policy in the areas of healthcare reform and the adoption of HIT. Lastly, nurse leaders need to acknowledge the strong link between HIT and its ability to innovate and transform clinical practice, and embrace the challenges of data analytics so that nurses provide evidence-based practice in all circumstances. The most direct contribution that HIT can make to improving healthcare is to provide clinicians with better information about the patient at the point of care, and the most significant contribution that nursing can make is to use HIT effectively in order to optimise evolving care delivery models and deliver safe and evidence-based care to every patient.

REFLECTIVE EXERCISE

1. What strategies could nurse executives deploy to increase support for HIT amongst the clinical nurse workforce?

2. What strategies could healthcare management deploy to encourage the clinical nurse workforce to achieve HIT competency assessment, credentialling of health informatics skills or enrolment in postgraduate health informatics programs?

3. What strategies could a nurse leader deploy to ensure he/she influences policy in relation to HIT implementation?

4. How would you evaluate whether a nurse leader has embraced the value of HIT within the healthcare delivery process?

5. How would a nurse leader evaluate whether the nursing workforce is supporting innovation?

6. What are the likely challenges of embedding data analytics into nursing practice?

Recommended Readings

Makar, E. V. (2012). The alliance for nursing informatics emerging leaders program: Reflections from the 2010–2012 emerging leader in nursing informatics. *CIN: Computers, Informatics, Nursing, 29*(1), 66–67.

Padavano, C., & Morton, A. (2011). The evolving national informatics landscape. In M. J. Ball, J. V. Douglas, P. Hinton Walker, D. DuLong, B. Gugerty, K. J. Hannah, et al. (Eds.), *Nursing informatics: Where caring and technology meet* (4th ed., pp. 193–205). London: Springer-Verlag.

Skiba, D. J., DuLong, D., & Newbold, S. K. (2010). TIGER collaborative and diffusion. In M. J. Ball, J. V. Douglas, P. Hinton Walker, D. DuLong, B. Gugerty, K. J. Hannah, et al. (Eds.), *Nursing informatics: Where caring and technology meet* (4th ed., pp. 35–50). London: Springer-Verlag.

Swindle, C. G., & Bradley, V. M. (2010). The newest O in the C-suite: CNIO. *Nurse Leader, 8*(3), 28–30.

TIGER Initiative Advisory Council (2009). *Collaborating to integrate evidence and informatics into nursing practice and education: An executive summary.* Technology Informatics Guiding Education Reform. Retrieved from <http://www.tigersummit.com/Home_Page.php>.

Tupper, S. R., & Alexander, D. (2012). Leading from the future: The nursing informatics executive. *CIN: Computers, Informatics, Nursing, 30*(3), 123–125.

References

Amarasingham, R., Plantinga, L., Diener-West, M., Gaskin, D. J., & Powe, N. R. (2009). Clinical information technologies and inpatient outcomes: A multiple hospital study. *Archives of Internal Medicine, 169*(2), 108–114.

Bates, D. W. (2002). The quality case for information technology in healthcare. *BMC Medical Informatics and Decision Making, 2*(7), 1–9.

Bichel-Findlay, J., & Doran, C. (2014). Nursing and informatics: A transformational synergy. In J. Daly, S. Speedy, & D. Jackson (Eds.), *Contexts of nursing* (4th ed., pp. 287–304). Chatswood, NSW: Churchill Livingstone.

Bowens, F. M., Frye, P. A., & Jones, W. A. (2010). Health information technology: Integration of clinical workflow into meaningful use of electronic health records. *Perspectives in Health Information Management, 7*(Fall), 1d.

Brennan, T. A., Leape, L. L., Laird, N. M., Herbert, L., Localio, A. R., Lawthers, A. G., et al. (1991). Incidence of adverse events and negligence in hospitalized patients. Results of the Harvard Medical Practice Study I. *New England Journal of Medicine, 324*(6), 370–376.

Carayon, P., Karsh, B.-T., & Cartmill, R. S. (2010). *Incorporating health information technology into workflow redesign—summary report.* Rockville, MD: Agency for Healthcare Research and Quality.

Committee on Quality of Health Care in America (2001). *Crossing the quality chasm: A new health system for the 21st century.* Washington, DC: National Academy Press.

Cusack, C. M. (2008). Electronic health records and electronic prescribing: Promise and pitfalls. *Obstetrics & Gynecology Clinics of North America, 35*(1), 63–79.

Department of Health (2012). Driving the data: The role of the chief clinical information officer. *Chief Nursing Officer Bulletin.* Retrieved from <http://webarchive.nationalarchives.gov.uk/20130402150017/http:/cno.dh.gov.uk/2012/09/10/driving-the-data-the-role-of-the-chief-clinical-information-officer/>.

DuLong, D. B., & Ball, M. J. (2010). TIGER: Technology Informatics Guiding Educational Reform—a nursing imperative. In C. A. Weaver, C. W. Delaney, P. Weber, & R. L. Carr (Eds.), *Nursing informatics for the 21st century: An international look at practice, education and EHR trends* (2nd ed., pp. 17–24). Chicago, IL: Health Information and Management Systems Society (HIMSS).

Grain, H. (2005). Information systems in the new world: An emerging national approach. *Australian Health Review, 29*(3), 292–296.

Graves, J. R., & Corcoran, S. (1989). The study of nursing informatics. *Journal of Nursing Scholarship, 21*(4), 227–231.

Greiner, A. C., & Knebel, E. (Eds.), (2003). *Health professions education: A bridge to quality.* Washington, DC: National Academies Press.

Gugerty, B., & Sensmeier, J. (2010). Informatics competencies for nurses across roles and international boundaries. In C. A. Weaver, C. W. Delaney, P. Weber, & R. L. Carr (Eds.), *Nursing informatics for the 21st century: An international look at practice, education and EHR trends* (2nd ed., pp. 129–143). Chicago, IL: Health Information and Management Systems Society (HIMSS).

Hammel-Jones, D. (2012). Nursing informatics: Improving workflow and meaningful use. In D. McGonigle & K. G. Mastrian (Eds.), *Nursing informatics and the foundation of knowledge* (2nd ed., pp. 264–279). Burlington, MA: Jones and Bartlett Learning.

Hanson, D. (2011). Evidence-based clinical decision support. In M. J. Ball, J. V. Douglas, P. Hinton, D. Walker, B. DuLong, B. Gugerty, et al. (Eds.), *Nursing informatics: Where caring and technology meet* (4th ed., pp. 243–258). London: Springer-Verlag.

Health Informatics Society of Australia (HISA) (2013). *Providing leadership in e-health.* Retrieved from <http://www.hisa.org.au/?page=CHIA>.

Health Information and Management Systems Society (HIMSS) (2011). *HIMSS position statement on transforming nursing practice through technology and informatics.* Retrieved from <http://www.himss.org/News/NewsDetail.aspx?ItemNumber=3973>.

HealthWorkforce Australia (2013). *Health informaticians speciality workforce studies.* Retrieved from <http://www.hwa.gov.au/work-programs/information-analysis-and-planning/health-workforce-planning/health-informaticians-spec>.

Hebda, T., & Czar, P. (2013). *Handbook of informatics for nurses and healthcare professionals* (5th ed., pp. 367–378). Boston, MA: Pearson.

Hillestad, R., Bigelow, J., & Bower, A. (2005). Can electronic medical record systems transform health care? Potential health benefits, savings, and costs. *Health Affairs, 24*(5), 1103–1117.

Holroyd-Leduc, J. M., Lorenzetti, D., Straus, S. E., Sykes, L., & Quan, H. (2011). The impact of the electronic medical record on structure, process, and outcomes within primary care: A systematic review of the evidence. *Journal of the American Medical Informatics Association, 18*(6), 732–737.

Hunt, E. C., Sproat, S. B., & Kitzmiller, R. R. (2004). *The nursing informatics implementation guide.* New York City, NY: Springer-Verlag.

Institute of Medicine (IOM) (2011). *The future of nursing: Leading change, advancing health.* Washington, DC: National Academies Press.

Institute of Medicine (IOM) (2012). *Health IT and patient safety: Building safer systems for better care.* Washington, DC: National Academies Press.

International Medical Informatics Association—Nursing Informatics Special Interest Group (IMIA-NI SIG) (2013). *Welcome to IMIA NI.* Retrieved from <http://imia-medinfo.org/ni/>.

Jha, A. K., & Classen, D. C. (2011). Getting moving on patient safety—harnessing electronic data for safer care. *New England Journal of Medicine, 365*(19), 1756–1758.

Kohn, L. T., Corrigan, J. M., & Donaldson, M. S. (Eds.), (1999). *To err is human: Building a safer health system.* Washington, DC: National Academy Press.

Leape, L. L., Brennan, T. A., Laird, N. M., Lawthers, A. G., Localio, A. R., Barnes, B. A., et al. (1991). The nature of adverse events in hospitalized patients. Results of the Harvard Medical Practice Study II. *New England Journal of Medicine, 324*(6), 377–384.

Lorenzi, N. M., Kouroubali, A., Detmer, D. E., & Bloomrosen, M. (2009). How to successfully select and implement electronic health records (EHR) in small ambulatory practice settings. *BMC Medical Informatics and Decision Making, 9*(15). Retrieved from <http://www.biomedcentral.com/1472-6947/9/15>.

Minelli, M., Chambers, M., & Dhiraj, A. (2013). *Big data big analytics: Emerging business intelligence and analytic trends for today's businesses.* Hoboken, NJ: John Wiley & Sons.

Murphy, J. (2010a). Nursing informatics: The intersection of nursing, computer, and information sciences. *Nursing Economics, 28*(3), 204–207.

Murphy, J. (2010b). The nursing informatics workforce: Who are they and what do they do? *Nursing Economics, 29*(3), 150–152.

Murphy, J., & Alexander, D. (2011). Leadership collaborative. In M. J. Ball, J. V. Douglas, P. Hinton, D. Walker, B. DuLong, B. Gugerty, et al. (Eds.), *Nursing informatics: Where caring and technology meet* (4th ed., pp. 133–154). London: Springer-Verlag.

Murphy, L. S., Wilson, M. L., & Newhouse, R. P. (2013). Data analytics: Making the most of input with strategic output. *Journal of Nursing Administration, 43*(7/8), 367–370.

Nagle, L. M. (2012). Information and knowledge needs of nurses in the 21st century. In D. McGonigle & K. G. Mastrian (Eds.), *Nursing informatics and the foundation of knowledge* (2nd ed., pp. 147–160). Burlington, MA: Jones and Bartlett Learning.

Nahm, E. S., & Wilson, M. L. (2011). Nursing curriculum reform and healthcare information technology. In V. K. Saba & K. A. McCormick (Eds.), *Essentials of nursing informatics* (5th ed., pp. 603–631). New York City, NY: McGraw-Hill.

Nickitas, D. M., & Kerfoot, K. (2010). Nursing informatics: Why nurse leaders need to stay informed. *Nursing Economics, 28*(3), 141–142.

Ortiz, E., & Clancy, C. M. (2003). Use of information technology to improve the quality of health care in the United States. *Health Services Research, 38*(2), xi–xxii.

Padavano, C., & Morton, A. (2011). The evolving national informatics landscape. In M. J. Ball, J. V. Douglas, P. Hinton Walker, D. DuLong, B. Gugerty, K. J. Hannah, et al. (Eds.), *Nursing informatics: Where caring and technology meet* (4th ed., pp. 193–205). London: Springer-Verlag.

RAND Health (2005). *Health information technology: Can HIT lower costs and improve quality?* Santa Monica, California: RAND Research Briefs, RAND Corporation.

Runciman, W. B., Coiera, E. W., Day, R. O., Hannaford, N. A., Hibbert, P. D., Hunt, T. D., et al. (2012). Towards the delivery of appropriate health care in Australia. *Medical Journal of Australia, 197*(2), 78–81.

Sensmeier, J. E. (2010). Nursing informatics: Designing the healthcare of the future. *Nursing Management, 41*(12), 52–53.

Sensmeier, J. (2011). Transforming nursing practice through technology and informatics. *Nursing Management, 42*(11), 20–23.

Simpson, R. L. (2006). Evidence-based practice: How nursing administration makes IT happen. *Nursing Administration Quarterly, 30*(3), 291–294.

Simpson, R. L. (2011). Challenging leadership status quo. In M. J. Ball, J. V. Douglas, P. Hinton Walker, D. DuLong, B. Gugerty, K. J. Hannah, et al. (Eds.), *Nursing informatics: Where caring and technology meet* (4th ed., pp. 155–165). London: Springer-Verlag.

Skiba, D. J., DuLong, D., & Newbold, S. K. (2010). TIGER collaborative and diffusion. In M. J. Ball, J. V. Douglas, P. Hinton Walker, D. DuLong, B. Gugerty, K. J. Hannah, et al. (Eds.), *Nursing informatics: Where technology and caring meet* (4th ed., pp. 35–50). London: Springer-Verlag.

Swindle, C. G., & Bradley, V. M. (2010). The newest O in the C-suite: CNIO. *Nurse Leader, 8*(3), 28–30.

Technology Informatics Guiding Education Reform (TIGER) (2013). *TIGER initiative working on phase III*. Retrieved from <http://www.tigersummit.com/>.

TIGER Initiative Advisory Council (2009). *Collaborating to integrate evidence and informatics into nursing practice and education: An executive summary*. Technology Informatics Guiding Education Reform. Retrieved from <http://www.tigersummit.com/Home_Page.php>.

Tupper, S. R., & Alexander, D. (2012). Leading from the future: The nursing informatics executive. *CIN: Computers, Informatics, Nursing, 30*(3), 123–125.

Walker, A. M. (2011). Shaping nursing informatics through the public policy process. In V. K. Saba & K. A. McCormick (Eds.), *Essentials of nursing informatics* (5th ed., pp. 279–287). New York City, NY: McGraw-Hill.

Wilson, R. M., Runciman, W. B., & Gibberd, R. W. (1995). The quality in Australian health care study. *Medical Journal of Australia, 163*(9), 458–471.

Woodill, G. (2012). Too big to know … too much to train. *Training Industry Quarterly, Summer*, 11.

World Health Organization (2013). *E-health*. Retrieved from <http://www.who.int/trade/glossary/story021/en/>.

CHAPTER NINE

Leading contemporary approaches to nursing practice

Gerard Fealy, Martin McNamara & Mary Casey

LEARNING OBJECTIVES

At the completion of this chapter, the reader will be able to:

▲ appreciate the range of levels of contemporary practice;
▲ recognise the value of effective clinical leadership in promoting quality care at micro, meso and macro levels of influence;
▲ discuss the enablers and barriers to effective clinical leadership development;
▲ discuss the methods and interventions for developing leaders for their individual and service-level effectiveness within contemporary practice.

KEY WORDS

Practice, clinical leadership, practice roles, interventions, enablers and barriers

INTRODUCTION

Contemporary nursing practice occurs in a number of contexts such as direct nurse–patient interactions, in the planning and organisation of nursing service and in wider dimensions of 'practice', such as education, research and professional policy and regulation. Within the context of healthcare, leading contemporary nursing practice necessarily involves engagement at micro, meso and macro levels of healthcare activity. At the micro level of the practicum, contemporary practice is ideally conducted on the basis of the individual practitioner's repertoire of knowledge and skills, agreed professional standards, best evidence and the particular needs of the individual patient or community in which the practitioner is working. It is conducted through a variety of professional nursing and midwifery roles and grades, including expanded roles of clinical special-ists and advanced practitioners. Beyond the individual professional–client interface, contempo-rary practice occurs at the organisation–community interface and is expressed in the way that nursing service is configured and integrated with other services; this meso level of practice takes place in contexts like tertiary care hospitals and primary care teams. Contemporary practice also takes place in the conduct of preparatory training and continuing professional development, the conduct of clinical and social research and the practice of policy development in health and professional practice and in activities associated with professional regulation. While not directly related to the care and treatment of patients, activities at this macro level of practice are none-theless influential in the content and quality of care proffered by nurses. For the purpose of this chapter, we consider that leading contemporary practice necessarily involves leading at micro, meso and macro levels of activity. We will focus on the role of clinical leadership development as a means of achieving leadership in practice. We define 'leadership' as a social process in which an individual influences others to attain a particular goal or set of goals. 'Clinical leadership' is a particular variant of leadership that is concerned with influencing clinicians to achieve the goal of improving the effectiveness of care.

LEADING CONTEMPORARY PRACTICE

Clinical leadership in contemporary nursing practice involves not only taking respon-sibility for the quality and outcomes of direct patient care but also monitoring the impact on patient care and professional practice of broader contextual influences on the delivery of nursing services (Carryer, Gardner, Dunn, & Gardner, 2007; Davidson, Elliot, & Daly, 2006; Hix, McKeon, & Walters, 2009). Hence, clinical leadership is con-cerned with both the minutiae of the everyday planning and delivery of direct patient care and the wider goals of service planning and organisational development (Casey, 2006). In modern health systems, these two aspects of leadership require a judicious balance between power sharing and control and between interpersonal trust and formalised procedures (Alexander, Comfort, Weiner, & Bogue, 2001). In nursing, clini-cal leadership is thus strongly related to both interpersonal and interdisciplinary processes and its development must be related to the development of both individual leader competences and explicit service improvements.

That aspect of clinical leadership concerned with everyday planning and care delivery incorporates individual intrapersonal and interpersonal human capacities; these capacities are necessary for the effective conduct of intra- and interdisciplinary working that are essential for the provision of quality care. The relationship between leadership quality and care quality has been shown to be critical and the absence of effective clinical leadership can have serious consequences for the quality of care, the most striking example being the serious failings in care that resulted from ineffective or absent leadership at the Mid-Staffordshire Hospital in the UK (Francis, 2013).

As providers of front-line clinical care, nurses are ideally placed to offer clinical leadership and leadership in nursing involves individual nurses taking responsibility for direct patient care and for monitoring service quality more generally (Carryer et al., 2007). Leadership is a process that involves identifying a goal, motivating others to act in particular ways and supporting and motivating others to achieve mutually negotiated goals (Davidson et al., 2006). The ways in which the clinical leader role is expressed determine clinical leadership effectiveness in monitoring and improving patient care (Gopee & Galloway, 2013). The leader's role is expressed through an assemblage of both intrapersonal and interpersonal capacities, acting across several, often interrelated, layers of influence, including other individuals, the team, the organisation and the wider health system, in areas such as education, management of service, research, policy and regulation.

Multidisciplinary working

We were struck by ... the great difficulty that nurses and midwives seem to experience in clearly articulating their discipline-specific or differentiated contribution to care in the multidisciplinary context (McNamara & Fealy, 2010).

Clinical leadership is especially relevant in contexts involving multidisciplinary teams working closely together, such as in modern tertiary hospitals or primary care teams, and clinical leader influence is a function of the extent to which the leader can articulate the particular and distinct disciplinary contribution to care (McNamara et al., 2011; McNamara & Fealy, 2010). Representing the nursing contribution to care is a function of nurses' ability to engage in effective teamwork, change management and conflict resolution, which is, in turn, linked to the capacity of nurses to clearly articulate and differentiate their respective roles in care (McNamara et al., 2011).

McNamara et al. (2011, p. 3509) write that 'an essential condition for clinical leadership in nursing is the ability to represent the profession at both an intra- and interprofessional level in the organisation ... [that is] the ability to articulate credibly and convincingly nurses' contribution to patient outcomes'. This implies that nursing has a clear disciplinary discourse with which to speak about the focus and content of its everyday work and to differentiate it from the work of other disciplines. Where the distinct nursing contribution is not visible in the multidisciplinary context, either because it is not clearly articulated by nurses or because it is ignored or undervalued by others, then a prerequisite for clinical leadership is absent. The capacity to represent nursing is therefore a foundational prerequisite for clinical leadership, since it underpins other key clinical leader and leadership roles and functions, notably effective teamwork, challenging, changing and innovating and conflict resolution (McNamara et al., 2011). Representing the nursing contribution can only come from nurses' professional formation and, more generally, from the way that nurses conceptualise their practice and speak about it to each other and to other disciplines. This is, in turn, influenced by nurses' professional training and formation as professionals and by both disciplinary and organisational cultures and practices that give rise to particular forms of interdisciplinary working.

Leading contemporary approaches to practice require that nurses bring their specialised and differentiated expert contribution to the table, in whatever professional context they are operating. In practice, clearly and credibly articulating the discipline-specific or differentiated contribution to care in the practicum involves both words and actions on the part of nurses and, in this same regard, it is their clinical expertise that delimits the scope of their clinical practice and, at the same time, confers on them their disciplinary identity for multidisciplinary working (McNamara & Fealy, 2010). Developing this capacity for true multidisciplinary working, whereby nurses contribute their unique expertise to care planning and/or policy formulation, should form a central part in any training initiative for clinical leadership development.

LEADING PRACTICE: IDENTIFYING PRACTITIONERS' LEADERSHIP NEED

While leadership is something that resides with individuals, according to Day (2001) it can also be considered as a shared and distributed property residing in organisations, and hence the development of individual leaders may be achieved through approaches that enable the acquisition of both the social resources that underpin interpersonal competences and the human resources that are realised as intrapersonal competences. Both sets of competences are expressed through key leader roles and functions and it is through these roles and functions that leaders can lead contemporary practice and also have an impact on the organisation. Day's (2001) model of leadership development emphasises how organisational systems, structures and culture facilitate or constrain the ability of leaders to impact positively on the quality of nursing services by mediating relationships between human and social resources, interpersonal and intrapersonal competences, and leader roles and functions.

Roberts and Coghlan (2011) suggest that developing skills in individual leaders is only one aspect of effective leadership development; there should also be a concomitant emphasis on the development of the organisation's social capital. It is the social capital within an organisation's networks that enables collective action. Storey and Holti (2013) have proposed a new leadership model for the English National Health Service (NHS) that highlights the importance of power dynamics and a clear sense of purpose and contribution; motivation of teams and individuals to work effectively, and improving system performance. Each of these categories embodies both intrapersonal and interpersonal competency development. The first category embraces behaviours and skills that focus on the needs and experiences of the users of health services, continually reinforcing an inspiring vision of the mission and social contribution of the healthcare organisation or a unit within the organisation. The second category refers to the wider ability to work in collaboration with other organisations and the third category focuses on service improvement based on compelling evidence for transformational change. On closer analysis, this framework also incorporates social and human capital development through these distinct aspects, although this is more implicit than explicit.

In our work on aspects of clinical leadership development in Ireland (Fealy et al., 2010; Fealy et al., 2012) we have taken as our starting point the premise that clinical leadership is not the preserve of any one disciplinary or occupational group in healthcare and nor is it the exclusive domain of those in formal leadership or management positions. We found that clinical leadership development need exists at the micro, meso and macro levels of contemporary practice. In our national study to investigate the clinical leadership development needs of nurses and midwives in Ireland, we categorised need as relating to five key aspects of clinical leadership development, as follows: 'managing the clinical area', 'managing patient care', 'developing the individual', 'developing the profession' and '[developing] skills for leadership' (Casey, McNamara, Fealy, & Geraghty, 2011).

A noteworthy finding from our analysis of clinical leadership development need was the fact that need was greatest with reference to those aspects of the nurse's role not associated with direct clinical care, but with the wider organisation and with policy development (Fealy et al., 2010; Casey et al., 2011). Specifically, clinical leadership development need was perceived as greatest in relation to those aspects of the professional role involving interdisciplinary interactions, organisational and interdisciplinary working and influencing decision making and health policy more generally. Conversely, clinical leadership development need was lowest in relation to those aspects of the professional role associated with the management of direct care, including the micro-system of care within which the practitioner operated and for which the practitioner was directly responsible. This micro-system of activity included such critical tasks as: protecting patients' dignity and confidentiality; involving patients in their own care; contributing to the development of clinical practice guidelines; and ensuring that the outcomes of care and other interventions are documented. We also found that the more senior grades among our national sample of nurses and midwives reported less clinical leadership development need in relation to interdisciplinary and organisational working and representing the interests of the profession at policy-making levels. Managers who are somewhat removed from the practitioner–patient interface perceived their influence on organisational and wider policy as being greater than their bedside practitioner counterparts.

Based on these findings, we concluded that clinical nurses operating at the micro level are less assured in their ability to influence, as the focus of their work shifts from the micro-system of the bedside towards the meso- and macro-systems, which demands more interdisciplinary, organisational and managerial engagement. Hence, while nurses can exert influence and thereby demonstrate clinical leadership through practice excellence (Davidson et al., 2006), their scope of clinical leadership is, perhaps unsurprisingly, influenced by their hierarchical position and relative status within the organisation (Casey et al., 2011). Therefore, a critical factor in leading contemporary practice is enabling nurses, who work at the micro-system, to develop clinical leadership competences for working in situations and contexts beyond the bedside, notably for those aspects of the professional role associated with interdisciplinary working and with the development of the organisation and the wider discipline. These competences naturally involve skills related to the interpersonal dimension of clinical leadership development and also contextually relate to the practitioner's organisational work environment within which these competences are to be demonstrated.

The conditions in the practice setting that can influence clinical leadership development constitute either enablers or barriers to effective clinical leadership for contemporary practice. The conditions that act as barriers include: the level of organisational support for nurses' clinical decision making; skill mix; lack of negotiated multidisciplinary care planning; nurses' perceived level of influence in decision making; fragmentation of clinical care; professional tensions among members of the interdisciplinary team and ineffective workplace communication (Fealy et al., 2011). Other barriers include managers' lack of authority at the level of the organisation and a lack of representation of nursing or midwifery interests at the organisational level. In our analysis of clinical leadership development needs of nurses and midwives we observed that, similar to self-reported clinical leadership development need, self-reported barriers to clinical leadership development were greater with reference to those aspects of nurses' and midwives' work that were associated with organisational dimensions of the professional role and with interdisciplinary working. We also found that certain grades differed in their self-perceived barriers to their clinical leadership development, with specialist and advanced practitioner grades and senior manager grades experiencing fewer barriers to their clinical leadership development than their more junior counterparts.

Differences in both self-reported clinical leadership development need and perceived barriers to clinical leadership development would appear to be related to the relative influence that nurses and midwives consider they have in decision making at the micro, meso and macro levels. In contemporary practice, when nurses and midwives are able to directly influence care through such activities as patient advocacy and attending to issues of safety, dignity and privacy, they have more influence, albeit within a narrow scope of practice activity. This level of influence has particular relevance for leading practice at the micro level, since patient advocacy and promoting quality of care are key clinical leadership competences. Their influence is also through the coordination and orchestration of the activities of others, including other health-care professionals in the care setting. Paradoxically, engaging in these kinds of 'compensatory activities' constrains nurses and midwives in their ability to engage in the work for which they are directly responsible and this, in turn, influences their ability to demonstrate and articulate the nursing or midwifery contribution to care (McNamara et al., 2011). Accordingly, leading practice at the micro level is best achieved when the practitioner is engaged in direct clinical care within an environment that supports both intra- and interpersonal development.

DEVELOPING THE LEADERS TO LEAD CONTEMPORARY PRACTICE: INTERVENTIONS AND THEIR EFFECTIVENESS

Leading contemporary practice requires explicit efforts to develop the leaders, particularly those working at the micro level of the clinician–client interface, but also those operating at all levels of the organisation and the wider health system. The outcomes of clinical leadership development can be represented in the well-defined and time-bound actions of practitioners, the actions taken by practitioners in particular challenging situations or in the more fundamental changes in practitioners' patterns of behaviour, in which actions and efforts are redirected to achieve particular practice goals (Grove et al., 2007). These outcomes represent, respectively, the episodic, developmental and transformative outcomes of leadership development (Grove, Barry, & Haas, 2007).

Leadership development training has been shown to be the most significant factor contributing to increased leadership practices in nursing (Cummings et al., 2008). Leadership and clinical leadership development initiatives can impact on practitioners' leadership effectiveness at the personal, organisational, wider community and disciplinary levels of leader roles (Woltring, Constantine, & Schwarte, 2003) and can promote significant improvements in leadership practices of both established and aspirant leaders (Tourangeau, 2003). The findings from studies reporting the effectiveness of leadership development initiatives show evidence of changes in leadership behaviours following interventions and a number of researchers have reported statistically significant self-reported and other-reported increases in leadership practices following educational interventions for clinical leadership development in nursing (Duygulu & Kublay, 2011; Krugman & Smith, 2003).

Several clinical leadership development strategies can be deployed to develop particular leader competences for particular nursing roles and situations (Fealy et al., 2012). Clinical leadership development interventions can include short-term attendance taught courses or more sustained experiential interventions that are provided over a period of weeks or months. The latter type is held to be more effective, particularly when the intervention is focused on the development of an explicit clinical leadership skill or a constellation of clinical leadership competences. Targeted and bespoke interventions like mentoring are especially effective for developing clinical leadership in context (Fealy et al., 2012). Mentoring is defined as a committed, long-term relationship in which a senior person supports the personal and professional development of a junior person, or protégé, and is used as an intervention in leadership development. Similarly, coaching places the individual in real situations in which they experience at first hand the unique problems that occur in particular clinical settings (Byrne, 2007). Coaching is focused on developing an individual's personal and professional goals and self-awareness as well as skills like self-management and interpersonal communication (Byrne, 2007) and is reported to be effective in improving individual and organisational effectiveness through helping nurses to identify and correct behaviours that hamper their performance (Reid Ponte, Gross, Galante, & Glazer, 2006).

In addition to mentoring and coaching, other experiential interventions include 360-degree feedback, involving direct peer and subordinate ratings and self-evaluation, and action learning (Day, 2001). An action learning approach to leadership development is a means of marrying the development of the individual as a leader along with developing the organisation's social capital. It is a method of working in small groups to tackle organisational issues or problems, in order to learn from the efforts of engaging in and effecting organisational change (Pedler, 2008). In this way action learning is a competence-based intervention for leader development, which focuses on particular individually relevant leadership and clinical leadership skills and practice problems in the real world and explores actionable solutions to the problems. As a leadership development mechanism, it is used increasingly as a primary method for building leadership skills and behaviours and has been shown to be effective in the development of specific critical leader competences, such as communication, team building and decisiveness (Leonard & Lang, 2010). The intervention can also build analytical, creativity and change management skills, and skills for influencing, engaging, collaborating and creating open communication (Leonard & Lang, 2010). Both action learning and coaching are reported to be more effective than the more traditional attendance programs, in developing individual-level leadership outcomes in areas like insight, skill development and leading in real-world practice (Leonard & Lang, 2010). Clinical leadership development interventions, such as mentoring, are likely to have a greater impact if they are delivered within a supportive organisational culture and targeted on transformational change (Stol, Foster-Turner, & Glen, 2010).

In our own work to evaluate interventions in a national clinical leadership development initiative in Ireland, we studied the impact of bespoke interventions designed to develop self-diagnosed, individual clinical leadership competences. We evaluated the mentoring, coaching and action learning with reference to individual and service outcomes, as well as workshops that addressed specific clinical leadership competences like communication, teamwork and patient advocacy (Fealy et al., 2013; Patton et al., 2013). Over the course of the six-month clinical leadership development program, participants in a clinical leadership development initiative provided us with detailed accounts of how they had developed and displayed particular clinical leadership competences.

Corroborated by mentors and coaches and their line managers, nurses and midwives were asked to provide structured self-reports of their own behaviours and dispositions, which indicated the attainment of particular clinical leadership competences like self-awareness, communication, and team working. The accounts referred to new competences and/or improved capabilities for developing their own practice and the wider service in which they worked and included particular instances of clinical leadership development through their behaviours and dispositions. Several participants in the program offered examples of how they had changed their own practices or altered their approach to certain situations, one remarking on the development of improved communication skills: '[I am] more prone to not dismissing people or I am more open or I will be more accepting of very different viewpoints.'

We found that coaching and action learning sets provided nurses and midwives with opportunities to share experiences of everyday practice problems and explore solutions to them through group processes (Fealy et al., 2012). With its focus on sharing ideas and concerns about practice and the action orientation of group discussions, action learning was particularly beneficial in helping practitioners to find solutions to real everyday problems. Many participants experienced the mentoring intervention as positive and supportive and it enabled individuals to clarify their clinical leadership development needs with their mentor and examine and prioritise their needs in the context of their own professional role.

Experiential interventions are not without challenges, which can include misinterpretations of roles and responsibilities in the coach–coachee or mentor–mentee relationship, an imbalance between challenge and support in mentoring, and the emergence of personal and/or emotional issues in the process of coaching (Fealy et al., 2013). Accordingly, the precise role of the coach or mentor needs to be made explicit to the coachee or mentee, role boundaries and temporal limits in the mentoring or coaching process need to be established and agreed at the outset, and coaches and mentors need to self-monitor their practice when acting in the role.

The elements of clinical leadership are underpinned by 'making a difference to patients', as indicated by quality improvement service initiatives (Stoddart, Bugge, Shepherd, & Farquharson, 2014). Specific service improvements can result from clinical leadership development initiatives; for example Large, MacLeod, Cunningham, and Kitson (2005) reported improvements in infection control, noise levels and service–user privacy, and Lunn, MacCurtain, and McMahon (2008) reported enhanced clinical leadership skills that resulted in novel methods of care delivery. In addition to individual leadership development needs, the various clinical leadership development interventions that we evaluated were also closely associated with service development, whereby individuals were required to develop service initiatives and/or improvements in the culture of their working environment. In this way the clinical leadership development initiatives focused on both the acquisition of the social resources that underpin interpersonal competences and the human resources that are realised as intrapersonal competences. Service initiatives that resulted from the mentoring, coaching and action learning interventions included improvements in precise clinical interventions and practices to more general service developments aimed at improving safety, service quality or the patient experience at the service–user interface. Several examples of service improvements were proffered, including improved chronic disease care and improved infection prevention practices, demonstrating the importance of linking clinical leadership development initiatives to service and practice development.

CONCLUSION

Nurses' and midwives' clinical leadership development needs reside in a range of dimensions of clinical leadership, from the intrapersonal to the departmental and the interdisciplinary to the wider organisational dimension. Our study of nurses' and midwives' clinical leadership development needs suggests that needs are related to their spheres of influence at two levels: their immediate professional practice and the organisations in which they work. At the micro level of their professional role where they manage direct care, nurses and midwives appear more self-confident in their ability to influence care. However, as they move further away from the clinician–client interface to the meso (departmental) and the macro (organisational and wider policy) levels their influence becomes somewhat more diffuse and dissipated. These spheres of influence give rise to particular areas of development need and to particular barriers to clinical leadership development, which are associated with the organisational and interprofessional domains of clinical leadership. Leading contemporary practice is achieved by paying attention to the various levels of leader influence when developing leaders' competences.

REFLECTIVE EXERCISE

1. What is clinical leadership?
2. a. List three aspects of your professional role that are distinct to nursing (or midwifery). (Be precise and avoid vague and non-specific phrases like 'provide holistic care', 'provide patient-centred care' or 'patient communication'.)
   b. Write down a key skill that is required for each of the three aspects that you list.
3. Consider your own practice situation and reflect on the following questions:

   Am I leading practice through the roles that I perform?

   In what way am I leading practice?

   In interdisciplinary contexts (e.g. case conference), what distinctive contribution do I make to the discussion?

   Am I advocating for patients at a point removed from direct patient care?

   Do I engage in wider debates about the role of nursing and the development of nursing policy?
4. Identify three attributes or characteristics of your clinical leadership role and then identify the behaviours that could be used as indicators of this attribute or characteristic. Consider if each characteristic could be used as an indicator of competence in clinical leadership.

Recommended Readings

Casey, M., McNamara, M., Fealy, G. M., & Geraghty, R. (2011). Nurses' and midwives' clinical leadership development needs: A mixed methods study. *Journal of Advanced Nursing, 67*(7), 1502–1513.

Cummings, G., Lee, H., MacGregor, T., Davey, M., Wong, C., Paul, L., et al. (2008). Factors contributing to nursing leadership: A systematic review. *Journal of Health Services Research & Policy, 13*(4), 240–248.

Fealy, G. M., McNamara, M., Casey, M., Geraghty, R., Butler, M., Halligan, P., et al. (2011). Barriers to clinical leadership development: Findings from a national survey. *Journal of Clinical Nursing, 20*(13–14), 2023–2032.

Fealy, G. M., McNamara, M. S., Casey, M., O'Connor, T., Patton, D., Doyle, L., et al. (2013). Service impact of a national clinical leadership development programme: Findings from a qualitative study. *Journal of Nursing Management*, doi:10.1111/jonm.12133.

Hix, C., McKeon, L., & Walters, S. (2009). Clinical nurse leader impact on microsystems outcomes. *Journal of Nursing Administration, 39*, 71–76.

McNamara, M., Fealy, G. M., Casey, M., Geraghty, R., Butler, M., Halligan, P., et al. (2011). Boundary matters: Clinical leadership and the distinctive disciplinary contribution of nursing to multidisciplinary care. *Journal of Clinical Nursing, 20*(23–24), 3502–3512.

Storey, J., & Holti, R. (2013). *Towards a new model for leadership in the NHS*. London: NHS Leadership Academy.

References

Alexander, J. A., Comfort, M. E., Weiner, B. J., & Bogue, R. (2001). Leadership in collaborative community health partnerships. *Nonprofit Management and Leadership, 12*, 159–175.

Byrne, G. (2007). Unlocking potential: Coaching as a means to enhance leadership and role performance in nursing. *Journal of Clinical Nursing, 16*(11), 1987–1988.

Carryer, J., Gardner, G., Dunn, S., & Gardner, A. (2007). The core role of the nurse practitioner: Practice, professionalism and clinical leadership. *Journal of Clinical Nursing, 16*, 1818–1825.

Casey, M. (2006). *Developing a framework for partnership between organizations that provide nursing and midwifery education*. Unpublished PhD Thesis, School of Business, University of Dublin, Trinity College, Dublin.

Casey, M., McNamara, M., Fealy, G. M., & Geraghty, R. (2011). Nurses' and midwives' clinical leadership development needs: A mixed methods study. *Journal of Advanced Nursing, 67*(7), 1502–1513.

Cummings, G., Lee, H., MacGregor, T., Davey, M., Wong, C., Paul, L., et al. (2008). Factors contributing to nursing leadership: A systematic review. *Journal of Health Services Research & Policy, 13*(4), 240–248.

Davidson, P., Elliot, D., & Daly, J. (2006). Clinical leadership in contemporary clinical practice: Implications for nursing in Australia. *Journal of Nursing Management, 14*, 180–187.

Day, D. V. (2001). Leadership development: A review in context. *Leadership Quarterly, 11*(4), 581–613.

Duygulu, S., & Kublay, G. (2011). Transformational leadership training programme for charge nurses. *Journal of Advanced Nursing, 67*(3), 633–642.

Fealy, G. M., McNamara, M., Casey, M., Doyle, L., O'Connor, T., Patton, D., et al. (2012). *The National Clinical Leadership Development Project Pilot Evaluation*. Dublin: Health Service Executive/University College Dublin.

Fealy, G. M., McNamara, M., Casey, M., Geraghty, R., Butler, M., Drennan, J., et al. (2010). *The National Clinical Leadership Needs Analysis Study*. Dublin: Health Service Executive.

Fealy, G. M., McNamara, M., Casey, M., Geraghty, R., Butler, M., Halligan, P., et al. (2011). Barriers to clinical leadership development: Findings from a national survey. *Journal of Clinical Nursing, 20*(13–14), 2023–2032.

Fealy, G. M., McNamara, M. S., Casey, M., O'Connor, T., Patton, D., Doyle, L., et al. (2013). Service impact of a national clinical leadership development programme: Findings from a qualitative study. *Journal of Nursing Management*, doi:10.1111/jonm.12133.

Francis, R. (2013). *Report of the Mid Staffordshire NHS Foundation Trust Public Inquiry: Executive Summary*. London: The Stationery Office.

Gopee, N., & Galloway, J. (2013). *Leadership and management in healthcare* (2nd ed.). London: Sage.

Grove, J. T., Barry, M. K., & Haas, T. (2007). EvaluLEAD: An open-systems perspective on evaluating leadership development. In K. M. Hannum, J. W. Martineau, & C. Reinelt (Eds.), *The handbook of leadership development evaluation* (pp. 71–110). San Francisco: Jossey-Bass.

Hix, C., McKeon, L., & Walters, S. (2009). Clinical nurse leader impact on microsystems outcomes. *The Journal of Nursing Administration, 39*, 71–76.

Krugman, M., & Smith, V. (2003). Charge nurse leadership development and evaluation. *Journal of Nursing Administration, 33*, 284–292.

Large, S., MacLeod, A., Cunningham, G., & Kitson, A. (2005). *A multiple-case study: Evaluation of the RCN Clinical Leadership Programme in England.* London: RCN.

Leonard, H. S., & Lang, F. (2010). Leadership development via action learning. *Advances in Developing Human Resources, 12*, 225–240.

Lunn, C., MacCurtain, S., & McMahon, J. (2008). *Clinical Leadership Pilot Evaluation Report.* Dublin: Health Services Executive.

McNamara, M., & Fealy, G. M. (2010). Lead us not again: Clinical leadership and the disciplinary contribution (Guest editorial). *Journal of Clinical Nursing, 19*, 3257–3259.

McNamara, M., Fealy, G. M., Casey, M., Geraghty, R., Butler, M., Halligan, P., et al. (2011). Boundary matters: Clinical leadership and the distinctive disciplinary contribution of nursing to multidisciplinary care. *Journal of Clinical Nursing, 20*(23–24), 3502–3512.

Patton, D., Fealy, G. M., McNamara, M., Casey, M., O Connor, T., Doyle, L., et al. (2013). Individual-level outcomes from a national clinical leadership development programme. *Contemporary Nurse, 45*(1), 56–63.

Pedler, M. (2008). *Action learning for managers* (2nd ed.). Aldershot: Gower.

Reid Ponte, P., Gross, A. H., Galante, A., & Glazer, G. (2006). Using an executive coach to increase leadership effectiveness. *Journal of Nursing Administration, 36*, 319–324.

Roberts, C., & Coghlan, D. (2011). Concentric collaboration: A model of leadership development for healthcare organizations. *Action Learning: Research and Practice, 8*(3), 231–252.

Stoddart, K., Bugge, C., Shepherd, A., & Farquharson, A. B. (2014). The new clinical leadership role of senior charge nurses: A mixed methods study of their views and experience. *Journal of Nursing Management, 22*(1), 49–59.

Stol, L., Foster-Turner, J., & Glen, M. (2010). *Mind shift: An evaluation of the NHS London 'Darzi' Fellowships in Clinical Leadership Programme.* London: NHS.

Storey, J., & Holti, R. (2013). *Towards a new model for leadership in the NHS.* London: NHS Leadership Academy.

Tourangeau, A. E. (2003). Building nurse leader capacity. *Journal of Nursing Administration, 33*(12), 624–626.

Woltring, C., Constantine, W., & Schwarte, L. (2003). Does leadership training make a difference? The CDC/UC Public Health Leadership Institute: 1991–1999. *Journal of Public Health Management and Practice, 9*(2), 103–122.

CHAPTER TEN

Governance of nursing practice: Steps for the quality and safety of healthcare

Patricia M. Davidson, Cheryl Dennison-Himmelfarb, & Nourah Alsadaan

LEARNING OBJECTIVES

At the completion of this chapter, the reader will be able to:

▲ demonstrate the importance of optimising a culture of quality improvement and the role of governance and monitoring in ensuring optimal patient outcomes;

▲ appreciate the role of nursing leadership in ensuring the quality and safety of patient outcomes;

▲ describe the role and importance of interprofessional education and practice in ensuring health outcomes;

▲ identify and critique the mechanism for ensuring quality and safety in your workplace.

KEY WORDS

Governance, nursing, leadership, interdisciplinary practice, quality and safety

INTRODUCTION

Challenges in delivering healthcare in contemporary environments

A constellation of factors such as technological innovation; increased demand for services; heightened consumer expectations; financial pressures; and identification of serious flaws in health delivery has led to an increased focus on not just how we deliver nursing care but how we monitor and address patient outcomes (Aiken et al., 2012). Of concern, in spite of advancement in clinical care, favourable patient outcomes are not universally experienced. Thousands of patients die unnecessarily every year from healthcare-acquired infections; diagnostic errors; teamwork errors; pressure sores; and a failure to receive evidence-based treatments (Magill et al., 2014; Pronovost & Weisfeldt, 2012). For example, catheter-related bloodstream infections (CRBSI) are responsible for substantial morbidity and mortality. Annually, an estimated 250,000 potentially preventable bacteraemia attributable to intravascular catheters occur in United States (US) hospitals resulting in a cost of 2.3 billion US dollars to the healthcare system and 31,000 deaths annually. Many of these deaths from CRBSI and others, as well as disability and distress, can be prevented by often simple measures (Marsteller et al., 2012; Pronovost et al., 2006; Pronovost et al., 2004).

Within this chapter the importance of adhering to evidence-based recommendations, forces moderating clinical practice and methods of evaluating practice and intervening to ensure optimal patient outcomes are discussed. Importantly, the role of nursing leadership in influencing healthcare organisations and promoting a safety culture are discussed.

Despite massive financial expenditures, healthcare delivery systems across the globe are failing to deliver safe, high-quality healthcare. The Institute of Medicine in the United States, over a decade ago, established a platform to increase the focus on healthcare safety and quality and this report cast a lens internationally on how we ensure the safety of patients (Leape & Berwick, 2005). In spite of the numerous tales of system failure that are regularly reported, some strides have been made in improving healthcare as a consequence of this increased scrutiny, systems engineering and accountability.

Healthcare today is best characterised as showing pockets of excellence on specific measures, such as CRBSI, or in particular services at individual healthcare facilities. Maintaining consistently high levels of quality over time and across all healthcare services and settings remains a challenge and is increasingly linked to the level and quality of nursing care as well as teamwork and cohesion (Drenkard, 2012).

Although promoting quality and safety through governance of practice, processes and procedure is the responsibility of all members of the healthcare team, nurses play a critical role, as they are often the 'safety net' in monitoring care and advocating for patients. Moreover, many nursing tasks, overtly perceived to be simplistic, are by no means trivial and contribute to patient safety—hand washing, pressure care, oral hygiene to name just a few (Berry & Davidson, 2006).

Nurses play an important role in monitoring, surveillance and governance of clinical practice within the context of interdisciplinary teams and often complex organisations, with each role critical in promoting the quality and safety of patient care. As a consequence, nurses need a range of skills in collecting and interpreting data and leveraging change in the healthcare team (Yoder-Wise, Scott, & Sullivan, 2013).

As advocates for patient care, nurses play a critical role in this agenda—both from the perspective of their independent and collaborative practice. The function of nurses and their leadership is also associated with favourable patient outcomes

(Stimpfel, Rosen, & McHugh, 2014). Importantly, our ways of organising nursing care, such as extended nursing shifts, can both help and hinder favourable patient outcomes (Stimpfel & Aiken, 2013). For example, 12-hour shifts may lead to decreased errors associated with care hand-offs due to fewer hand-offs as well as improved nurse work–life balance and scheduling flexibility. Conversely, extended shifts combined with overtime, shifts that rotate between day and night duty, or consecutive shifts, may place nurses at risk for fatigue and burnout, which may compromise patient care (Stimpfel, Sloane, & Aiken, 2012).

What does governance mean?

The word *governance* is derived from the Greek verb *to steer*. This is an important metaphor for considering what governance means in clinical practice. Although there is limited consensus on the definition of clinical governance and it is more commonly used in the United Kingdom, this term refers to an integrated approach to data-driven quality improvement; and links administrative and clinical staff in a framework for accountability (Brennan & Flynn, 2013). This role of accountability is critical in leveraging executive, clinical and administrative support and responsibility for ensuring optimal patient outcomes. Basically, it means more than just monitoring, it means action and accountability.

As you can imagine, there is a need for systems, processes and structures to enable this process to function effectively and efficiently and 'steer' clinical systems and processes in a direction that enables not just favourable patient outcomes but ensures the welfare of employees and financial viability. There is a need to ensure that organisations value this activity and promote a culture that allows critical reflection of practice and makes individuals and systems accountable for patient outcomes (DiCuccio, 2014). Regulation, audit and oversight are important considerations to ensure there is monitoring and vigilance of patient care. Depending on the healthcare system, this supervision can be provided by a governing board or council or in some instances government and funding bodies (Bismark, Walter, & Studdert, 2013).

Models of governance also have important implications for existing nurse leaders and those of the future. These approaches not only increase our accountability but our control over our practice and practice environment. They also give us an important voice at the decision-making table. This has important implications for nursing leadership.

The importance of functional interdisciplinary teams

The Robert Wood Johnson /Institute of Medicine (IOM) report, *The Future of Nursing: Leading Change, Advancing Health*, has emphasised that collaboration between health professionals and preparation of nurse leaders is critical to improving the coordination and quality of care and increasing access to healthcare services. This report has also called for nurses to practise to their capabilities and also rise to the challenge of contemporary health systems (Davidson, Daly, & Hill, 2013; National Research Council, 2011).

Not only do collaborative, interprofessional practice environments foster improved patient outcomes for patients, they also increase the satisfaction of nurses and their engagement in the workplace (Clavelle, Drenkard, Tullai-McGuinness, & Fitzpatrick, 2012). As a consequence there is a call for nurses to achieve higher levels of education and training in preparing as leaders in redesigning the healthcare system. It is also likely that nurses will need new skills in entrepreneurship and innovation as well as the courage and resilience to have a voice at the table and to advocate for changes in healthcare systems and lead teams (Davidson et al., 2013).

The role that effective interprofessional teamwork plays in improving healthcare quality and practice environments has been increasingly recognised and, over a decade ago, the IOM urged academic institutions to begin educating health professionals to work collaboratively (Zorek & Raehl, 2013). Core competencies for interprofessional collaborative practice have been established:

▲   values and ethics for interprofessional practice;

▲   roles and responsibilities;

▲   interprofessional communication;

▲   teams and teamwork (Interprofessional Education Collaborative Expert Panel, 2011).

Though interprofessional education and collaborative practice are essential to improving healthcare quality advances these approaches remain in their infancy and effective models of effective and efficient collaborative practice in healthcare are lacking. But there are glimpses of hope through the advocacy of peak bodies (Zorek & Raehl, 2013). Effective interdisciplinary teamwork is important in ensuring cohesion, monitoring and governance of patient outcomes. As cadres of healthcare workers diversify, there will be an increasing number of nurses with varying levels of educational preparation and increasingly the registered nurse will be leading teams of nurses, other healthcare professionals, and unlicensed care assistants as well as working in interprofessional teams.

THE IMPORTANCE OF MONITORING AND GOVERNANCE OF PRACTICE

The concept of governance of practice has long been associated with the professions and the professional role (Scally & Donaldson, 1998). Increased autonomy, particularly, associated with advanced practice nursing roles, is accompanied by an increased measure of professional responsibility and accountability (Brooten et al., 2002). Licensure and professional standards, as well as increasing expectations at government and local institutional level, regulate this accountability. Yet it is only generally catastrophic events that come to the attention of licensing and professional boards and therefore much of the governance of practice occurs at the unit and institutional level.

This obligation carries with it the need for health professionals to be responsible for controlling the quality of their practice through oversight and monitoring, so as to ensure high-quality care. A variety of models of governance have emerged to assist professionals meet this obligation and play an important role in healthcare planning, improving care delivery and ensuring quality care.

To implement a mechanism of governance, organisational changes and mechanisms for participation in the decision-making process need to be established. In healthcare organisations that implement these processes nurses are able to share information and opinions, increase responsibilities and improve their education, thereby increasing the opportunity to provide better patient care.

Interprofessional dysfunction contributes not only to workplace dissatisfaction and low retention rates but also inferior patient outcomes. Efforts to evaluate and improve healthcare safety and quality must be conducted within a framework of systems and contextual factors in which errors and adverse events occur and where the solutions are present. Among the factors that influence clinical practice are organisational factors such as safety climate and morale, work environment factors such as staffing levels and managerial support, team factors such as teamwork and supervision, and staff factors such as overconfidence and being overly self-assured. Health professionals' attitudes about these and related factors are one component of an organisation's safety culture (Guldenmund, 2000). Safety culture refers to the integration of individual and group values, knowledge, attitudes, perceptions, competencies and behaviour that determine a commitment to an organisation's health and safety strategy (Singer et al., 2003). Implicit in this statement is the level of accountability and commitment to governance of practice.

GOVERNANCE AND LEADERSHIP DEVELOPMENT

Leadership is a construct that has gained attention worldwide due to the strong correlation with organisational outcomes. Leadership can be viewed from a relational standpoint or as a trait or behaviour. There are diverse definitions of leadership (Stodgill, 1974). Despite the varying ways that leadership has been conceptualised, Northouse (2012) argues that there are four components to leadership: leadership is a process, involves influence, occurs in groups and involves the achievement of goals. You can readily see how these factors are important in clinical practice. For example, nurses can influence their colleagues in upholding policies, such as the checking of medications, or achieving targets of screening and surveillance, such as monitoring falls.

Leadership has been defined as a power relationship as well as an instrument of goal achievement. Bass (1990) and Burns (1978) defined leadership as the degree to which the leader creates a vision for the future for the organisation and articulates new ways for the followers to accomplish the organisational goals. To accept leadership as a complex and multifaceted phenomenon, it is necessary to be familiar with a variety of perspectives from theorists and researchers (Marriner-Tomey, 1993).

The varying conceptualisations of leadership have been associated with references to individual attributes and traits, leadership behaviours, role relationships, patterns of interaction, exertion of influence over others, or having influence over tasks. More recently, the definition of leadership has also been linked to the importance of being able to transform an organisation and/or bring about a positive influence on followers (DeRue, Nahrgang, Wellman, & Humphrey, 2011). It is easy to see that in healthcare settings this is important in defining and shaping standards.

There is a positive relationship between effective leadership styles and organisational outcomes such as productivity, staff recruitment and retention, willingness to undertake additional efforts, and job satisfaction. In Magnet hospitals studies, transformational leadership style was the most reported style (Clavelle et al., 2012; Schwartz, Spencer, Wilson, & Wood, 2011). Also, The Magnet Recognition Program® recognises healthcare organisations for quality patient care, nursing excellence and innovations in professional nursing practice (McHugh et al., 2013).

This certification, developed by the American Nurses Credentialing Center, is a global source of successful nursing practices and strategies. Importantly, this process of promoting excellence has articulated critical elements of professional practice environments and governance of practice (Lankshear, Kerr, Laschinger, & Wong, 2013). The links between these qualities and patient outcomes including mortality is an impressive achievement (McHugh et al., 2013).

As discussed above, Magnet hospitals studies indicate that the transformational leadership approach significantly contributes to the creation of a culture of excellence and the establishment of an appropriate vision and mission for organisations

(Upenieks, 2003). Notably, leaders who adopt the transformational style in their roles usually identify a particular vision and mission in their organisations. However, some authors argue that solely focusing on this leadership style can ignore aspects of leadership that are critical, such as integrity and engagement (Hutchinson & Jackson, 2013).

The vision and mission of these leaders are able to be communicated to and understood by staff and can help in the development of staff to a higher level of ability and potential. These factors are also important in directing a workplace culture where there is critical evaluation and governance of practice.

PREPARING NURSE LEADERS AND CLINICAL CHAMPIONS OF THE FUTURE

As nursing leaders at all levels of the organisation we must engage in the mentoring and coaching of students and new graduate nurses (Sherwood & Drenkard, 2007). We need to provide opportunities that encourage and help them participate in reflective practice and clinical decision making as well as monitoring practice and being accountable for patient outcomes. This also requires a skill set beyond clinical knowledge to metrics to assess performance and leadership strategies for driving organisational change.

All nurses must play an active role in retaining new graduates in the profession to build a strong workforce that will be able to secure a positive future of healthcare (Laschinger & Leiter, 2006). Part of our professional obligation as registered nurses is to participate in the activities that have the potential to have an impact on our professional practice.

Organisational involvement should occur at both the unit and system levels and may focus on such issues as adherence to standards, the impact of diversity on clinical practice, the need for education to develop the knowledge and skill of the workforce and to create mechanisms to ensure standards-based practice (Nieva & Sorra, 2003). Through this work we are able to provide an enhanced perspective based on our knowledge, education and experience in providing quality, effective patient care.

Internationally, some cultural factors limit the voice of nurses and their confidence and ability to address quality and safety issues and to have control over their professional practice environment (Soh, Soh, & Davidson, 2013). This underscores the role of education and leadership in promoting the effectiveness of patient safety initiatives. Response to errors and the capacity to question authority is an important determinant of safety culture in healthcare organisations. This also includes eliminating a fear of blame and creating mechanisms for open communication and disclosure (Alahmadi, 2010).

PRACTICE PERFORMANCE AND OUTCOMES

For the most part, the measurement of outcomes in health has been limited to a negative focus, such as morbidity, mortality and adverse events. A more dynamic, proactive measurement outcome approach focuses on patient-reported outcomes (Chang et al., 2011). Trends exist to include positive outcomes, such as improved health status, functional ability, patient satisfaction and quality of life. These data can provide guidance in how to develop and monitor services to better meet patient needs (Chang et al., 2012).

An exciting development in the United States has been the establishment of the Patient-Centered Outcomes Research Institute (PCORI) (Selby & Lipstein, 2014).

PCORI has developed a model for research that engages individuals and organisations representing patients, caregivers, clinicians, delivery systems, payers and purchasers, researchers, policy makers and industry. This is an exciting approach to increase not only the utility and application of research findings but also accountability to multiple stakeholders (Selby, Beal, & Frank, 2012).

NURSES TAKING CONTROL OF PRACTICE PERFORMANCE AND OUTCOMES

There are many opportunities and forums to enhance our professional practice. Nurses should continually be critically evaluating practice in relation to patient outcomes and asking if what they are doing is best for the patient. There is also an important agenda for systematic research and evaluation of practice. Implicit in the definition of a profession is the commitment of each individual nurse to being involved in enhancing professional practice. There is a role for every nurse, whether it is as a member of a local quality committee, discussing ideas about nursing practice with members at handover or participation in a national committee. The need to help identify issues and offer potential solutions and feedback is the responsibility of every nurse. The more nurses are involved in the decision-making process, the more supported the decision will be.

A CASE STUDY FROM JOHNS HOPKINS UNIVERSITY SCHOOL OF NURSING, BALTIMORE, USA

The Helene Fuld Leadership Program for the Advancement of Patient Safety and Quality (The Fuld Fellows Program) at the Johns Hopkins University School of Nursing is designed to prepare a select group of nursing undergraduates for future leadership at the bedside and in other care settings, who have exceptional competencies for promoting quality and safety, particularly among older patients. This program provides academic support for students who have a special interest in developing quality and safety skills beyond those ensured by the current curriculum. These selected students, Fuld Fellows, are given unique opportunities to capitalise on the intellectual and institutional resources that distinguish Johns Hopkins as a leader in healthcare quality and safety. The Fuld Fellows Program provides each Fellow with the following: 1) broad, evidence-based, quality/patient safety interprofessional education; 2) practical quality/patient safety learning experiences with Johns Hopkins improvement teams; and 3) mentoring to bridge theory and practice. This program helps to strengthen nursing education globally by offering an exemplary academic model and innovative curricula models for building competencies in quality and safety that can be replicated in other clinical settings.

Many of these projects use the Armstrong Institute Model for Translating Evidence into Practice (Pronovost & Bo-Linn, 2012). This model embeds an explicit method for knowledge translation in a collaborative model for broader dissemination of knowledge into practice. It is intended for collaborative projects, in which centralised researchers support the technical development (for example, summarise the research evidence for transitional care best practices and develop measures) and local teams throughout a hospital (or more broadly) perform the adaptive work (engage staff in the project, tailor interventions to fit the local work processes and identify how to modify work so that all patients can receive the intervention). This implementation framework is summarised as the 6Es: engage, educate, execute, evaluate, endure and expand. These are excellent strategies for facilitating the governance of practice. Further engaging executive support and strategies for promoting accountability is another critical step in this process.

This tailored and targeted program is designed to build knowledge, skills and attitudes as well as leadership skills to enable them to be nurse leaders of the future. Almost 100 students have been in this program since 2012 enabling them to engage in active partnerships with leaders in the field and programs such as: Preventing venous thromboembolism, deep vein thrombosis and pulmonary embolism and the use of radio frequency identification to promote improved hand hygiene compliance. These projects involve not only evidence-based principles related to the subject area but also state-of-the-art and rigorous principles for quality and safety, including interprofessional education and teamwork as well as governance and leadership of practice.

CASE STUDY FROM THE LITERATURE

Alexandrou et al. (2012). Nurse-led central venous catheter insertion—Procedural characteristics and outcomes of three intensive-care-based catheter placement services. *International Journal of Nursing Studies, 49*(2), 162–168

Central line associated bacteraemia (CLAB) are responsible for up to 60% of nosocomial acquired infections in an intensive care unit. Traditionally the role of medical practitioners, the insertion of central lines are increasingly carried out by advance practice nurses (Alexandrou et al., 2010).

The New South Wales (NSW) Central Line Associated Bacteraemia Intensive Care Units (CLAB-ICU) project was a successful 'top down, bottom up' initiative aimed at reducing the incidence of CLAB in NSW coordinated by the NSW Clinical Excellence Commission (CEC) in Australia. This represents an interesting model in driving practice change and governance of practice (Burrell et al., 2011).

All adult and paediatric intensive care units (ICUs) in NSW participated in this program, which is a demonstration of governance and accountability of practice. Alexandrou and colleagues reviewed the characteristics and outcomes of the three nurse-led central venous catheter insertion services and compared these to the total data set (Alexandrou et al., 2012).

Between March 2007 and June 2009, 760 vascular access devices were inserted by hospitals with nurse-led services. Hospital A inserted 520 catheters; Hospital C 164; and Hospital B 76. Over the study period, only one pneumothorax (1%), one arterial puncture (1%) and a single CLAB (1%) were noted. The CLAB rate in the nurse-led services was lower in comparison with the aggregated CLAB data set [1.3 per 1000 catheters (95% CI = 0.03–7.3) vs. 7.2 per 1000 catheters (95% CI = 5.9–8.7)].

This study demonstrated safe patient outcomes with nurse-led CVC insertion as compared with published data. Nurses who are formally trained and credentialled to insert CVCs can improve organisational efficiencies. This study adds to emerging data that developing clinical roles focusing on skills, procedural volume and competency rather than professional designation is an important strategy in improving patient outcomes (Alexandrou et al., 2012; Alexandrou et al., 2013).

GOVERNANCE OF PRACTICE: A KEY TO OUR CREDIBILITY AND PLACE AT THE TABLE

It is only through data-based approaches to evaluating interventions and monitoring patient outcomes that nurses can demonstrate their valuable contribution to the healthcare system (Royal, Smeaton, Avery, Hurwitz, & Sheikh, 2006). An emerging number of nurse scientists have demonstrated their value in improving health outcomes. High levels of professional satisfaction are related to recruitment and retention (Lu, While, & Louise Barriball, 2005). Nurses need to be responsible and accountable for their professional practice and be willing to embrace the responsibility and implications of governance of practice.

A combination of forces—healthcare reform, demographic trends, technological advances and a focus on population-based strategies to both prevent and manage health conditions—are driving an unprecedented rise in the need for credible, credentialled and competent nurse leaders. In parallel, there is an increased scrutiny on factors that contribute to the quality and safety of patient care, as well as drivers of effectiveness and efficiencies in the healthcare system.

Undeniably, nurses play a crucial role in patient outcomes, not only through the care they deliver but the role they play in monitoring and evaluating patient outcomes. Ensuring that nurses are at the decision-making table where decisions are made to influence patient outcomes and ensuring accountability is an important dimension of our professional role.

CONCLUSION

This chapter has underscored the importance of not merely measuring and monitoring patient outcomes but ensuring models of governance and accountability. It has also emphasised that leadership across all levels of the organisation is critical in optimising patient outcomes and nursing leadership at all levels of an organisation is of critical importance in driving safety cultures.

Without the scaffolding and safeguards of governance enveloping clinical outcome assessment it is difficult to leverage the changes in practice and resources to improve patient outcomes. Healthcare delivery systems increasingly depend on interdisciplinary and collaborative practice to achieve optimal patient, healthcare worker and organisational outcomes. Monitoring the quality and safety of clinical care and governing clinical practice is of essential importance in ensuring that the work of nurses and their colleagues optimises patient and organisational outcomes.

REFLECTIVE EXERCISE

In the organisation in which you work or you have had experience, identify the mechanisms for monitoring the quality and safety and governance of clinical outcomes. This may be a clinical council, a quality and safety committee or a similar structure. Take the time to appraise the strategic goals of this group; the representation of health professionals, consumers and executives in this structure; the mechanisms for engaging with the organisation and the methods for ensuring accountability for practice.

As you undertake this exercise also reflect on the value placed on the professional practice environment and the role of nursing in promoting efficient and effective patient outcomes in this organisation.

1. Describe the mechanism for clinical governance in this setting; how is it organised, what is the process of engaging with the broader community including consumers?

2. Identify the membership of this organisation—what are their roles internal and external to this organisation?

3.   What are the mechanisms for information dissemination with clinicians and staff in the facility as well as consumers and regulatory bodies?

4.   What are the barriers and facilitators for leveraging accountability for practice in this organisation?

5.   Can you identify strategies for improving the mechanism of governance and models of professional practice evaluation at your institution?

Recommended Readings

Cummings, G. G., MacGregor, T., Davey, M., Lee, H., Wong, C. A., Lo, E., et al. (2010). Leadership styles and outcome patterns for the nursing workforce and work environment: A systematic review. *International Journal of Nursing Studies, 47*(3), 363–385.

Curtis, E. A., Sheerin, F. K., & de Vries, J. (2011). Developing leadership in nursing: The impact of education and training. *British Journal of Nursing, 20*(6), 344–352.

Kelly, L. A., McHugh, M. D., & Aiken, L. H. (2011). Nurse outcomes in Magnet® and non-magnet hospitals. *Journal of Nursing Administration, 41*(10), 428–433.

Naylor, M. D., Aiken, L. H., Kurtzman, E. T., Olds, D. M., & Hirschman, K. B. (2011). The importance of transitional care in achieving health reform. *Health Affairs, 30*(4), 746–754.

Stimpfel, A. W., Rosen, J. E., & McHugh, M. D. (2014). Understanding the role of the professional practice environment on quality of care in Magnet® and Non-Magnet hospitals. *Journal of Nursing Administration, 44*(1), 10–16.

References

Aiken, L. H., Sermeus, W., Van den Heede, K., Sloane, D. M., Busse, R., McKee, M., et al. (2012). Patient safety, satisfaction, and quality of hospital care: Cross sectional surveys of nurses and patients in 12 countries in Europe and the United States. *BMJ (Clinical Research Ed.), 344.*

Alahmadi, H. (2010). Assessment of patient safety culture in Saudi Arabian hospitals. *Quality and Safety in Health Care, 19*(5), e17–e17.

Alexandrou, E., Murgo, M., Calabria, E., Spencer, T. R., Carpen, H., Brennan, K., et al. (2012). Nurse-led central venous catheter insertion—Procedural characteristics and outcomes of three intensive care based catheter placement services. *International Journal of Nursing Studies, 49*(2), 162–168.

Alexandrou, E., Spencer, T. R., Frost, S. A., Mifflin, N., Davidson, P. M., & Hillman, K. M. (2013). Central venous catheter placement by advanced practice nurses demonstrates low procedural complication and infection rates—a report from 13 years of service. *Critical Care Medicine, 42*(3), 536–543.

Alexandrou, E., Spencer, T. R., Frost, S. A., Parr, M. J., Davidson, P. M., & Hillman, K. M. (2010). A review of the nursing role in central venous cannulation: Implications for practice policy and research. *Journal of Clinical Nursing, 19*(11–12), 1485–1494.

Bass, B. M. (1990). *Bass & Stogdill's handbook of leadership: Theory, research and managerial applications.* New York: Free Press.

Berry, A. M., & Davidson, P. M. (2006). Beyond comfort: Oral hygiene as a critical nursing activity in the intensive care unit. *Intensive and Critical Care Nursing, 22*(6), 318–328.

Bismark, M. M., Walter, S. J., & Studdert, D. M. (2013). The role of boards in clinical governance: Activities and attitudes among members of public health service boards in Victoria. *Australian Health Review, 37*(5), 682–687.

Brennan, N. M., & Flynn, M. A. (2013). Differentiating clinical governance, clinical management and clinical practice. *Clinical Governance: An International Journal, 18*(2), 114–131.

Brooten, D., Naylor, M. D., York, R., Brown, L. P., Munro, B. H., Hollingsworth, A. O., et al. (2002). Lessons learned from testing the quality cost model of advanced practice nursing (APN) transitional care. *Journal of Nursing Scholarship*, *34*(4), 369–375.

Burns, J. (1978). *Leadership*. New York: Harper & Row.

Burrell, A. R., McLaws, M.-L., Murgo, M., Calabria, E., Pantle, A. C., & Herkes, R. (2011). Aseptic insertion of central venous lines to reduce bacteraemia. *Medical Journal of Australia*, *194*(11), 583.

Chang, S., Gholizadeh, L., Salamonson, Y., DiGiacomo, M., Betihavas, V., & Davidson, P. M. (2011). Health span or life span: The role of patient-reported outcomes in informing health policy. *Health Policy*, *100*(1), 96–104.

Chang, S., Newton, P. J., Inglis, S., Luckett, T., Krum, H., Macdonald, P., et al. (2012). Are all outcomes in chronic heart failure rated equally? An argument for a patient-centred approach to outcome assessment. *Heart Failure Reviews*, 1–10.

Clavelle, J. T., Drenkard, K., Tullai-McGuinness, S., & Fitzpatrick, J. J. (2012). Transformational leadership practices of chief nursing officers in Magnet® organizations. *Journal of Nursing Administration*, *42*(4), 195–201.

Davidson, P. M., Daly, J., & Hill, M. N. (2013). Editorial: Looking to the future with courage, commitment, competence and compassion. *Journal of Clinical Nursing*, *22*(19–20), 2665–2667.

DeRue, D. S., Nahrgang, J. D., Wellman, N., & Humphrey, S. E. (2011). Trait and behavioral theories of leadership: An integration and meta-analytic test of their relative validity. *Personnel Psychology*, *64*(1), 7–52.

DiCuccio, M. H. (2014). The relationship between patient safety culture and patient outcomes: A systematic review. *Journal of Patient Safety, February*.

Drenkard, K. (2012). The transformative power of personal and organizational leadership. *Nursing Administration Quarterly*, *36*(2), 147–154.

Guldenmund, F. W. (2000). The nature of safety culture: A review of theory and research. *Safety Science*, *34*(1), 215–257.

Hutchinson, M., & Jackson, D. (2013). Transformational leadership in nursing: Towards a more critical interpretation. *Nursing Inquiry*, *20*(1), 11–22.

Interprofessional Education Collaborative Expert Panel (2011). *Core competencies for interprofessional collaborative practice: Report of an expert panel*. Interprofessional Education Collaborative. Washington, DC.

Lankshear, S., Kerr, M. S., Laschinger, H. K. S., & Wong, C. A. (2013). Professional practice leadership roles: The role of organizational power and personal influence in creating a professional practice environment for nurses. *Health Care Management Review*, *38*(4), 349–360.

Laschinger, H. K. S., & Leiter, M. P. (2006). The impact of nursing work environments on patient safety outcomes: The mediating role of burnout engagement. *Journal of Nursing Administration*, *36*(5), 259–267.

Leape, L., & Berwick, D. (2005). Five years after To Err Is Human: what have we learned? *The Journal of the American Medical Association*, *293*(19), 2384–2390.

Lu, H., While, A. E., & Louise Barriball, K. (2005). Job satisfaction among nurses: A literature review. *International Journal of Nursing Studies*, *42*(2), 211–227.

Magill, S. S., Edwards, J. R., Bamberg, W., Beldavs, Z. G., Dumyati, G., Kainer, M. A., et al. (2014). Multistate point-prevalence survey of health care-associated infections. *New England Journal of Medicine*, *370*(13), 1198–1208.

Marriner-Tomey, A. (1993). *Transformational leadership in nursing*. St Louis, MO: Mosby Inc.

Marsteller, J. A., Sexton, J. B., Hsu, Y.-J., Hsiao, C.-J., Holzmueller, C. G., Pronovost, P. J., et al. (2012). A multicenter, phased, cluster-randomized controlled trial to reduce central line-associated bloodstream infections in intensive care units. *Critical Care Medicine*, *40*(11), 2933–2939.

McHugh, M. D., Kelly, L. A., Smith, H. L., Wu, E. S., Vanak, J. M., & Aiken, L. H. (2013). Lower mortality in magnet hospitals. *Medical Care*, *51*(5), 382–388.

National Research Council (2011). *The future of nursing: Leading change, advancing health.* Washington DC: National Academies.

Nieva, V., & Sorra, J. (2003). Safety culture assessment: A tool for improving patient safety in healthcare organizations. *Quality and Safety in Health Care, 12*(Suppl. 2), ii17–ii23.

Northouse, P. J. (2012). *Leadership: Theory and practice* (6th ed.). Thousand Oaks: Sage.

Pronovost, P. J., & Bo-Linn, G. (2012). Preventing patient harms through systems of care. *The Journal of the American Medical Association, 308*(8), 769–770.

Pronovost, P., Needham, D., Berenholtz, S., Sinopoli, D., Chu, H., Cosgrove, S., et al. (2006). An intervention to decrease catheter-related bloodstream infections in the ICU. *New England Journal of Medicine, 355*(26), 2725–2732.

Pronovost, P., Rinke, M. L., Emery, K., Dennison, C., Blackledge, C., & Berenholtz, S. M. (2004). Interventions to reduce mortality among patients treated in intensive care units. *Journal of Critical Care, 19*(3), 158–164.

Pronovost, P., & Weisfeldt, M. (2012). Science-based training in patient safety and quality. *Annals of Internal Medicine, 157*(2), 141–143.

Royal, S., Smeaton, L., Avery, A., Hurwitz, B., & Sheikh, A. (2006). Interventions in primary care to reduce medication related adverse events and hospital admissions: Systematic review and meta-analysis. *Quality and Safety in Health Care, 15*(1), 23–31.

Scally, G., & Donaldson, L. J. (1998). Looking forward: Clinical governance and the drive for quality improvement in the new NHS in England. *BMJ: British Medical Journal, 317*(7150), 61.

Schwartz, D. B., Spencer, T., Wilson, B., & Wood, K. (2011). Transformational leadership: implications for nursing leaders in facilities seeking magnet designation. *AORN Journal, 93*(6), 737–748.

Selby, J., Beal, A., & Frank, L. (2012). The Patient-Centered Outcomes Research Institute (PCORI) national priorities for research and initial research agenda. *The Journal of the American Medical Association, 307*(15), 1583–1584.

Selby, J. V., & Lipstein, S. H. (2014). PCORI at 3 Years—Progress, Lessons, and Plans. *New England Journal of Medicine, 370*(7), 592–595.

Sherwood, G., & Drenkard, K. (2007). Quality and safety curricula in nursing education: Matching practice realities. *Nursing Outlook, 55*(3), 151–155.

Singer, S. J., Gaba, D., Geppert, J., Sinaiko, A., Howard, S., & Park, K. (2003). The culture of safety: Results of an organization-wide survey in 15 California hospitals. *Quality and Safety in Health Care, 12*(2), 112–118.

Soh, K. L., Soh, K. G., & Davidson, P. M. (2013). The role of culture in quality improvement in the intensive care unit: A literature review. *Journal of Hospital Administration, 2*(2).

Stimpfel, A. W., & Aiken, L. H. (2013). Hospital staff nurses' shift length associated with safety and quality of care. *Journal of Nursing Care Quality, 28*(2), 122–129.

Stimpfel, A. W., Rosen, J. E., & McHugh, M. D. (2014). Understanding the role of the professional practice environment on quality of care in Magnet® and Non-Magnet Hospitals. *Journal of Nursing Administration, 44*(1), 10–16.

Stimpfel, A. W., Sloane, D. M., & Aiken, L. H. (2012). The longer the shifts for hospital nurses, the higher the levels of burnout and patient dissatisfaction. *Health Affairs, 31*(11), 2501–2509.

Stodgill, R. M. (1974). *Handbook of leadership: A survey of theory and research.* Collier Macmillan: Free Press.

Upenieks, V. V. (2003). What constitutes effective leadership?: Perceptions of magnet and nonmagnet nurse leaders. *Journal of Nursing Administration, 33*(9), 456–467.

Yoder-Wise, P. S., Scott, E. S., & Sullivan, D. T. (2013). Expanding leadership capacity: Educational levels for nurse leaders. *Journal of Nursing Administration, 43*(6), 326–328.

Zorek, J., & Raehl, C. (2013). Interprofessional education accreditation standards in the USA: A comparative analysis. *Journal of Interprofessional Care, 27*(2), 123–130.

CHAPTER ELEVEN

Indigenous leadership in nursing: Speaking life into each other's spirits

Tamara Power, Juanita Sherwood,
Lynore K. Geia & Roianne West

LEARNING OBJECTIVES

At the completion of this chapter, and with further reading, the reader will be able to:

▲ reflect on their own cultural worldviews and explore how they impact upon their clients and peers;

▲ describe further the impact of the normalisation of Whiteness within the nursing profession;

▲ demonstrate insight into the challenges and barriers created in nursing that Indigenous people must deal with regularly;

▲ discuss the impact of colonisation on the health and wellbeing of Indigenous peoples;

▲ express awareness of the need to be culturally competent in the workplace.

KEY WORDS

Aboriginal and Torres Strait Islander peoples, Indigenous, racism, colonisation, cultural competency

ACKNOWLEDGEMENT

We wish to acknowledge and pay respect to the traditional owners of this land, past and present. We are grateful for the wisdom and traditions passed down by our Elders and buoyed by the resilience of our people and culture. This is the spirit in which we write. As four Indigenous women, we can only write from women's perspectives. However, we also pay our respect to men who are Indigenous leaders and acknowledge men in nursing.

In this chapter we will use the terms Indigenous and Aboriginal and Torres Strait Islander peoples interchangeably when referring to Australia's first people. While we write as a group of Australian Indigenous nurses, the purpose of this chapter is to raise awareness of some of the issues that affect Indigenous people globally. Whilst each Indigenous group has its own stories of leadership to tell, international literature suggests that there are commonalities (Donovan et al., 2012; Keltner, Kelley, & Smith, 2004; Nichols, 2004).

INTRODUCTION

The literature on nursing leadership reads as a list of exemplary personal traits. However, a leader's ability to shape the healthcare environment and contribute to positive outcomes for patients is undeniable (Mannix, Wilkes, & Daly, 2013). The impact that nursing leaders have on patient outcomes means that leadership needs to be scrutinised (Jackson & Watson, 2009). Leadership in nursing explored from an Australian Aboriginal and Torres Strait Islander perspective is a story that is vital to all health professionals. Our work has often gone unnoticed and unrecorded, yet we have made significant differences to the health, wellbeing and safety of our people. Leadership is a mantle taken on by all Indigenous women and men entering this workforce. We have been the warriors of our people in the academy, hospitals, community health and primary healthcare settings.

We begin this chapter with Lynore's story, which exemplifies some of the challenges of being an Indigenous nurse leader. These challenges include racist assumptions about ability, the Whiteness of the Australian healthcare system, and ownership of Indigenous issues. Other issues that will be discussed include the nature of Indigenous leadership and some of the intrinsic challenges to Indigenous leadership. Throughout the chapter as you read, we ask that you set aside any preconceived assumptions about Aboriginal and Torres Strait Islander peoples and open your mind to the possibility of alternative worldviews.

LYNORE'S STORY

My assumption of a leadership role was expected by my parents and my community. I was fortunate that throughout my life I have been encouraged and nurtured by various nursing and non-nursing individuals. Thus, the progression into nursing leadership was a natural one in my eyes, but for many non-Aboriginal and Torres Strait Islander people, the fact that I have come so far was perceived as a remarkable achievement.

The impact of colonisation has distorted the concept of Aboriginal and Torres Strait Island leadership, which has been progressively re-defined by western constructs of professionalism (Geia, 2012). What was once a very natural and accepted standpoint of recognition of leadership from the Aboriginal and Torres Strait Island community perspective is now often seen as an extraordinary feat of accomplishment through the non-Indigenous Australian hegemonic philosophy. Thus it has been my experience that it is non-Indigenous people who question our progression in nursing asking, 'How did we do this, how did we get this far?'

Hence, I argue, therein lies the major contemporary issue that we face on a daily basis in nursing leadership.

On the one hand, as Indigenous women, we are naturally accepted as leaders in our communities; on the other hand, as Indigenous nursing leaders we are an oddity in the system. More often than not, Indigenous nurse leaders have to prove their worth in the eyes of the 'White system', including proving our ability to non-Indigenous nursing colleagues (Mapedzahama, Rudge, West, & Perron, 2012; Puzan, 2003). It became even more complex, when as a nursing leader, employed by a government health service, I returned to my own community to work at a nursing leadership level. I was welcomed home with open arms by my people like a celebrated homecoming queen. However, not so by non-Aboriginal nursing colleagues who considered me a collegial threat to 'their' nursing domain in my own community. This is what I call the sophisticated walk, where we have one foot in each world (Geia, 2012; West, Geia, & Power, 2013). We walk with ease in the community where our professionalism is an accepted physical and metaphysical, familial, cultural, community expectation. Yet, we also walk in the physical domain of the western paradigms of nursing and academia, which we all easily do, but with the awareness that we carry a certain expectation of having to prove oneself with the mainstream domain.

INDIGENOUS LEADERSHIP

Indigenous leadership is informed by a tradition that pre-dates western notions of leadership by tens of thousands of years (Myers, 1986; Smallacombe et al., 2007). It is this tradition that provides the essential framework for the way we take up our roles within the health workforce (Sherwood, 2009). Our ways of knowing leadership have been handed down to us through our Elders. 'Elders are scholars in their own right within First Nation knowledge systems' (Ermine, Sinclair, & Browne, 2005), and although often discounted, our Aboriginal knowledge systems continue to be vital and necessary in this contemporary world. Our ways of knowing have developed through our unique connection with and cognition of the spiritual, physical, spatial, relational, ecological, social and emotional Indigenous world (Battiste, 2002).

Our Elders have authority in relation to moral and ethical matters relating to Aboriginal law, society and culture. They continue to hold responsibility in the jurisdiction of all key components of law. They have been in the past the lawmakers, law keepers and judges of the law. This standing in our community is not gender specific and therefore both women and men are considered to be equal in importance in taking up these roles (Sherwood, 2010). As alluded to in Lynore's story there is the expectation that we will be the bridge between our culture and the culture we work within.

Mick Dodson asserted that [Indigenous]:

Leaders are essentially creatures of habit. They don't really do extraordinary things that often. They do ordinary things often and consistently and persistently ... Good leaders keep turning up, they're there, ... at the coalface, they want to take on the challenges, they want to fight the fight, regardless of how overwhelming the opposition seems, from both in and outside (Reconciliation Australia, 2011a, 4.0.1).

It is important to stress that Australian Indigenous values and protocols for leadership are not shared by the western mainstream. Challenges for Indigenous leaders stem from trying to unite Indigenous ways of leadership with western organisations and management systems. Working within organisations that are funded and governed by government departments means Indigenous leaders are accountable for funding and upholding the values of the organisation to stakeholders. However, Indigenous leaders are simultaneously accountable to their communities to uphold the interests of family networks, community and laws of culture (Reconciliation Australia, 2010). Our way of leadership rejects an independent leader speaking on behalf of all. Instead, it encourages us to remember and celebrate our culture and collective agency. However, a major challenge for us is:

> the difficult balance between 'looking after' and being directly accountable to their own families and 'own mob', at the same time as fulfilling their wider responsibilities of working for their nations, communities and organisations, and with governments and other stakeholders (Reconciliation Australia, 2011b, 4.2).

This very high and two-level graded accountability is beyond the normal western manager's obligations; however, it ensures that we acknowledge, maintain and sustain our responsibility to our communities.

Indigenous leaders of today have had the opportunity to reflect on the strengths, knowledge and wisdom of those who came before, and appreciate that the struggle for self-determination requires many approaches. Respecting every Aboriginal and Torres Strait Islander peoples and their communities' unique experiences remains a mandate of moving forward (West, Geia, & Power, 2013). Indigenous leaders belong to their communities and work with and within them to find pragmatic solutions that all can agree on and work towards together. It is only through Indigenous collaboration, that Indigenous problems can be fully understood and addressed (Taylor, 2013).

There 'are vast differences amongst and within Indigenous Australia' (Elston, Saunders, Hayes, Bainbridge, & McCoy, 2013, p. 8) and Indigenous leaders face unique challenges. Indigenous leaders are few in number and often have competing priorities (Reconciliation Australia, 2010). Western leadership styles where one person speaks on behalf of many are not compatible with Aboriginal culture. Too often Indigenous people that step into a leadership role find themselves criticised by their own people (Reconciliation Australia, 2010). Disempowerment, dispossession (Saunders, 2003) and racism have all been named as the root causes of infighting and disagreement in the Aboriginal community (Tim, 2002). We need to stop imbibing the negative stereotypes about our people and instead showcase and celebrate the positives about our culture, and the resilience, cleverness and diversity of our people (Tim, 2002). Here in this chapter, Murri and Koori women have come together to write and show that the way forward is to walk together hand in hand. We acknowledge that we come from different countries and have had vastly different experiences, yet we share and celebrate our commonalities.

'WHITENESS' AND INSTITUTIONALISED RACISM IN NURSING

Lynore stated that as an Indigenous nurse leader she was an 'oddity in the system'. An Aboriginal woman with clinical skills and a PhD is considered an aberration. This stance by her non-Indigenous colleagues represents racist assumptions that as an Aboriginal woman she was less capable of succeeding in higher education and the nursing profession than non-Indigenous people. This is not surprising when you consider the 'Whiteness' of nursing as a profession.

In 2011, the nursing and midwifery workforce in Australia was predominantly female (90.1%) and middle aged (average 43.7 to 44.5 years old) (Australian Institute of Health and Welfare, 2012). Of the 283,577 nurses and midwives employed in

Australia that year, only 2212 (0.8%) identified as being of Aboriginal or Torres Strait Islander descent (Australian Institute of Health and Welfare, 2012). Although data regarding how many nurses and midwives have been internationally trained is fragmented, it has been estimated that one in six nurses in Australia was trained overseas (Buchanan, Naccarella, & Brooks, 2011). Even taking into account the heavy reliance on international health professionals, these figures indicate that the vast majority of nurses and midwives in Australia are White.

We do not draw attention to the Whiteness of nursing lightly, but rather to make visible the often-unconsidered power differentials that exist. 'Being White confers structural advantage, usually invisible to those who are White, and operates through a set of cultural practices that shape both the lives of the privileged and the marginalised' (Durey & Thompson, 2012, p. 3). Durey and Thompson (2012) drew attention to the phenomenon of 'racialisation' in which marginalised racial groups internalised the deficit view of their culture, whereas those who are White accepted their privilege and entitlement as evidence of their superiority.

The normalisation of Whiteness in the nursing profession begins during nursing education (Allen, 2006; Puzan, 2003). Nursing education and practice aligns itself with scientific hegemony that dictates which knowledge systems are worthy, therefore discounting Indigenous knowledges. Australian nursing students are taught about cultural diversity in regards to how non-White patients may not comply or 'fit' with the Eurocentric medical model of the Australian healthcare system. It is the expectation that patients from diverse cultures, races and classes conform to standardised care that marks the authority of White privilege in the system (Puzan, 2003).

A predominantly White workforce represents challenges for Indigenous nurses. In the past, the health system and profession were not welcoming. Many of our Elders in nursing were trailblazers who fought difficult battles to even participate within the profession. They perceived that they had to work twice as hard as their non-racialised sisters who enjoyed the privilege of Whiteness and the authority that went with this 'invisible' attribute. Stories shared within the text *In Our Own Right: Black Australian Nurses' Stories* (Goold, 2007) emphasised just how difficult it has been for many Indigenous men and women to enter the profession. This was not a result of their skill base but rather their ethnicity, being excluded from the general hospital-based training programs offered throughout the country due to their Aboriginality (Goold, 2007b, p. 195). This approach fostered genuine class hierarchies within the health setting that continue today, and are experienced by many Aboriginal and Torres Strait Islander health professionals. Puzan (2003) argued that non-White nurses must act White if they are to fit within the profession without ridicule or harassment. Goold (2007a) similarly contended that Indigenous nurses must be better than their peers if they are to survive and make a difference. All health professionals bring their own experiences, histories and values to the bedside. While seeking to increase the Aboriginal workforce it has to be acknowledged that Aboriginal health professionals themselves are likely to carry the burden of colonisation and trans-generational trauma (Sherwood, 2009). Furthermore, we are working in an arena that discounts Indigenous knowledge, beliefs and values (Durey & Thompson, 2012).

The Australian nursing profession is beset by issues of horizontal violence and bullying (Hutchinson, Vickers, Wilkes, & Jackson, 2010). It is therefore not surprising that racism is also an issue. Being Indigenous in a White profession means being exposed to relentless and frequent episodes of racism both personally as a health professional and vicariously through Indigenous patients. As Olga Kanitsaki (2007, p. v) wrote in the foreword of *In Our Own Right: Black Australian Nurses' Stories*:

Each of the stories told in this book exposes the nasty and dehumanising effects of racism even in the 'caring' environments. What is particularly confronting about this expose is that individual nurses, and the nursing profession as a whole, were complicit in this racism and its soul-destroying consequences to Indigenous nurses—whose stories are only now being told, for the first time.

Racism is not always overt and not always intended, but rather can stem from ignorance and stereotyping (Coulthard, 2010), and growing up with a colonised view of Australian history (Sherwood, 2009). Morbidity and mortality is strongly correlated with racism and it is a common experience for many Australian Indigenous people within the health service, both as patients and health professionals (Brondolo, Brady, Libby, & Pencille, 2011; Larson, Gillies, Howard, & Coffin, 2007; Paradies, Harris, & Anderson, 2007). Although it is acknowledged that there are numerous individuals and organisations striving to make a difference, in many cases there is still a paternalistic and deficit-based approach to Aboriginal health (Pyett, Waples-Crowe, & van der Sterren, 2008) that fails to acknowledge the ongoing legacy of trauma that stems from colonisation (Sherwood, 2009). A misguided focus on 'lifestyle' diseases, education and health promotion fails to address the real problem, which is the social determinants of health (Durey & Thompson, 2012). Furthermore, there has been a focus on Aboriginal culture as a social determinant of health (Dion Stout & Downey, 2006). Aboriginal culture is not the problem; it is the disruption to culture and its knowledge systems stemming from colonisation that is culpable.

RESEARCH INFORMED BY INDIGENOUS EXPERTS

Nursing research involving Indigenous people is also contested terrain in need of strong Indigenous leaders. We have been endlessly examined and are the most researched people in Australia (Martin-McDonald & McCarthy, 2007). Yet mainstream solutions have not solved the marked health disparities between Indigenous and non-Indigenous people (Durey & Thompson, 2012). Indigenous people are aware that they have been exploited as subjects in research by non-Indigenous investigators and more recently as token members of research groups and now demand to be engaged in the process (Elston et al., 2013). Scholars have called for increasing Indigenisation of research, where the data collected about Indigenous people is owned, controlled and possessed by those Aboriginal people (Dion Stout & Downey, 2006; Rigney, 2002). Lynore's PhD thesis (Geia, 2012) embodies the possibilities of Indigenous-led research with Indigenous people. For her doctoral study, Lynore explored intergenerational child-rearing practices and strengths in her own community. One of the intrinsic strengths of her method was employing counter-story, which rejects 'western ways of understanding and allows for an Aboriginal reclamation of research processes and outcomes; privileging to voices of Aboriginal and Torres Strait Island people' (Geia, 2012, p. xvii).

In addition to the small numbers of Indigenous people graduating from higher degrees, a barrier to Indigenous-led research is the need for Indigenous people to compete for funding and approval from institutions against large numbers of White academics who have proven track records and understand the 'concomitant overt and covert rules and ways of succeeding' (Martin-McDonald & McCarthy, 2007, p. 129). This barrier exists despite agreement that Indigenous health research should be autonomous and self-sufficient (Elston et al., 2013; NHMRC, 2005). What is essential to improving Indigenous health in Australia is growing the Indigenous academic workforce (Elston et al., 2013). This can be achieved through funding for professional development, refining Indigenous methodologies and providing opportunities for Indigenous leaders to invest in mentoring Indigenous scholars (Elston et al., 2013).

Having carved their careers in the area of Indigenous health, it may be difficult for non-Indigenous researchers to relinquish control of budgets and research agendas to Indigenous researchers (Pyett, Waples-Crowe, & van der Sterren, 2008). In order to avoid perpetuating White hegemony in Indigenous research, non-Indigenous researchers working in Indigenous health should closely examine their motivations and honour the knowledge and expertise of their Indigenous co-investigators (Martin-McDonald & McCarthy, 2007; Pyett, Waples-Crowe, & van der Sterren, 2008). When confronted with their own Whiteness and position of privilege Martin-McDonald and McCarthy (2007, p. 131) stated that 'their emotions and worldviews were in disarray'. These non-Indigenous researchers struggled with shame as they confronted their own privilege and preconceptions of Indigenous people. Previously believing themselves to be 'enlightened and culturally sensitive' they recognised their well-meaning ignorance. Having experienced an epiphany of Whiteness themselves, these researchers urged all nurses to examine their own 'cultural norms and expectations; establish symmetry with people who are culturally different; and, explore practice, education, research and leadership issues from multiple worldviews' (Martin-McDonald & McCarthy, 2007, p. 131). Pyett, Waples-Crow, and van der Sterren (2008) also advised researchers to give proper acknowledgement to Aboriginal and Torres Strait Islander co-researchers, consultation groups and participants and to be careful of the terms they use to describe them. It is heartening to see White investigators examine their own positioning in Indigenous health and this gives us hope for a shared future. Otherwise we will continue to see inappropriate Indigenous health solutions dictated by non-Indigenous health professionals who do not recognise the system as part of the problem (Durey & Thompson, 2012).

PROMOTING AND EVALUATING CULTURAL COMPETENCY

Over the decades we have demonstrated and mentored cultural competency and have been the voices behind the importance of cultural competency in all health and academic settings. This praxis of care is instrumental to shifting the inequity experienced by the Aboriginal and Torres Strait Islander population across Australia. We have been effective in having this message heard, and recognised, along with our Indigenous sisters and brothers across the seas. However, we must continue to encourage our peers and future students to take up this skill base and teaching pedagogy of care.

'Cultural safety and competence' has been a contested term simply to shift the agenda from what is not occurring. Even where there is an organisational commitment to ensure health professionals can provide culturally competent care, this can often be a token exercise such as a single educational session addressing cultural safety (Durey & Thompson, 2012). Cultural safety approaches need to be evaluated to see if they truly support Indigenous people's needs as opposed to being 'another form of paternalistic control disguised as a panacea' (Rigney, 2002, p. 331). Despite the many social and health issues affecting Indigenous people, it has to be acknowledged that we have survived over 200 years of colonisation and attempts to eradicate us. This resilience needs to be acknowledged and Indigenous people consulted about our health needs and strategies (Dion Stout & Downey, 2006). This includes incorporating and valuing Indigenous beliefs about health in Indigenous healthcare and moving past the Eurocentric assumption that any non-White interventions are unscientific and meaningless (Puzan, 2003).

Durey and Thompson (2012, p. 9) asked the questions:

If the institutional requirements are for health care providers to practise in culturally safe ways when working with Indigenous patients, what criteria are put in place to inform the assessment of culturally safe care and who deems a service provider is delivering health care in culturally safe ways?

However, the argument behind such pedagogy of care is vital to improving the workplace for Aboriginal and Torres Strait Islander health professionals and most importantly the health and wellbeing of our Indigenous clients (Ranzijn, McConnochie, & Nolan, 2009; Smith, 2004; Taylor & Guerin, 2010). Furthermore, health professionals must be made to understand that the health inequities experienced by Aboriginal people in Australia do not stem from a deficit culture but rather are directly attributable to generations of social injustices brought about by colonisation (Pyett, Waples-Crowe, & van der Sterren, 2008; Sherwood, 2013).

CONCLUSION

Each of us as Aboriginal women comes from a different country and lived experiences which has shaped us as individuals—all of us have experienced the legacies of past government policies and practices in our respective Murri and Koori communities. All of us have made choices in our life that have propelled us along in our nursing careers. We are now nurses and midwives and each of us holds a Doctor of Philosophy, the highest academic degree a university confers upon an individual scholar. Little did we know as girls growing up in our communities amongst our own people that we would find ourselves in this place and position. We have become hybrid creatures that can navigate both the Indigenous and western worlds.

Our task as leaders is to encourage our people to participate in what can be a very rewarding career. We have, as our story outlines, held out our hands to be partners, shared stories to demonstrate injuries resulting from unsafe work practices and cultural 'unsafety', participated in research and teaching praxis to improve levels of knowledge for all, and have mentored goodwill. We would like to see this reciprocated today, rather than tomorrow. However, to protect those that follow us, it is incumbent upon us to endeavour to make tertiary degree institutions more culturally safe places (West, Usher, & Foster, 2010; West, Usher, Foster, Buettner, & Stewart, 2013), educate non-Indigenous students and nurses about our history and culture (Jackson, Power, Sherwood, & Geia, 2013), and clear the way for others to follow (West, Geia, & Power, 2013).

It is also up to us to shape the Australian research on Indigenous health through adding an Indigenous perspective to the pool of nursing literature and research methodology (Geia, Hayes, & Usher, 2013; Power, West, & Geia, 2013), that is community led, community directed and sensitive (Pyett, Waples-Crowe, & van der Sterren, 2008). Research methodologies and ethics will need to be adapted to accommodate the wishes of the community.

As Indigenous women in prominent positions it is up to us to not promulgate the deficit view of our communities but instead promote the strength and resilience of Indigenous people. In many cases we acknowledge that White control of organisations has come about due to a dearth of qualified Indigenous people ready to assume the management mantle. However, we are here, and we are increasing. Prepare to step aside and watch us transform the rhetoric of self-determination into a reality as we work together and speak life into each other's spirits.

REFLECTIVE EXERCISE

1. At the start of this chapter, we acknowledged the traditional owners of this land, past and present. Discuss the importance of acknowledging country and why it is relevant to you as a health professional.
2. Consider how racism impacts upon Indigenous patients and health professionals.
3. Explore why the concept of Indigenous leadership in nursing should be considered separately from nursing leadership generally.
4. Reflect upon your own cultural background, and how it might influence your interactions with Indigenous peoples.
5. Outline the key points you have learned about Indigenous leadership in nursing.
6. Reflect on the concept of leaving a legacy in your nursing practice. From your reading of this chapter write a personal goal of the professional and/or personal legacy you would like to leave in your nursing practice in relation to Indigenous health and/or Indigenous patient care. It will be useful to revisit this goal at regular intervals in your nursing career as part of your ongoing reflective nursing practice.

Recommended Readings

Ahmed, S. (2012). *On being included: Racism and diversity in institutional life*. London: Duke University Press.

Jackson, D., Power, T., Sherwood, J., & Geia, L. (2013). Amazingly resilient Indigenous people! Using transformative learning to facilitate positive student engagement with sensitive material. *Contemporary Nurse, 46*(1), 105–112.

Mapedzahama, V., Rudge, T., West, S., & Perron, A. (2012). Black nurse in white space? Rethinking the in/visibility of race within the Australian nursing workplace. *Nursing Inquiry, 19*(2), 153–164.

Puzan, E. (2003). The unbearable whiteness of being (in nursing). *Nursing Inquiry, 10*(3), 193–200.

Sherwood, J. (2013). Colonisation—it's bad for your health: The context of Aboriginal health. *Contemporary Nurse, 46*(1), 28–40.

References

Allen, D. G. (2006). Whiteness and difference in nursing. *Nursing Philosophy, 7*(2), 65–78.

Australian Institute of Health and Welfare (2012). *Nursing and midwifery workforce 2011*. Canberra: AIHW. National health workforce series no. 2, Cat. no. HWL 48.

Battiste, M. (2002). *Indigenous knowledge and pedagogy in First Nations education: A literature review with recommendations: Prepared for the National Working Group on Education and the Minister of Indian Affairs Indian and Northern Affairs Canada (INAC) Ottawa*. Ottawa: Indigenous Education, Apamuwek Institute.

Brondolo, E., Brady, N., Libby, D., & Pencille, M. (2011). Racism as a psychosocial stressor. In R. Contrada & A. Baum (Eds.), *The handbook of stress science: Biology, Psychology, and Health* (pp. 167–184). New York: Springer Publishing Company.

Buchanan, J. M., Naccarella, L., & Brooks, P. M. (2011). Is health workforce sustainability in Australia and New Zealand a realistic policy goal? *Australian Health Review, 35*(2), 152–155.

Coulthard, R. (2010). A little story about racism in nursing. *Aboriginal and Islander Health Worker Journal, 34*(1), 12.

Dion Stout, M., & Downey, B. (2006). Nursing, Indigenous peoples and cultural safety: So what? Now what? *Contemporary Nurse, 22*(2), 327–332.

Donovan, D. J., Diers, D., Goodrich, A. W., & Carryer, J. (2012). Perceptions of policy and political leadership in nursing in New Zealand. *Nursing Praxis in New Zealand, 28*(2), 15–25.

Durey, A., & Thompson, S. C. (2012). Reducing the health disparities of Indigenous Australians: Time to change focus. *BMC Health Services Research, 12*(151). Retrieved from <http://www.biomedcentral.com/1472-6963/12/151>.

Elston, J. K., Saunders, V., Hayes, B., Bainbridge, R., & McCoy, B. (2013). Building Indigenous Australian research capacity. *Contemporary Nurse, 46*(1), 6–12.

Ermine, W., Sinclair, R., & Browne, M. (2005). *Kwayask itotamowin: Indigenous Research Ethics: Report of the Indigenous Peoples' Health Research Centre to the Institute of Aboriginal Peoples' Health and the Canadian Institutes of Health Research.* Saskatoon, SK: Indigenous Peoples' Health Research Centre.

Geia, L. K. (2012). *First steps, making footprints: Intergenerational Palm Island families' Indigenous stories (narratives) of childrearing practice strengths.* Australia: James Cook University.

Geia, L. K., Hayes, B., & Usher, K. (2013). Yarning/Aboriginal storytelling: Towards an understanding of an Indigenous perspective and its implications for research practice. *Contemporary Nurse, 46*(1), 13–17.

Goold, S. (2007a). Keep your eye on the prize! In S. Goold & K. Liddle (Eds.), *In our own right: Black Australian nurses' stories* (pp. 82–92). Sydney: eContent Management Pty Ltd.

Goold, S. (2007b). Preface. In S. Goold & K. Liddle (Eds.), *In our own right: Black Australian nurses' stories* (p. viii). Sydney: eContent Management Pty Ltd.

Hutchinson, M., Vickers, M. H., Wilkes, L., & Jackson, D. (2010). A typology of bullying behaviours: The experiences of Australian nurses. *Journal of Clinical Nursing, 19*(15–16), 2319–2328.

Jackson, D., Power, T., Sherwood, J., & Geia, L. (2013). Amazingly resilient Indigenous people! Using transformative learning to facilitate positive student engagement with sensitive material. *Contemporary Nurse, 46*(1), 105–112.

Jackson, D., & Watson, R. (2009). Editorial: Lead us not. *Journal of Clinical Nursing, 18*(14), 1961–1962.

Kanitsaki, O. (2007). Foreword. In S. Goold & K. Liddle (Eds.), *In our own right: Black Australian nurses' stories* (pp. v–vi). Sydney: eContent Management Pty Ltd.

Keltner, B., Kelley, F. J., & Smith, D. (2004). Leadership to reduce health disparities: A model of nursing leadership in American Indian communities. *Nursing Administration Quarterly, 28*(3), 181–190.

Larson, A., Gillies, M., Howard, P. J., & Coffin, J. (2007). It's enough to make you sick: The impact of racism on the health of Aboriginal Australians. *Australian and New Zealand Journal of Public Health, 31*(4), 322–328.

Mannix, J., Wilkes, L., & Daly, J. (2013). Attributes of clinical leadership in contemporary nursing: An integrative review. *Contemporary Nurse, 45*(1), 10–21.

Mapedzahama, V., Rudge, T., West, S., & Perron, A. (2012). Black nurse in white space? Rethinking the in/visibility of race within the Australian nursing workplace. *Nursing Inquiry, 19*(2), 153–164.

Martin-McDonald, K., & McCarthy, A. (2007). 'Marking' the white terrain in Indigenous health research: Literature review. *Journal of Advanced Nursing, 61*(2), 126–133.

Myers, F. R. (1986). *Pintupi country, Pintupi self: Sentiment, place, and politics among Western Desert Aborigines.* Washington, DC: Smithsonian Institution Press.

NHMRC. (2005). Keeping research on track: A guide for Aboriginal and Torres Strait Islander peoples about health research ethics. Retrieved from <http://www.nhmrc.gov.au/guidelines/publications/e65>.

Nichols, L. (2004). Native American nurse leadership. *Journal of Transcultural Nursing, 15*(3), 177–183.

Paradies, Y., Harris, R., & Anderson, I. (2007). *The impact of racism on Indigenous health in Australia and Aotearoa: Towards a research agenda.* Darwin: CRCAH. No. 4.

Power, T., West, R., & Geia, L. K. (2013). Epilogue: Indigenous special editions—Benefiting a community of scholars. *Contemporary Nurse, 46*(1), 143–144.

Puzan, E. (2003). The unbearable whiteness of being (in nursing). *Nursing Inquiry, 10*(3), 193–200.

Pyett, P., Waples-Crowe, P., & van der Sterren, A. (2008). Challenging our own practices in Indigenous health promotion and research. *Health Promotion Journal of Australia, 19*(3), 179–183.

Ranzijn, R., McConnochie, K., & Nolan, W. (2009). *Psychology and Indigenous Australians foundations of cultural competence.* South Yarra, Victoria: Palgrave Macmillan.

Reconciliation Australia (2010). *Sharing Success Workshop Workbook, Sharing Success Workshop: Building good governance and strong leadership.* Port Augusta: Reconciliation Australia.

Reconciliation Australia (2011a). *Indigenous Governance Toolkit: 4.0.1 What is leadership and why is it important?* Retrieved from <http://www.reconciliation.org.au/governance/toolkit/4-0-your-governing-body-and-leadership>.

Reconciliation Australia (2011b). *Indigenous Governance Toolkit: 4.2 The challenges of leadership.* Retrieved from <http://www.reconciliation.org.au/governance/toolkit/4-2-evaluating-your-leadership>.

Rigney, L. I. (2002). Indigenous education and treaty: Building Indigenous management capacity. *Balayi: Culture, Law and Colonialism, 4,* 73–82.

Saunders, M. (2003). Indigenous health, Indigenous men: Leadership and other bad medicine. *Aboriginal and Islander Health Worker Journal, 27*(6), 10–13.

Sherwood, J. (2009). Who is not coping with colonisation? Laying out the map for decolonisation. *Australiasian Psychiatry, 17*(1), S24–S27.

Sherwood, J. (2010). *Do no harm: Decolonising Aboriginal health research.* Sydney: UNSW.

Sherwood, J. (2013). Colonisation—it's bad for your health: The context of Aboriginal health. *Contemporary Nurse, 46*(1), 28–40.

Smallacombe, S., Davis, M., Quiggin, R., Christie, M., Craig, D., Cronin, D., et al. (2007). *Desert knowledge CRC: Final report of the Scoping Project on Aboriginal Traditional Knowledge.* Alice Springs: Desert Knowledge CRC.

Smith, J. D. (2004). *Australia's rural and remote health: A social justice perspective.* Croydon, Victoria: Tertiary Press.

Taylor, K., & Guerin, P. (2010). *Health care and Indigenous Australians: Cultural safety in practice.* Malayasia: Palgrave Macmillan.

Taylor, R. (2003). Indigenous Community Capacity Building and the relationship to sound governance and leadership. Paper presented to the *National Native Title Conference. June 2003,* Darwin, June 2003. Retrieved from <http://www.aiatsis.gov.au/ntru/nativetitleconference/conf2003/papers/russell.pdf>.

Tim, K. (2002). Leading with courage and integrity. *Aboriginal and Islander Health Worker Journal, 26*(3), 23–26.

West, R., Geia, L. K., & Power, T. (2013). Finding strength in our Indigeneity: Indigenous perspectives in nursing and midwifery leadership. *Contemporary Nurse, 46*(1), 3–5.

West, R., Usher, K., & Foster, K. (2010). Increased numbers of Australian Indigenous nurses would make a significant contribution to 'closing the gap' in Indigenous health: What is getting in the way? *Contemporary Nurse, 36*(1–2), 121–230.

West, R., Usher, K., Foster, K., Buettner, P., & Stewart, L. (2013). Indigenous Australians' participation in pre-registration tertiary nursing courses: A mixed methods study. *Contemporary Nurse, 46*(1), 123–134.

CHAPTER TWELVE

Leadership and its influence on patient outcomes

Carol Wong & Lisa Giallonardo

LEARNING OBJECTIVES

At the completion of this chapter, the reader will be able to:

▲ describe current challenges facing leaders working to improve patient outcomes;
▲ identify the major leadership theories that have been linked to patient outcomes;
▲ explain key processes that link leadership behaviours to patient outcomes;
▲ summarise key findings on the relationship between leadership and patient outcomes;
▲ discuss the current role of leadership in the patient safety movement;
▲ describe some practical implications for influencing patient outcomes.

KEY WORDS

Relational and task-oriented leadership, patient outcomes, transformational, patient safety, adverse events

INTRODUCTION

In this chapter, we explore the influence of nursing leadership on patient outcomes. First an overview of some factors that contribute to current leadership challenges related to improving and sustaining quality patient care and outcomes is presented. Then the current state of the research evidence supporting connections between leadership and patient outcomes based on findings from current literature is described. Some newer leadership theories and the patient safety movement are briefly explored in relation to outcomes. The chapter concludes with a discussion of some practical ways in which leaders can influence patient outcomes and safety in healthcare settings.

CURRENT CONTEXT FOR LEADERSHIP AND PATIENT OUTCOMES

Healthcare in many countries has undergone significant and rapid change over the past three decades. Hospitals have merged into large regional corporations and many healthcare services have moved out of the hospital into the community. In hospitals there is increasing emphasis on managing programs based on a business model that emphasises fiscal and organisational efficiencies. This leads to shorter hospital stays and waiting times for procedures, integration of services to reduce duplication, and computerised information management systems. The result is a more complex care environment with an increase in the acuity and complexity of patients remaining in hospital, which may increase risks to provision of quality care.

In addition, the changes reflected in restructuring and downsizing of healthcare organisations have contributed to the redeployment of many front-line nurses and the elimination of nursing management positions. In some new management models, nursing leaders are replaced with non-nursing managers responsible for multiple clinical programs with larger numbers of staff reporting to them (Laschinger et al., 2008). Studies examining the impact of such restructuring changes reveal it produces an environment of increased mistrust and a reduction in nurse satisfaction (Aiken, Clarke, & Sloane, 2000; Baumann et al., 2001; Cummings & Estabrooks, 2003; Davidson, Folcarelli, Crawford, Duprat, & Clifford, 1997).

From these studies substantial evidence has emerged in the last decade linking nursing work environment characteristics, such as nurse staffing, to patient outcomes (Aiken, Clarke, Sloane, Lake, & Cheney, 2008; Blegen, Goode, Spetz, Vaughn, & Park, 2011; Cho, Ketefian, Barkauskas, & Smith, 2003; Duffield et al., 2011; Estabrooks, Midodzi, Cummings, Ricker, & Giovannetti, 2005; Kovner & Gergen, 1998; McGillis Hall et al., 2003; Needleman et al., 2011; Tourangeau, Giovannetti, Tu, & Wood, 2002). Despite strong empirical support for the relationship between nurses' work environments and patient outcomes, there is much less research examining the effects of nursing leadership on patient outcomes.

In practice, we know that effective nurse leaders strive to ensure adequate staff and other resources are in place to achieve high-quality care. At higher levels in organisations, senior nurse executives influence how nursing is practised and valued through their role in policy making (Huston, 2008; Wong, Laschinger, Cummings, Vincent, & O'Connor et al., 2010). At ward or unit levels, managers include nurses in care and staffing decisions, quality improvement activities, and learning opportunities to advance overall care delivery (Page, 2004; Thompson et al., 2011; Tregunno et al., 2009). Ongoing economic pressures in organisations, health and safety concerns associated with stressful work environments, a large number of leaders nearing retirement and other projected workforce shortages are some additional challenges facing current healthcare leaders in maintaining and improving the level of patient care. Effective nursing leadership is critical to advance agendas for change to make care practices cost-effective, improve patient outcomes and attract and retain staff (Fine, Holden, Hannam, & Morra, 2009; Lowe, 2005; Page, 2004).

BROAD LENS FOR EXAMINING THE INFLUENCE OF LEADERSHIP ON OUTCOMES

Relational versus task-oriented approaches

There are many definitions of leadership but consistently there is agreement on the key elements of leadership: 'Leadership is a process whereby an individual influences a group of individuals to achieve a common goal' (Northouse, 2013, p. 5). There are also many leadership styles and theories that have been used to study leadership but one broad way to categorise leadership is by the focus of attention leaders have on either the task to be accomplished or the quality of their relationships with others (Bass & Stogdill, 1990). That is, leadership behaviours can be categorised as either relational or task-oriented (see Table 12.1). Relational leaders focus on people and work to maintain supportive relations with followers (Bass & Stogdill, 1990.) For example, transformational leadership is a relational leadership style in which followers have trust and respect for the leader and are motivated to go above and beyond normal work expectations to achieve organisational goals (Bass & Avolio, 1994).

Leaders also differ on the degree to which they focus on goals and tasks and the ways to achieve them (Bass & Stogdill, 1990). Task-oriented leaders tend to define and organise the roles of followers, focus on goals and procedures, and are likely to keep emotional distance from their followers. An example of a task-oriented style is transactional leadership which emphasises the transaction or economic exchange that takes place among leaders and followers to accomplish work (Bass & Avolio, 1994). The transactional leader's role is primarily that of recognising follower needs and monitoring their work (Bono & Judge, 2004).

A systematic review of research studies linking leadership practices, styles and behaviours with patient outcomes used the broad categorisation of relational and task-oriented leadership to describe and organise leadership styles (Wong, Cummings, & Ducharme, 2013). Findings from this review will be used to describe leadership and its influence on patient outcomes in this chapter.

Table 12.1 Leader behaviours from task and relational perspectives

Task orientation—focuses on group goals and means to achieve them	Relations orientation—focuses on relationships
Creates structures and procedures that promote goal achievement	Facilitates a positive social and emotional work climate
Sets clear performance expectations	Adopts a supportive communication style
Allocates resources to ensure work production	Attends to follower needs and concerns
Defines communication channels	Works to establish mutual trust with others
Focuses on short- and long-term planning and goals	Coaches and mentors for effective performance
Determines the ways to accomplish work	Promotes participative approaches to decision making

Processes of influence

Evidence supporting the influence of nurses in leadership and management roles on staff nurse outcomes such as job satisfaction, retention and empowerment is significant (Cummings, MacGregor et al., 2010), but much less is known about the link between nursing leadership and patient outcomes. The mechanisms of action by which nursing leaders influence patient outcomes are often viewed as a 'black box' in which the processes or methods of operation are not known (Wong & Cummings, 2009). It has been proposed that even though leaders may directly impact outcomes at multiple levels (individual nurses, groups or units and organisations), their influence on patient outcomes is indirect, working through others and occurring over time (Lord & Dinh, 2012). For example, indirect processes of influence may include facilitating working conditions that promote optimal patient care, creating open communication with staff that supports changing quality care standards, or promoting positive relationships with staff that encourage their motivation and engagement in work (Cummings, MacGregor et al., 2010).

Patient outcomes

Outcomes consider the measurable results of care; however, patient outcomes are the specific focus of this chapter. Patient outcomes are defined as outcomes describing patient mortality, patient safety outcomes such as the incidence of adverse events involving patients (e.g. falls, nosocomial infections, or complications during hospitalisation), patient perceptions of satisfaction with care, and healthcare utilisation such as length of stay (Doran & Pringle, 2011).

STATE OF THE EVIDENCE ON THE RELATIONSHIP BETWEEN LEADERSHIP AND PATIENT OUTCOMES

In 2007, Wong and Cummings published a systematic review of the research literature to identify the state of knowledge on the relationship between nursing leadership and patient outcomes. Only seven studies that examined whether the leadership styles of nurses in management roles were related to better patient outcomes were found. While evidence was not conclusive given the small number of studies, it did show a beginning trend towards higher patient satisfaction and lower adverse outcomes when leaders employed a positive, relational leadership style (Wong & Cummings, 2007). Wong et al. (2013) recently updated this systematic review and located 13 additional studies published since 2007 (for a total of 20). These findings represent an increased interest in the topic of leadership and patient outcomes. Additionally, the trend in findings (greater patient satisfaction, and lower mortality, adverse events and complications) is strengthening. The following sections describe the highlights of this review.

In this review, Wong et al. (2013) searched eight bibliographic databases for studies that met the following inclusion criteria: leadership styles or practices of formal nurse leaders/managers in healthcare organisations were measured; patient outcomes were reported as direct observations of patient outcomes or extracted from administrative databases; and the relationships between leadership and patient outcomes(s) were measured quantitatively and tested statistically. All 20 studies meeting these criteria were published between 1999 and 31 July 2012. Fifteen studies were conducted in the United States, four in Canada and one in Norway. The majority of studies represented acute care units of hospitals and to a lesser extent nursing homes and home healthcare agencies. Findings were combined despite the variety of settings.

The quality of the research methods used in the studies were rated as strong (85%) and moderate (15%). All studies used a cross-sectional design, meaning that data was collected at only one point in time. This prevents researchers from making definitive cause and effect inferences from findings. Strengths of the studies included the fact that the majority used sound measures, multi-sited data collection techniques, acceptable sample sizes, and reported correlations of multiple effects. In all but one study, leadership was measured by asking followers to rate the leadership style of their formal leader. Six (30%) studies used only self-report measures for patient outcomes, specifically satisfaction with care. All other patient outcome measures were collected prospectively in the study or extracted from administrative databases. Weaknesses of studies included lack of an explicit conceptual or theoretical framework, lower (less than 60%) response rates, and reliance on non-random sampling methods.

Leadership theories tested in relation to patient outcomes

A variety of leadership styles were tested across all studies and were primarily relational in focus. Transformational/transactional leadership was examined in one-third of the studies (Capuano, Bokovoy, Hitchings, & Houser, 2005; Doran et al., 2004; Houser, 2003; Larrabee et al., 2004; McNeese-Smith, 1999; Raup, 2008). Another third of studies used other leadership approaches, which included participative leadership practices (Anderson, Issel, & McDaniel, 2003; Castle & Decker, 2011; Kroposki & Alexander, 2006), task- or relationship-oriented leadership (Havig, Skogstad, Kjekshus, & Romoren, 2011), resonant leadership (Cummings, Midodzi, Wong, & Estabrooks, 2010), trust in leadership (Vogus & Sutcliffe, 2007), and positive perceptions of leaders (Taylor et al., 2012). The final third of studies measured leadership as the leader's ability and support (Boyle, 2004; Flynn, Liang, Dickson, & Aiken, 2010; Gardner, Thomas-Hawkins, Fogg, & Latham, 2007; Hansen, Williams, & Singer, 2011; Paquet, Courcy, Lavoie-Tremblay, Gagnon, & Maillet, 2013; Pollack & Koch, 2003; Tourangeau et al., 2007).

The prominent leadership theory examined in relation to patient outcomes was transformational leadership, specifically Bass and Avolio's (1994) transformational/transactional leadership theory or Kouzes and Posner's (1995) transformational leadership practices model. A number of different tools were used to measure leadership but the most frequently used tools were Bass and Avolio's (1994, 2000) Multifactor Leadership Questionnaire (MLQ), and Kouzes and Posner's (1995) Leadership Practices Inventory (LPI). Leadership was measured using a component or subscale of a larger measure of the work context in 35% of studies. In these studies the most commonly used measures were the manager ability and support subscale of Aiken and Patrician's (2000) Nursing Work Index-Revised (NWI-R) or the manager support subscales of various patient safety climate measures.

Processes: how leadership influences outcomes

Leadership influences patient outcomes indirectly through making changes in nurses' work context and influencing staff attitudes, behaviour or performance. In order to understand the mechanisms or processes by which leadership indirectly affects patient outcomes, advanced statistical techniques are sometimes used to explicitly test this complex relationship. For example, transformational leadership practices were positively related to staff expertise and negatively related to staff turnover, both of which contributed to reduced patient mortality, hospital-acquired infections, medication errors and patient falls (Houser, 2003). Capuano et al. (2005) added to these findings by showing that transformational leadership practices were also associated with staff expertise, which in turn decreased the same adverse patient outcomes. In both studies, the authors stated that strong leaders might retain higher numbers of skilled staff. The indirect effect of manager support on patient outcomes (decreased medication errors and patient length of stay) through reduced absenteeism, overtime and nurse/patient ratios has also been demonstrated (Paquet et al., 2013). Furthermore, trust in the manager has been shown to increase the strength of the relationship between staff safety organising behaviours (e.g. discussing errors, questioning current practices) and the incidence of medication errors (Vogus & Sutcliffe, 2007). When trust in the leader is high, nurses participate more actively in safety organising behaviours, which in turn contributes to fewer medication errors. These findings suggest the key role of supportive leadership styles in facilitating positive work conditions, which contribute to better patient outcomes.

In other studies where the direct effect of leadership on patient outcomes is explored, the authors discuss possible processes by which leadership may have influenced outcomes. Cummings, Midodzi, et al. (2010) suggest staff performance and ultimately patient outcomes are improved when leaders present well-defined leadership styles and communicate clear expectations. Other researchers report that relational leadership behaviours may contribute to more effective teamwork and a clear vision for quality care (Anderson et al., 2003; Doran et al., 2004; McNeese-Smith, 1999; Pollack & Koch, 2003) or support increased staff participation in care decision making (Boyle, 2004; Castle & Decker, 2011; Cummings, Midodzi et al., 2010; Kroposki & Alexander, 2006). Finally, several studies have examined the effect of work climate factors, including leadership and staff safety organising behaviours, on patient safety outcomes (Hansen et al., 2011; Taylor et al., 2012; Vogus & Sutcliffe, 2007).

Patient outcomes related to leadership

Patient outcome variables found in the studies were grouped into four categories considering the relationship between leadership and: (1) patient satisfaction, (2) patient mortality, (3) patient safety outcomes including adverse events and complications and (4) patient healthcare utilisation (Doran & Pringle, 2011). In a third of studies reviewed, patient or family satisfaction ratings were collected, while in the remainder of studies patient outcomes were extracted from administrative databases of the organisations participating in the studies. Patient mortality and medication errors were the most frequently examined outcomes. Over all studies, a total of 43 relationships between leadership and patient outcomes were examined and 63% (n = 27) of these were significant.

Patient satisfaction

Patient satisfaction is broadly described as a patient's overall perceptions of the total healthcare experience and in relation to specific aspects of care such as nursing or medical care or admission or discharge processes (Laschinger, Gilbert, & Smith, 2011). Researchers often report statistically significant relationships between leadership and increased patient satisfaction. Relational leadership has been associated with increased patient satisfaction (Kroposki & Alexander, 2006; McNeese-Smith, 1999). Similarly, task-orientated leadership of nursing home ward managers has been positively related to family satisfaction with care (Havig et al., 2011) and transactional leadership style has been associated with increased patient satisfaction in acute care settings (Doran et al., 2004). Perhaps task-oriented or transactional leaders facilitate patient care by providing clear work expectations and procedures for quality care.

There is an important trend suggesting that both relational and task-oriented leadership styles increase patient satisfaction. This finding may indicate that some elements of each style are needed to ensure care processes that contribute to satisfied patients such as clear standards of care and role expectations as well as collaborative working relationships.

Patient mortality

A significant relationship may exist between leadership and patient mortality. Transformational and resonant leadership styles have been related to lower patient mortality (Capuano et al., 2005; Cummings, Midodzi et al., 2010; Houser, 2003) while contrary to what was expected leadership was associated with higher mortality in one study (Tourangeau et al., 2007). Both Houser and Capuano et al. have shown that transformational leadership of unit managers contributed to lower patient mortality through increased retention and expertise of staff. This suggests that positive and inspirational managers at the unit level and senior nurse leaders at the organisational level may influence mortality through the creation of working conditions that promote satisfied staff who are able to perform optimally. Specifically, these leaders may ensure that appropriate staffing levels, resources and care processes are in place that support nurses in preventing unnecessary deaths (Wong & Cummings, 2007).

Patient safety outcomes: adverse events and complications

Adverse patient outcomes or events are defined as unintended injuries or complications caused by healthcare management, rather than the patient's underlying condition, leading to death or disability or prolonged hospital length of stay (Baker et al., 2004). Almost 50% of studies in Wong et al.'s (2013) review addressed adverse patient events. These events include nosocomial infections, medication errors, patient falls or pressure ulcers. The strongest relationship was between leadership and medication errors as four of five studies showed significant negative relationships. Transformational leadership (Capuano et al., 2005; Houser, 2003), manager support (Paquet et al., 2013) and trust in leadership (Vogus & Sutcliffe, 2007b) were all associated with lower medication errors. Results linking leadership to patient falls were mixed as were results for pressure ulcers. Participative leadership styles were related to lower restraint use in nursing homes (Anderson et al., 2003; Castle & Decker, 2011). Transformational leadership has been associated with lower hospital-acquired infections; specifically, pneumonia and urinary tract infections (Capuano et al., 2005; Houser, 2003).

Patient healthcare utilisation

Healthcare utilisation measures reflect services or resources consumed in managing patients' health-related needs, such as number of hospitalisations, hospital readmissions and hospital length of stay (Clarke, 2011). Wong et al. (2013) found three studies that measured these outcomes (Gardner et al., 2007; Hansen et al., 2011; Paquet et al., 2013) but only one study had significant results. Paquet et al. (2013) found that manager support was associated with lower patient length of stay through the human resource indicators of lower absenteeism, overtime and nurse to patient ratio, again suggesting some processes in which leadership may influence patient outcomes.

Summary of the evidence

Overall, findings from studies testing the relationship between leadership and patient outcomes reflect positive trends in research design and methods. Most studies were multi-sited, used advanced statistical procedures to assess results and examined the relationship between leadership and patient outcomes in a wide variety of clinical settings, although the majority was conducted in acute care. Results (summarised in Figure 12.1) show key relationships between relational leadership and the reduction of adverse events; specifically, medication errors. This relationship may be due to leaders' influence on increased staff expertise and lower turnover, absenteeism, overtime and nurse-to-patient ratios. There are also promising trends in findings for restraint use and hospital-acquired infections. Findings on mortality outcomes are also strong, showing a significant relationship between relational leadership and lower patient mortality in three of six studies. Finally, there are significant relationships between both relational and task-oriented leadership and higher patient satisfaction.

OTHER LEADERSHIP APPROACHES AND OUTCOMES

Leader-member exchange (LMX) theory is a relational leadership approach that describes leadership as a process centred on the quality of interactions (also called exchanges) between leaders and followers (Graen & Uhl-Bien, 1995). Higher LMX quality has been related to increased job satisfaction and performance through workplace empowerment in a large study of acute care nurses in Ontario, Canada (Laschinger, Finegan, & Wilk, 2009). Similarly, results from a survey of staff in 34 inpatient units in an American academic medical centre revealed that when leaders demonstrate relational leadership (LMX), staff on their units report more positive patient

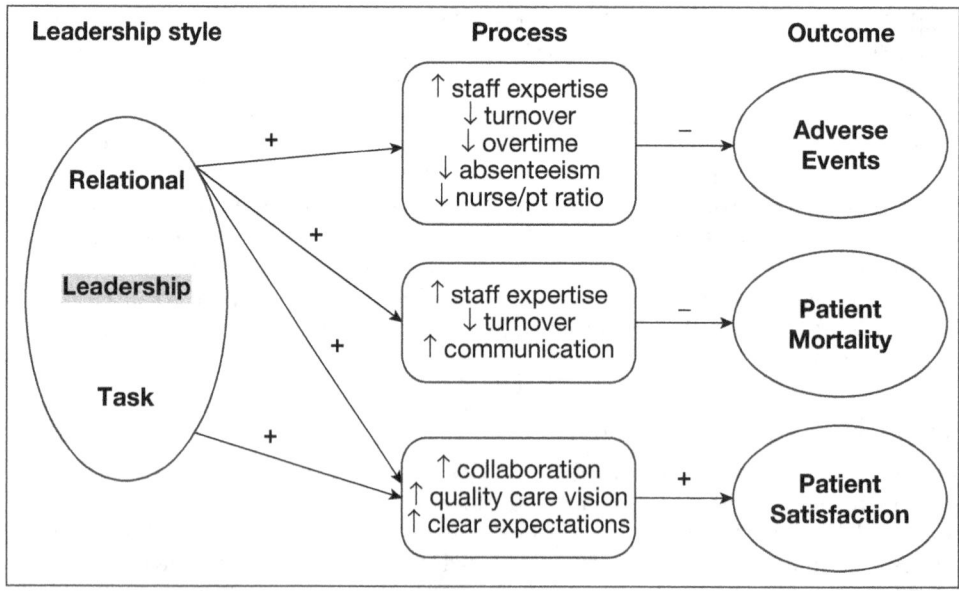

FIGURE 12.1

Relationships between leadership, process and outcome suggested by review findings

Source: Wong et al., 2013, p. 717

safety climates (Thompson et al., 2011). Despite these promising findings linking LMX to positive outcomes, research on LMX in nursing is limited.

Authentic leadership (Avolio, Gardner, Walumbwa, Luthans, & May, 2004) is a relatively new leadership theory from the field of positive organisational psychology. Authentic leadership focuses on the authenticity or genuineness of leaders and suggests that leadership is transparent, grounded in ethical values and responsive to others' needs and values (Avolio et al., 2004; Wong & Cummings, 2009). In this relational leadership style, authentic leadership (AL) is a collective process created by leaders and followers together. Work outcomes have been linked to authentic leadership in research studies reported in both management and nursing literature. In management literature, findings included evidence of positive relationships between authentic leadership and performance, trust in leaders, job satisfaction and work engagement. In nursing, authentic leadership has been linked to greater trust in management, empowerment, work engagement, job satisfaction, higher ratings of patient care quality and lower ratings of burnout and adverse patient outcomes (Giallonardo, Wong, & Iwasiw, 2010; Laschinger, Wong, & Grau, 2013; Wong, Laschinger, & Cummings, 2010; Wong & Giallonardo, 2013).

LEADERSHIP AND PATIENT SAFETY

Patient safety has been a leading theme in the literature and in healthcare organisations since the late 1990s. Defined as 'the absence of preventable harm to a patient during the process of health care' (WHO, 2013), the World Health Organization (WHO) recognises patient safety as an issue of global importance that requires much work and research. The patient safety movement emphasises the reporting, analysis and prevention of errors that often lead to adverse health events. Several studies in the United States, the United Kingdom, Australia and New Zealand have shown that adverse events may occur in anywhere from 3.7% to 16.6% of all hospital admissions and that a significant portion of these may be preventable (White, McGillis Hall, & Lalonde, 2011). A number of factors are reported to influence adverse patient outcomes including perceptions about error and system/organisational factors such as stressful work environments, inadequate communication, excessive workloads, ineffective care processes, staff shortages or stressful environments or poor communication (Ausserhofer et al., 2013; Duffield et al., 2011; Stone et al., 2007).

In a follow-up to a major report, *To Err is Human*, profiling adverse events in the American healthcare system (Kohn, Corrigan, & Donaldson, 2000), the Institute of Medicine (IOM) points to the critical role nursing plays in providing safe care and identifying healthcare management practices necessary to create a positive patient safety culture (Page, 2004). Identified practices include creating and maintaining trust throughout the organisation, deploying healthcare workers in adequate numbers, creating a culture of openness regarding reporting and prevention of errors, involving workers in decision making pertaining to work design and work flow, and actively managing the process of change. The report specifically targets the salient role of strong nursing leadership to implement effective management practices that create 'cultures of safety' (Page, 2004, p. 253) and improve patient outcomes. Reports in other countries also profile the need for safer patient care environments and echoed the call for leadership to make the required changes (Baker et al., 2004; Wilson et al., 1995). The IOM emphasised that quality of patient care is directly affected by the degree to which hospital nurses are active and empowered participants in decisions about their patients' plans of care and by the degree to which they have an active and central role in organisational decision making (Page, 2004). Patient safety has always been fundamental to nursing care and to healthcare more generally, across all settings and sectors (International Council of Nurses, 2012). Concern for safety and ultimately overall quality of care must be a fundamental driving force behind the work of nursing leaders and managers.

Recently, much of the research on patient safety has focused on patient safety climate (Singer et al., 2009; Taylor et al., 2012). Safety climate relates to the attitudes, values and beliefs about patient safety (Feng, Bobay, & Weiss, 2008) and is usually measured using items that describe the degree of staff participation in safety behaviours and perceptions of the importance of patient safety (Singer, Lin, Falwell, Gaba, & Baker, 2009; Sexton, Thomas, & Helmreich, 2000). In a review of safety literature, Lekka, Healey, and Hill (2012) found consistent associations between transformational leadership and staff safety outcomes (Lekka et al., 2012). Specifically, transformational leadership was positively related to a number of employee safety outcomes including fostering perceptions of a positive safety climate, encouraging higher levels of employee involvement in safety activities, compliance with safety measures and safety citizenship behaviours such as participating in safety committees and looking out for the safety of others. While findings have consistently linked patient outcomes to nurse work environment factors, the effect of patient safety climate on patient outcomes is mixed; thus, there is a need for more studies as well as studies linking leadership to safety climate and patient outcomes.

PRACTICAL IMPLICATIONS: LEADERSHIP ACTIONS FOR OPTIMISING PATIENT SAFETY AND OUTCOMES

Findings from research emphasise the value of relational leadership styles and, predominantly, transformational leadership, in healthcare workplaces. These findings also support other reviews where relational leadership styles are positively related to nurses' motivation to perform (Brady-Germain & Cummings, 2010), improved work environments and nurses' work outcomes (Cummings, MacGregor, et al., 2010), and nurse retention (Cowden, Cummings, & Profetto-McGrath, 2011). These findings suggest that a complex interaction between the relational practices of formal nursing leaders to provide vision, support and resources for positive practice environments and the health, knowledge, competencies and motivation of nurses contribute to quality care and optimal patient outcomes.

Positive work environments include those elements that foster strong nursing practice such as collaborative teamwork, autonomous decision making, professional development, adequate staffing and skill mix since these are the elements most closely aligned with patient safety, potential adverse events and patient outcomes (Estabrooks et al., 2005; Lake, 2002). These environments are created by the contributions of both unit leaders and staff. To create these supportive practice environments, leaders must have the vision, problem-solving abilities and the relationship-building and influencing skills to navigate the dynamic context and structure of organisations to obtain needed resources. They also need to engage staff in a way that instils a sense of accountability, confidence and professionalism. Transformational leaders motivate and inspire staff to be the best they can be and to exert extra effort to meet goals.

Transformational leadership is a relational leadership style where the focus of the relationship is on developing the individual and the leader to their fullest potential in line with the organisation's goals (Bass & Avolio, 1994). Four elements characterise transformational leadership as outlined in Table 12.2: (1) idealised influence occurs when leaders are perceived as having high ideals and a strong sense of ethics; (2) inspirational motivation which describes leaders who communicate high expectations and inspire commitment to a shared vision; (3) intellectual stimulation describes leader behaviours that promote innovation and new ways of approaching problems; and (4) individualised consideration that includes creating a supportive environment and attending to the needs and concerns of followers. Transactional leadership is a style of leadership in which leaders promote compliance of followers through reciprocal transactions aimed at achieving specified work objectives where rewards are

Table 12.2 Transformational and transactional leadership behaviours for optimising patient safety and outcomes

Transformational and transactional leadership dimensions	Behaviours for optimising patient outcomes
Idealised influence: the charismatic qualities of the leader and a leader's consistent conduct based on underlying principles, ethics and values	Displays visible commitment to patient care and safety Acts as role model for championing optimal patient care Promotes mutual trust through openness, honesty, integrity and behavioural consistency Communicates clear ethics and values as the basis for decision making Actively incorporates staff suggestions in patient care improvement activities Ensures appropriate staff and resources are in place to manage workload
Inspirational motivation: leader behaviours that generate optimism and hope in followers and promote commitment to a shared vision	Inspires and motivates staff for best performance and safety Articulates a clear vision for patient care and outcomes Fosters perceptions of a positive climate for optimal performance and safety Promotes high levels of participation in quality improvement and safety activities Creates opportunities for meaningful dialogue with staff on patient care issues that could impede patient safety Promotes staff citizenship behaviours in relation to patient care and safety
Intellectual stimulation: leader behaviours that challenge followers to be innovative by questioning assumptions, reframing problems, finding solutions and acting proactively	Challenges current knowledge and practices with a view to change and improvement Enhances knowledge and awareness of patient care issues Uses problems and errors as a learning opportunity to improve practice and evaluate changes Encourages creativity and innovation in improving care processes Engages staff in point-of-care problem solving

Table 12.2 cont

Transformational and transactional leadership dimensions	Behaviours for optimising patient outcomes
Individual consideration: gives personal attention to the individual needs of each staff member and strives to develop a supportive climate	Recognises good patient care and safety practices
	Expresses appreciation for staff contributions
	Openly discusses patient care problems and safety concerns
	Provides positive and constructive feedback
	Promotes a no-blame climate in response to errors
	Acts as a coach and mentor for quality patient care
	Creates a supportive learning environment where staff are developed to higher levels of achievement
Transactional: leader behaviours based on reciprocal 'transactions' aimed at achieving specified work objectives where rewards are usually contingent on performance	Clarifies role and performance expectations
	Monitors and recognises/rewards good performance
	Promotes compliance with safety rules and procedures and patient care standards and processes

usually dependent on performance. In Table 12.2 examples of leader behaviours or actions that can be purposely focused on improving patient outcomes and organised according to the four elements of transformational and transactional leadership styles are presented.

Effective leadership is vital to provide guidance for solving complex problems related to nursing care delivery. With a potential shortage of nursing leaders and nurses, it is increasingly important to find ways to recruit, develop and retain nursing leaders to ensure positive outcomes for the healthcare system (Laschinger et al., 2008). Relational leadership styles are grounded in the emotional intelligence (Goleman, Boyatzis, & McKee, 2002) competencies known as self-awareness, self-management, social awareness and relationship management. Thus, the hiring of leaders with relational skills, or providing training for existing leaders, becomes a priority consideration in organisations (Cummings, 2004; Young-Ritchie, Laschinger, & Wong, 2009). While clinical competencies are very important, leaders who are skilled in emotional intelligence have the ability to monitor their own and others' emotions, use this information to build solid working relationships with others and are assets to the system.

A relational approach to leadership contributes to healthy work environments through support, and genuine, open and honest communication. Leaders who create opportunities for meaningful dialogue with nurses to resolve patient care issues that risk patient safety and then follow through on staff suggestions for improvement role model their commitment to patient care. The research evidence found connecting supportive leadership styles and positive patient safety outcomes emphasises how important it is for unit leaders to understand and value patient care and the contributions of nurses and other care providers in promoting better outcomes (Thompson et al., 2011; Tregunno et al., 2009). The capacity of leaders to promote a safe workplace is governed by their knowledge of patient care needs, the quality of their relational skills and their competence to implement safe care.

CONCLUSION

In this chapter we provided an examination of the current state of the evidence describing the influence of nursing leadership on patient outcomes. Findings to date show a promising research foundation that supports the contribution of relational, transformational nursing leadership to positive patient outcomes. Specifically, the current evidence suggests a clear relationship between relational leadership styles and lower patient mortality and reduced medication errors, restraint use and hospital-acquired infections. Some examples of strategies leaders and managers can use in practice to build positive work environments that optimise patient safety and outcomes were discussed.

REFLECTIVE EXERCISE

1. Reflect on leaders and managers you have worked with who have had a positive influence on patient outcomes in your nursing practice setting.

    a. Reflect on what values, behaviours and actions they showed that most affected patient outcomes and how.

    b. Consider how your own values about patient care might influence your actions in a leadership role.

2. Think of a clinical/patient care issue or problem that you are passionate about and would like to see improved. Imagine you have a month to make a difference and create a plan identifying some leadership actions, the support needed from others and how you will evaluate results.

    a. What would you do if you could not get support from others for your issue?

    b. Reflect on why the issue might be important to you but not to others.

3. Visit the website of one of your local hospitals and search to see what information is available to the public about the patient outcomes tracked in that organisation. Do they report the incidence of adverse patient events? If so, what are your impressions of the information presented?

Recommended Readings

McCutcheon, A. S., Doran, D., Evans, M., McGillis Hall, L., & Pringle, D. (2009). Understanding nurse manager stress and work complexity: Factors that make a difference. *Nursing Leadership, 22*(3), 48–67.

Murphy, J. (2009). Role of clinical nurse leadership in improving patient care. *Nursing Management, 16*(8), 26–28.

Page, A. (2004). *Keeping patients safe: Transforming the work environment of nurses.* Washington, DC: National Academies Press.

Squires, M., Tourangeau, A., Laschinger, H. K., & Doran, D. (2010). The link between leadership and safety outcomes in hospitals. *Journal of Nursing Management, 18*, 914–925.

Thompson, D. N., Hoffman, L. A., Sereika, S. M., Lorenz, H. L., Wolf, G. A., Burns, H. K., et al. (2011). A relational leadership perspective on unit-level safety climate. *Journal of Nursing Administration, 41*(11), 479–487.

References

Aiken, L. H., Clarke, S. P., & Sloane, D. M. (2000). Hospital restructuring: Does it adversely affect care and outcomes? *Journal of Nursing Administration, 30*, 457–465.

Aiken, L. H., Clarke, S. P., Sloane, D. M., Lake, E. T., & Cheney, T. (2008). Effects of hospital care environment on patient mortality and nurse outcomes. *Journal of Nursing Administration, 38*(5), 223–229.

Aiken, L. H., & Patrician, P. A. (2000). Measuring organizational traits of hospitals: The Revised Nursing Work Index. *Nursing Research, 49*, 146–153.

Anderson, R. A., Issel, L. M., & McDaniel, R. R. (2003). Nursing homes as complex adaptive systems. *Nursing Research, 52*(1), 12–21.

Ausserhofer, D., Schubert, M., Desmedt, M., Blegen, M. A., De Geest, S., & Schwendimann, R. (2013). The association of patient safety climate and nurse-related organizational factors with selected patient outcomes: A cross-sectional survey. *International Journal of Nursing Studies, 50*(2), 240–252.

Avolio, B. J., Gardner, W. L., Walumbwa, F. O., Luthans, F., & May, D. R. (2004). Unlocking the mask: A look at the process by which authentic leaders impact follower attitudes and behaviours. *Leadership Quarterly, 15*, 801–823.

Baker, G. R., Norton, P. G., Flintoft, V., Blais, R., Brown, A., Cox, J., et al. (2004). The Canadian Adverse Events Study: The incidence of adverse events among hospital patients in Canada. *Canadian Medical Association Journal, 170*(11), 1678–1686.

Bass, B. M., & Avolio, B. J. (1994). *Improving organizational effectiveness through transformational leadership.* Thousand Oaks, CA: Sage.

Bass, B., & Avolio, B. (2000). *Multifactor Leadership Questionnaire.* Redwood City, CA: Mind Garden, Inc.

Bass, B. M., & Stogdill, R. M. (1990). *Bass and Stogdill's handbook of leadership: Theory, research and applications.* New York, NY: Free Press.

Baumann, A., Giovannetti, P., O'Brien-Pallas, L., Mallette, C., Deber, R., Blythe, J., et al. (2001). Healthcare restructuring: The impact of job change. *Canadian Journal of Nursing Leadership, 14*(1), 14–20.

Blegen, M. A., Goode, C. J., Spetz, J., Vaughn, T., & Park, S. H. (2011). Nurse staffing effects on patient outcomes: Safety-net and non-safety-net hospitals. *Medical Care, 49*(4), 406–414.

Bono, J. E., & Judge, T. A. (2004). Personality and transformational and transactional leadership: A meta-analysis. *Journal of Applied Psychology, 89*, 901–910.

Boyle, S. M. (2004). Nursing unit characteristics and patient outcomes. *Nursing Economics, 22*(3), 111–123.

Brady-Germain, P., & Cummings, G. G. (2010). The influence of nursing leadership on nurse performance: A systematic literature review. *Journal of Nursing Management, 18*, 425–439.

Capuano, T., Bokovoy, J., Hitchings, K., & Houser, J. (2005). Use of a validated model to evaluate the impact of the work environment on outcomes at a magnet hospital. *Health Care Management Review, 30*(3), 229–236.

Castle, N. G., & Decker, F. H. (2011). Top management leadership style and quality of care in nursing homes. *The Gerontologist, 51*(5), 630–642.

Cho, S. H., Ketefian, S., Barkauskas, V. H., & Smith, D. G. (2003). The effects of nurse staffing on adverse events, morbidity, mortality, and medical costs. *Nursing Research, 52*(2), 71–79.

Clarke, S. P. (2011). Healthcare utilization. In D. M. Doran (Ed.), *Nursing outcomes: The state of the science* (2nd ed., pp. 487–508). Sudbury MA: Jones & Bartlett Learning.

Cowden, T., Cummings, G., & Profetto-McGrath, J. (2011). *Journal of Nursing Management, 19,* 461–477.

Cummings, G. G. (2004). Investing relational energy: The hallmark of resonant leadership. *Canadian Journal of Nursing Leadership, 17*(4), 76–87.

Cummings, G. G., & Estabrooks, C. A. (2003). The effects of hospital restructuring that included layoffs on individual nurses who remained employed: A systematic review. *International Journal of Sociology & Social Policy, 8/9,* 8–53.

Cummings, G. G., MacGregor, T., Davey, M., Lee, H., Wong, C. A., Lo, E., et al. (2010). Leadership styles and outcome patterns for the nursing workforce and work environment: A systematic review. *International Journal of Nursing Studies, 47,* 363–385.

Cummings, G. G., Midodzi, W. K., Wong, C. A., & Estabrooks, C. A. (2010). The contribution of hospital nursing leadership styles to 30-day patient mortality. *Nursing Research, 59*(5), 331–339.

Davidson, H., Folcarelli, P., Crawford, S., Duprat, L., & Clifford, J. (1997). Effects of healthcare reforms on job satisfaction and voluntary turnover among hospital based nurses. *Medical Care, 35*(6), 634–645.

Doran, D., McCutcheon, A. S., Evans, M. G., MacMillan, K., McGillis-Hall, L., Pringle, D., et al. (2004). *Impact of the manager's span of control on leadership and performance.* Ottawa, Ontario: Canadian Health Services Research Foundation.

Doran, D. M., & Pringle, D. (2011). Patient outcomes as an accountability. In D. M. Doran (Ed.), *Nursing outcomes: The state of the science* (2nd ed., pp. 1–27). Sudbury MA: Jones & Bartlett Learning.

Duffield, C., Diers, D., O'Brien-Pallas, L., Aisbett, C., Roche, M., King, M., et al. (2011). Nursing staffing, nursing workload, the work environment and patient outcomes. *Applied Nursing Research, 24,* 244–255.

Estabrooks, C. A., Midodzi, W. K., Cummings, G. G., Ricker, K. L., & Giovannetti, P. (2005). The impact of hospital nursing characteristics on 30-day mortality. *Nursing Research, 54*(2), 74–84.

Feng, X., Bobay, K., & Weiss, M. (2008). Patient safety culture in nursing: A dimensional concept analysis. *Journal of Advanced Nursing, 63*(3), 310–319.

Fine, B. A., Golden, B., Hannam, R., & Morra, D. (2009). Leading lean: A Canadian healthcare leader's guide. *Healthcare Quarterly, 12*(3), 32–41.

Flynn, L., Liang, Y., Dickson, G. L., & Aiken, L. H. (2010). Effects of nursing practice environments on quality outcomes in nursing homes. *Journal of the American Geriatrics Society, 58*(12), 2401–2406.

Gardner, J. K., Thomas-Hawkins, C., Fogg, L., & Latham, C. E. (2007). The relationships between nurses' perceptions of the hemodialysis unit work environment and nurse turnover, patient satisfaction, and hospitalizations. *Nephrology Nursing Journal, 34*(3), 271–281.

Giallonardo, L., Wong, C. A., & Iwasiw, C. (2010). Authentic leadership of preceptors: Predictor of new graduate nurses' work engagement and job satisfaction. *Journal of Nursing Management, 18,* 993–1003.

Goleman, D., Boyatzis, R., & McKee, A. (2002). *The new leaders: Transforming the art of leadership into the science of results.* London, UK: Little Brown.

Graen, G., & Uhl-Bein, M. (1995). Relationship-based approach to leadership: Development of leader-member exchange (LMX) theory of leadership over 25 years: Applying a multi-level multi-domain perspective. *Leadership Quarterly, 6,* 219–247.

Hansen, L. O., Williams, M. V., & Singer, S. J. (2011). Perceptions of hospital safety climate and incidence of readmission. *Health Services Research, 46*(2), 596–616.

Havig, A. K., Skogstad, A., Kjekshus, L. E., & Romoren, T. I. (2011). Leadership, staffing and quality of care in nursing homes. *BMC Health Services Research, 11*(327), doi:10.1186/1472-6963-11-327. Retrieved from <http://www.biomedcentral.com/1472-6963/11/327>.

Houser, J. (2003). A model for evaluating the context of nursing care delivery. *Journal of Nursing Administration, 33*(1), 39–47.

Huston, C. (2008). Preparing nurse leaders for 2010. *Journal of Nursing Management, 16,* 905–911.

International Council of Nurses (ICN) (2012). Position statement on patient safety. Retrieved from <http://www.icn.ch/images/stories/documents/publications/position_statements/D05_Patient_Safety.pdf>.

Kohn, L. T., Corrigan, J. M., & Donaldson, M. S. (2000). *To err is human: Building a safer health system.* Institute of Medicine. A report of the Committee on Quality of Health Care in America.

Kouzes, J. M., & Posner, B. Z. (1995). *The leadership challenge: How to get extraordinary things done in organizations* (2nd ed.). San Francisco, CA: Jossey-Bass.

Kovner, C., & Gergen, P. (1998). Nurse staffing levels and adverse events following surgery in U.S. hospitals. *Image: Journal of Nursing Scholarship, 30*(4), 315–321.

Kroposki, M., & Alexander, J. W. (2006). Correlation among client satisfaction, nursing perception of outcomes, and organizational variables. *Home Healthcare Nurse, 24*(2), 87–94.

Lake, E. T. (2002). Development of the practice environment scale of the Nursing Work Index. *Research in Nursing and Health, 25*(3), 176–188.

Larrabee, J. H., Ostrow, C. L., Withrow, M. L., Janney, M. A., Hobbs, G. R., & Buran, C. (2004). Predictors of patient satisfaction with inpatient hospital nursing care. *Research in Nursing & Health, 27,* 254–268.

Laschinger, H. K. S., Finegan, J., & Wilk, P. (2009). Context matters: The impact of unit leadership and empowerment on nurses' organizational commitment. *Journal of Nursing Administration, 39*(5), 228–235.

Laschinger, H. K., Gilbert, S., & Smith, L. (2011). Patient satisfaction as a nurse-sensitive outcome. In D. M. Doran (Ed.), *Nursing outcomes: The state of the science* (2nd ed., pp. 359–408). Sudbury MA: Jones & Bartlett Learning.

Laschinger, H. K., Wong, C. A., & Grau, A. (2013). Authentic leadership, empowerment and burnout: A comparison in new graduates and experienced nurses. *Journal of Nursing Management, 21*(3), 541–552.

Laschinger, H. K., Wong, C. A., Ritchie, J., D'Amour, D., Vincent, L., Wilk, P., et al. (2008). A profile of the structure and impact of nursing management in Canadian hospitals. *Healthcare Quarterly, 11*(2), 85–94.

Lekka, C., Healey, N., & Hill, H. (2012). *A review of the literature on effective leadership behaviours for safety.* Report prepared by the Health and Safety Laboratory for the Health and Safety Executive. Retrieved from <http://www.hse.gov.uk/research/rrpdf/rr952.pdf>.

Lord, R. G., & Dinh, J. E. (2012). Aggregation processes and levels of analysis as organizing structures for leadership theories. In D. V. Day & J. Antonakis (Eds.), *The nature of leadership* (2nd ed., pp. 29–65). Thousand Oaks, CA: Sage.

Lowe, G. S. (2005). Raising the bar for people practices: Helping all health organizations become 'preferred employers'. *Healthcare Quarterly, 8*(1), 60–63.

McGillis Hall, L., Doran, D., Baker, R. G., Pink, G. H., Sidani, S., O'Brien-Pallas, L., et al. (2003). Nurse staffing models as predictors of patient outcomes. *Medical Care, 41*(9), 1096–1109.

McNeese-Smith, D. K. (1999). The relationship between managerial motivation, leadership, nurse outcomes and patient satisfaction. *Journal of Organizational Behavior, 20,* 243–259.

Needleman, J., Buerhaus, P., Pankratz, V. S., Leibson, C. L., Stevens, S. R., & Harris, M. (2011). Nurse staffing and inpatient hospital mortality. *New England Journal of Medicine, 364*(11), 1037–1045.

Northouse, P. G. (2013). *Leadership: Theory and practice* (6th ed.). Thousand Oaks, CA: Sage.

Page, A. (2004). *Keeping patients safe: Transforming the work environment of nurses.* Washington, DC: National Academies Press.

Paquet, M., Courcy, F., Lavoie-Tremblay, M., Gagnon, S., & Maillet, S. (2013). Psychosocial work environment and prediction of quality of care indicators in one Canadian health center. *Worldviews on Evidence-based Nursing, 10*(2), 82–94.

Pollack, M. M., & Koch, M. A. (2003). Association of outcomes with organizational characteristics of neonatal intensive care units. *Critical Care Medicine, 31*(6), 1620–1629.

Raup, G. H. (2008). The impact of ED nurse manager leadership style on staff nurse turnover and patient satisfaction in academic health center hospitals. *Journal of Emergency Nursing, 34*(5), 403–409.

Sexton, J. B., Thomas, E. J., & Helmreich, R. L. (2000). Error, stress, and teamwork in medicine and aviation: Cross sectional surveys. *BMJ, 320*(7237), 745–749.

Singer, S., Lin, S., Falwell, A., Gaba, D., & Baker, L. (2009). Relationship of safety climate and safety performance in hospitals. *Health Services Research, 44*(2), 399–421.

Stone, P. W., Mooney-Kane, C., Larson, E. L., Horan, T., Glance, L. G., Zwanziger, J., et al. (2007). Nurse working conditions and patient safety outcomes. *Medical Care, 45*(6), 571–578.

Taylor, J. A., Dominici, F., Agnew, J., Gerwin, D., Morlock, L., & Miller, M. R. (2012). Do nurse and patient injuries share common antecedents? An analysis of associations with safety climate and working conditions. *BMJ Quality & Safety, 21*(2), 101–111. doi:10.1136/bmjqs-2011-000082.

Thompson, D. N., Hoffman, L. A., Sereika, S. M., Lorenz, H. L., Wolf, G. A., Burns, H. K., et al. (2011). A relational leadership perspective on unit-level safety climate. *Journal of Nursing Administration, 41*(11), 479–487.

Tourangeau, A. E., Doran, D. M., McGillis Hall, L., O'Brien Pallas, L., Pringle, D., Tu, J. V., et al. (2007). Impact of hospital nursing care on 30-day mortality for acute medical patients. *Journal of Advanced Nursing, 57*(1), 32–44.

Tourangeau, A. E., Giovannetti, P., Tu, J. V., & Wood, M. (2002). Nursing-related determinants of 30-day mortality for hospitalized patients. *Canadian Journal of Nursing Research, 33*(4), 71–88.

Tregunno, D., Jeffs, L., McGillis Hall, L., Baker, R., Doran, D., & Bassett, S. (2009). On the ball— Leadership for patient safety and learning in critical care. *Journal of Nursing Administration, 39*(7/8), 334–339.

Vogus, T. J., & Sutcliffe, K. M. (2007). The impact of safety organizing, trusted leadership, and care pathways on reported medication errors in hospital nursing units. *Medical Care, 45*(10), 997–1002.

White, P., McGillis Hall, L., & Lalonde, M. (2011). Adverse patient outcomes. In D. M. Doran (Ed.), *Nursing outcomes: The state of the science* (2nd ed., pp. 241–284). Sudbury MA: Jones & Bartlett Learning.

Wilson, R. M., Runciman, W. B., Gibberd, R. W., Harrison, B. T., Newby, L., & Hamilton, J. D. (1995). The quality in Australian health care study. *Medical Journal of Australia, 163*(9), 458–476.

Wong, C. A., & Cummings, G. G. (2007). The relationship between nursing leadership and patient outcomes: A systematic review. *Journal of Nursing Management, 15*(5), 508–521.

Wong, C. A., & Cummings, G. G. (2009). Authentic leadership: A new theory for nursing or back to basics? *Journal of Health Organization and Management, 23*(5), 522–538.

Wong, C. A., Cummings, G. G., & Ducharme, L. (2013). The relationship between nursing leadership and patient outcomes: A systematic review update. *Journal of Nursing Management, 21*, 709–724.

Wong, C. A., & Giallonardo, L. (2013). Authentic leadership and nurse-assessed adverse patient outcomes. *Journal of Nursing Management, 21*, 740–752.

Wong, C. A., Laschinger, H. K., & Cummings, G. G. (2010). Authentic leadership and nurses' voice behaviour and perceptions of care quality. *Journal of Nursing Management, 18*, 889–900.

Wong, C. A., Laschinger, H. K., Cummings, G. G., Vincent, L., & O'Connor, P. (2010). Decisional involvement of senior nurse leaders in Canadian acute care hospitals. *Journal of Nursing Management, 18*(2), 122–133.

World Health Organization (WHO) (2013). *What is patient safety?* Retrieved from <http://www.who.int/patientsafety/about/en/index.html>.

Young-Ritchie, C., Laschinger, H. K. S., & Wong, C. (2009). The effects of emotionally intelligent leadership behaviour on emergency staff nurses' workplace empowerment and organizational commitment. *Nursing Leadership, 22*(1), 70–85.

CHAPTER THIRTEEN

Leadership and empowerment in nursing

Heather Laschinger, Christine Duffield
& Emily Read

LEARNING OBJECTIVES

At the completion of this chapter, the reader will be able to:

▲ give a comprehensive overview of the relationship between positive leadership practices and structural empowerment in nursing workplaces;

▲ describe and compare several different types of leadership theories and styles that foster nurses' empowerment;

▲ have an understanding of relationally focused and behaviourally focused leadership styles in relation to their influence on nurse empowerment;

▲ summarise the current body of evidence linking leadership and empowerment in nursing and will have received some directions for future research in this area;

▲ provide an overview of outcomes associated with structural empowerment that provide benefits to nurses, patients and healthcare organisations.

KEY WORDS

Empowerment, leadership, nursing work environment

INTRODUCTION

The nursing profession is facing a severe workforce shortage as many nurses near retirement and greater attention is paid to recruitment and retention of nursing staff in healthcare organisations. Leadership plays a key role in ensuring that employees are able to optimise their performance in healthcare settings. For nurses, the ability to provide high-quality patient care is a key determinant of work satisfaction and perceptions of patient care quality (Blegen, Goode, & Reed, 1998; Dignam, Duffield, Stasa, Gray, Jackson, & Daly, 2012; Duffield, Diers et al., 2011; Irvine & Evans, 1995). Leadership is often defined as the ability to influence others to accomplish common goals and this is achieved by making sure that conditions are in place to enable the accomplishment of work in meaningful ways.

For many years empowering leadership has been linked to a wide array of factors that influence the retention of staff nurses (Laschinger, Leiter, Day, & Gilin, 2009; McNeese-Smith, 1995). According to Kanter (1977, 1993) basic social structures in the workplace create necessary conditions to empower employees to accomplish meaningful work. From this perspective, empowerment is a fundamental leadership strategy that fosters high-quality nursing practice and ultimately high-quality patient care. Research has demonstrated the essential role of nursing leadership in creating empowering work environments that engage nurses and enrich their work lives in order to retain a satisfied nursing workforce (Duffield, Roche, O'Brien-Pallas, Catling-Paull, & King, 2009; Duffield, Baldwin, Roche, & Weiss, 2013; Force, 2005; Tuckey, Bakker, & Dollard, 2012; Weberg, 2010).

Kanter's structural empowerment theory

Kanter (1977, 1993) describes four key organisational empowerment structures: access to information, support, resources needed to do the job, and opportunities to learn and grow. Access to information means having knowledge of organisational decisions, policies and goals, as well as data, technical knowledge, and expertise that enable one to be effective within the broader context of the organisation. For example, being provided with access to reference material for technical procedures that are not performed regularly can remind nurses of the step-by-step process involved and ensure they gather the correct supplies before entering a patient's room. Information provides employees with a sense of purpose and meaning, while enhancing their ability to make informed decisions, provide high-quality patient care and contribute to organisational goals. Access to support includes informal and formal feedback and guidance received from superiors, peers and subordinates. Leaders can provide support in a multitude of ways. For example, a leader may provide support for others' ideas by including others' feedback in their decision-making processes or show empathy and compassion to a nurse who is having a tough day. Access to resources refers to individuals' capability to access the materials, money, supplies, time and equipment required to accomplish organisational goals. Limited resources constrain nurses' ability to be effective in their work, though it can lead to innovation and creative problem solving. For example, if a patient requires a special wound dressing that is expensive or unavailable, it may be more difficult for the nurse to provide ideal care to that patient. Opportunity to learn and grow includes access to challenging work, rewards and professional development opportunities, such as ongoing training and attending educational workshops.

Formal and informal job characteristics facilitate employee access to these empowerment structures. Formal power is the ability to exercise control over one's job and make decisions at work. It is enhanced by flexible jobs central to the organisation's goals that allow employees to implement creativity and discretionary decision making. Informal power describes an employee's level of social influence at work that comes from developing effective relationships and communication channels both within and outside the organisation (Kanter, 1977, 1993). According to Kanter (1993), employees who have access to these conditions are empowered to accomplish their work in meaningful ways; that is, they work in structurally empowering workplaces. Empowered individuals have control and influence over conditions that make their actions possible, resulting in improved overall organisational functioning. Those with access to the power and opportunity structures within an organisation are highly motivated and are able to motivate and empower others by sharing their sources of power. Importantly, empowered nurses may also be a source of patient empowerment by sharing this power with patients. Recently, Laschinger, Gilbert, Smith, and Leslie (2010) proposed an expanded version of Kanter's model that links nurses' workplace empowerment to patient empowerment, although this model has yet to be tested empirically.

Structural empowerment has been linked to numerous positive organisational outcomes in nursing settings including higher job satisfaction (Cicolini, Comparcini, & Simonetti, 2013; Ning, Zhong, Libo, & Qiujie, 2009; Wong & Laschinger, 2012), organisational commitment (Smith, Andrusyszyn, & Laschinger, 2010; Yang, Liu, Huang, & Zhu, 2013), feelings of trust and respect in the workplace (Laschinger, Wong, & Cummings, in press), and higher ratings of patient care quality (Laschinger et al., 2010) and performance (Wong & Laschinger, 2012). Structural empowerment has also been shown to be associated with lower levels of burnout, bullying and incivility in the workplace (Laschinger, Wong, & Grau, 2013), better mental and physical health (Wing, Regan, & Laschinger, in press), and lower job and career turnover intentions (Laschinger & Fida, 2013; Nedd, 2006).

Numerous studies have linked leadership practices to nurses' workplace empowerment and subsequent positive attitudes and behaviours (Laschinger, 2008; Laschinger, Finegan, & Wilk, 2011; Laschinger & Smith, 2013). This is logical because nurse managers are in a position to shape the conditions of the workplace that influence how employees experience their day-to-day work (Duffield, Roche, Blay, & Stasa, 2011). Empirical studies linking leadership to Kanter's notion of organisational empowerment are summarised in the following section.

RESEARCH LINKING LEADERSHIP TO STRUCTURAL EMPOWERMENT

A variety of leadership models have been used to investigate the relationships between leadership and structural empowerment of nurses. We divided these models into 1) relationally focused leadership and 2) behaviourally focused leadership categories in terms of their primary orientation. Table 13.1 summarises the empirical relationships between leadership and structural empowerment across this body of research.

Relationally focused leadership models

Leader member exchange theory

The Leader Member Exchange (LMX) model of leadership emphasises the importance of high-quality relationships between leaders and their employees (members) (Dansereau, Graen, & Haga, 1975; Liden & Maslyn, 1998). LMX theory is based on the idea that the quality of relationships between leader–follower dyads depends on both parties' perceptions of contribution (quality and quantity of work activities directed at achieving mutual goals), loyalty (the degree to which the leader and member provide support to each other publicly), professional respect (being considerate), and

Table 13.1 Empirical relationships between leadership and structural empowerment

Leadership	Empowerment				
	Total empowerment	Support	Resources	Information	Opportunity
Relational leadership					
Leader member exchange					
Laschinger, Finegan, & Wilk (2011)	.36	.35	.22	.19	.25
Bamford, Wong, & Laschinger (2012) JNM	.50	.34	.28	.39	.21
Davies, Wong, & Laschinger (2011)	.50	.34	.28	.39	13
Laschinger, Purdy, & Almost (2007)	.42	–	–	–	–
Authentic leadership					
Laschinger, Wong, & Grau (2012)	.40	.43	.31	.25	.14
Laschinger & Smith (2013)	.42	.42	.32	.25	.17
Resonant leadership					
Laschinger, Wong, & Grau (2013)	.47	.44	.34	.33	.33
Emotional intelligence					
Young-Ritchie, Laschinger, & Wong (2009)	.54	.53	.37	.35	.16
Lucus, Laschinger, & Wong (2008)	.62	.64	.41	.26	.31
Behavioural leadership					
Kouzes & Posner (Laschinger et al. 2012)	.34	.36	.20	.33	.18
Patrick, Laschinger, Wong, & Finegan (2011)	.69	–	–	–	–
Leader empowering behaviours					
Greco, Laschinger, & Wong (2006)	.71	.64	.36	.47	33
Laschinger & Wong (1999)	.61	.56	.47	.43	.51
Magnet hospital leadership					
Laschinger (2008)	.60	–	–	–	–
Manojlovich & Laschinger (2007)	.59	.38	.56	.32	.30

affect (how well the leader and member like each other as people) (Liden & Maslyn, 1998). High LMX quality refers to leader–follower relationships characterised by mutual trust, loyalty, support and respect.

From an LMX perspective, leaders and followers are more likely to invest resources into one another if they view each other as likable people who are working towards shared goals (Liden & Maslyn, 1998). Although there may be varying levels of LMX between leaders and individual nurses on a particular unit there is evidence that leaders may relate to followers in ways that colour the nature of overall leader–follower relationships on a work unit and promote positive outcomes. For example, Laschinger et al. (2011) found that nursing units with high LMX were likely to have higher levels of structural empowerment and that nurses who worked on these units experienced less burnout and higher job satisfaction. These studies show that leader–member relationships play an important role in creating a structurally empowering work environment. High LMX quality has been found to be significantly related to structural empowerment in studies of nurses at the individual level (Laschinger et al., 2011) and nurse managers (Laschinger, Almost, Purdy, & Kim, 2004).

Authentic leadership theory

More recently, structural empowerment of nurses has been linked to their immediate supervisors' authentic leadership behaviour (Laschinger, Wong, & Grau, 2013; Laschinger & Smith, 2013). Authentic leadership is a relatively new model of leadership that defines four fundamental leadership qualities necessary for leadership effectiveness. Characteristics of authentic leadership are: 1) self-awareness (having insight into one's abilities, strengths and weaknesses); 2) an internalised moral perspective (acting in accordance with one's inner values and beliefs); 3) balanced processing (considering multiple points of view when making decisions); and 4) relational transparency (being clear, upfront and honest in relationships with other people) (Avolio & Gardner, 2005). These authors contend that authentic leaders create conditions that foster trust and build employee confidence in accomplishing work goals thereby increasing both employee and organisational performance. Authentic leaders influence performance by purposely focusing on employees' strengths and encouraging them to derive a sense of meaning in their work to take a hopeful, optimistic and confident approach. In this way, nurse leaders who engage in authentic leadership behaviour cultivate the growth and development of followers (Wong & Cummings, 2009).

Providing access to Kanter's (1977, 1993) empowerment structures is one way in which authentic leaders contribute to nurses' success in achieving their work and professional development goals. Research has shown that staff nurses' perceptions of authentic leadership behaviours by their immediate supervisor are associated with higher levels of structural empowerment regardless of experience level (Laschinger, Wong, & Grau, 2013; Wong & Laschinger, 2012), suggesting that authentic leadership is important for fostering optimal performance of both new graduate and experienced nurses. Furthermore, structural empowerment has been found to mediate the relationships between authentic leadership and several positive outcomes such as increased nurse voice behaviour and nurses' ratings of high-quality patient care (Wong, Laschinger, & Cummings, 2010), low levels of burnout (Laschinger et al., 2013), and better job performance and job satisfaction (Wong & Laschinger, 2012). Although more research in this area is needed, early findings have shown that authentic leaders tend to support nurses to achieve positive personal and organisational outcomes by providing structurally empowering work environments.

Emotional intelligence leadership theories

Other relationship-focused models include Goleman, Boyatzis, and McKee's (2002) models of emotional intelligence (EI) and resonant leadership theory. Emotional intelligence is characterised by emotional self-awareness and self-management, as well as social awareness and effective relationship management with others (Goleman et al., 2002). According to this theory, leaders who exemplify emotionally intelligent leadership display high levels of these competencies in their behaviour with their followers. Resonant leadership styles reflect a leader's use of EI qualities in the workplace (Goleman et al., 2002). Goleman et al. (2002) defined resonant leadership as being 'attuned to people's feelings and moving them in a positive emotional direction' (p. 20). The resonant leader uses EI to read and manage the feelings of others to connect with others and help the group achieve common goals. According to Goleman et al. (2002), leaders can develop emotional intelligence competencies and learn when and how to use resonant leadership styles in different circumstances. Resonant leaders are sensitive to the thoughts and emotions of people working around them and are able to build strong and trusting relationships, enabling those around them to be the best they can be (Boyatzis & McKee, 2005).

Resonant leadership is particularly well suited to the discipline of nursing because key capabilities of EI, such as empathy, awareness of self and others through self-reflection and developing positive interpersonal relationships are essential elements of nursing practice. This leadership theory emphasises the emotional work of nurse leaders making it a valuable lens through which to examine leadership in nursing. Studies have linked resonant leadership styles to strong leader–nurse relationships, reduced medication errors, lower intention to leave (Squires, Tourangeau, Laschinger, & Doran, 2010), and lower patient mortality (Cummings, Midodzi, Wong, & Estabrooks, 2010), and higher levels of structural empowerment (Lucas et al., 2008). Resonant leadership has been shown to influence job satisfaction by creating a greater sense of empowerment in nursing settings (Laschinger et al., in press). Squires et al. (2010) also linked resonant leadership to workplace conditions that support professional nursing practice, providing additional support for Boyatzis and McKee's (2005) explanation of how resonant leaders create positive work environments that empower their followers.

Behaviourally focused leadership models

Leader empowering behaviours model

Conger and Kanungo (1998) describe five categories of leadership empowering behaviours. These include:

1. Enhancing the Meaningfulness of Work: Leader behaviours aimed at providing purpose and meaning to followers' work allowing them to identify themselves as important members of the organisation and increasing motivation to perform their work;

2. Fostering Participation in Decision Making: Leader behaviours aimed at soliciting inputs from followers in problem situations and inducing active involvement in decision-making processes;

3. Facilitating Goal Accomplishment: Leader behaviours aimed at maximising the likelihood that followers may achieve their performance goals by enhancing their skills and providing resources required for effective performance (including training followers in their areas of deficiencies, providing necessary resources and removing obstacles to performance);

4. Expressing Confidence in High Performance: Leader behaviours aimed at cultivating the confidence of, as well as showing confidence in, the follower's ability to perform at a high level; and

5. Providing Autonomy from Bureaucratic Constraints: Leader behaviours aimed at minimising administrative details and rule-mindedness so that followers can initiate task behaviours and perform their jobs with effectiveness and efficiency.

Research in this area has shown that leader-empowering behaviours are associated with structurally empowering work environments in nursing. For example, Laschinger, Wong, McMahon, and Kaufmann (1999) showed that staff nurses' perceived access to Kanter's (1977, 1993) empowerment structures were predicted by their manager's leader-empowering behaviours and resulted in lower job tension and enhanced work effectiveness. More recently, Dahinten et al. (2014) demonstrated that leader-empowering behaviours were associated with structural empowerment and organisational commitment among staff nurses. Greco et al. (2006) demonstrated that nurses' perceptions of leader-empowering behaviours were related to the extent to which they felt they had access to information, resources, support and opportunities to learn and grow, which positively influenced the fit between work expectations and their actual experiences of their workplace. More specifically, leader empowering behaviours created an environment in which they felt a greater sense of job autonomy and control, felt rewarded for their work achievements, that they were treated fairly, experienced a strong sense of community, and felt alignment between their personal values and those of the organisation (Greco et al., 2006). Consequently, nurses felt engaged with their work and reported lower levels of burnout. These studies reinforce the important role that leaders play in creating empowering work environments that engage nurses and enhance their worklife experience.

Leadership practices model

Kouzes and Posner's (1995) model of leadership consists of five fundamental leadership practices that enable leaders to be effective in organisations: (1) Challenging the Process, (2) Inspiring a Shared Vision, (3) Modelling the Way, (4) Enabling Others to Act, and (5) Encouraging the Heart. Each leadership practice is associated with specific observable behaviours or activities that, according to Kouzes and Posner (1995), effective leaders use all the time. Leaders who challenge the process think critically and creatively to solve problems, seek out opportunities to make change, and take calculated risks to improve current practices. Inspiring a shared vision involves communicating in an open and positive manner, creating a shared vision, and motivating others to work together to achieve group goals. Modelling the way is a leadership practice made visible in the core behaviours of setting an example, clarifying values, sustaining commitment, and planning. Leaders enable others to act by collaborating purposefully and respectfully with others, cultivating trusting relationships and sharing information and resources that allow people to engage in their job effectively. Finally, encouraging the heart is a leadership practice that emphasises employee appreciation by recognising contributions, providing feedback and celebrating accomplishments.

This model of leadership emphasises that leadership behaviours must be learned and developed, but most importantly, practised. Evidence shows that leaders can learn and develop these five exemplary leadership practices through professional development workshops (Krugman & Smith, 2003; Tourangeau, Lemonde, Luba, Dakers, & Alksnis, 2003). Research has linked managers' use of these five leadership practices to staff nurse workplace empowerment (Patrick et al., 2011), job satisfaction (McNeese-Smith, 1997), commitment to the organisation (McNeese-Smith, 1995), and higher levels of staff nurse expertise (Houser, 2003). More recent work has shown links between front-line and mid-level nurse managers' perceptions of immediate supervisors' use of these five practices and their perceptions of structural empowerment (Laschinger, Wong, Grau, Read, & Stam, 2012). Managers reporting higher levels of structural empowerment also reported higher levels of perceived organisational support, better quality patient care and lower intentions to leave their jobs (Laschinger, Wong, Grau et al., 2012). These studies provide support for the link between transformational leadership practices and the creation of work environments that empower nurses for optimal practice.

Transformational leadership can also influence nurses' satisfaction with their supervisory arrangements but consideration must be given to the span of control (number of reportees) and the amount of operational time leaders have to ensure there is sufficient contact with those they are to lead for influence to be possible (Meyer et al., 2011). This aspect is critical as organisations seek to flatten hierarchies, often at the expense of nursing leadership positions (Kearin, Duffield, & Johnston, 2007) at both the first-line and executive levels.

Linking leadership and empowerment to magnet hospital characteristics: the nursing worklife model

Empowering leadership is a key element of work environments that support professional nursing practice and attract and retain nurses. The Nursing Worklife Model (NWM), originally described by Leiter and Laschinger (2006), was derived from the Magnet Hospital research literature and describes how five worklife factors identified by Lake (1998) interact with each other to affect nurse and patient outcomes. The five interrelated worklife factors are: (1) effective nursing leadership; (2) staff participation in organisational affairs/policy; (3) adequate staffing resources for quality care; (4) support for a nursing (vs. medical) model of patient care; and (5) effective nurse/physician relationships. In this model, leadership is the starting point, with direct paths to (or influence on) staffing/resource adequacy and policy involvement, as well as the quality of nurse/physician relationships. Both policy involvement and nurse/physician relationships influence the extent to which a nursing model of care (in contrast to a medical model) is emphasised in the delivery of nursing care, which in turn influences perceived staffing/resource adequacy, and ultimately nurse and patient outcomes.

Leiter and Laschinger (2006) showed that nursing leadership is the driving force of the model, strongly influencing the other professional practice environment factors. These studies demonstrated how professional practice characteristics were related to burnout and nurse-assessed adverse events. Manojlovich and Laschinger (2008) extended the model to demonstrate the role of structural empowerment in promoting supportive professional practice environments and subsequent outcomes. Nurses who reported higher levels of structural empowerment were more likely to report better leadership on their units and subsequently greater access to elements of support for professional practice in their work environments. Laschinger (2008) found similar results in a Canadian sample by linking structural empowerment to unit leadership and other professional practice characteristics and ultimately job satisfaction and nurse-assessed patient care quality.

The results of these studies demonstrate the importance of empowerment and leadership in creating effective professional practice environments. Research has clearly demonstrated that empowering nursing work environments are fostered by a variety of leadership practices and behaviours. Taken together, the results of these studies add to the growing body of knowledge documenting the key role of leadership in creating empowering work environments that optimise nursing practice and promote nurses' satisfaction with their work and subsequent retention in their current workplaces. This is particularly important given the current nursing workforce shortage worldwide.

IMPLICATIONS FOR MANAGEMENT

Kanter's model of workplace empowerment provides a practical and actionable approach for leaders interested in optimising nurses' ability to provide high-quality patient care. Examples of empowering leadership behaviours based on components of Kanter's model are illustrated in Table 13.2 and described in detail elsewhere (Laschinger & Grau, 2012). Kanter's model has also been used by the Nursing Leadership Institute in British Columbia, Canada, to develop a year-long leadership development program for nursing leaders. Through workshops, mentoring, organisational

Table 13.2 Structurally empowering leadership behaviours

Component of Kanter's theory	Examples of nurse empowering leadership behaviours
Access to information	Engage in open, transparent communication
	Share information openly and in a timely manner
	Communicate management goals and plans effectively
	Communicate current state of the organisation and vision for the future
	Use multiple methods of communication (e.g. in person, bulletin boards, email, websites, online newsletters)
Access to support	Cultivate a collaborative, coaching and facilitating leadership style
	Provide specific and timely feedback that is constructive
	Provide recognition and applaud achievements
	Encourage autonomy and decision making within one's scope of practice
	Encourage collaboration and collegiality among staff
	Be visible and available to meet with employees
	Provide links to helpful people when needed
Access to resources	Provide adequate time and resources to accomplish work
	Assure supplies are accessible and responsibly used
	Involve nurses in evaluation of supplies to assure quality
	Develop a plan for equipment replacement and preventative maintenance strategies
	Develop proposals to obtain funding for new equipment and equipment sharing
	Request staff involvement in resource decision making
	Encourage interpretation of workload data as a necessary part of decision making

Table 13.2 cont

Component of Kanter's theory	Examples of nurse empowering leadership behaviours
Access to opportunity to learn and grow	Encourage/facilitate advanced educational preparation and lifelong learning
	Provide professional training and development opportunities for staff
	Encourage secondment or job exchange to expand skills
	Negotiate expanded role/function in current job to maximise scope of practice
	Establish career ladders based on skill rather than status
	Help employees develop a career vision that inspires them and work together to make it happen
	Participate in special task forces or important organisational committees
Informal power	Provide opportunities to network with colleagues through task forces, workgroups and social events
	Build networking skills initially at the unit level through team-building exercises
	Broaden networking to include agency-wide and extra-organisational contacts
	Develop interdisciplinary networking opportunities
	Encourage collegiality by being visible and friendly
Formal power	Increase the profile of staff nurse recognition at the unit and organisational levels
	Develop a comprehensive job analysis of professional nursing practice
	Define outcomes of nursing practice and align with organisational goals
	Encourage nurses to positively view their contribution to patient care and education
	Collect data on nurse-sensitive patient care outcomes to show empirical evidence of the influence nurses have on care quality and provide impetus for budget decisions
	Provide opportunities for nurses to showcase their skills
	Provide opportunities to develop skills
	Promote participative management and autonomous work units

Adapted from Laschinger & Grau (2012)

support, and virtual networking, this program helps empower leaders by changing behaviours, attitudes and values. MacPhee et al. (2012) have demonstrated that this program helps empower nurse leaders, helping them become more self-aware and confident in their leadership abilities (i.e. psychological empowerment), giving them project management skills, and providing them with access to support, tools and resources needed to be successful in their role, which in turn helps them empower the nurses on their units.

Recent work by Duffield, Baldwin, Roche, and Weiss (2013) also provides a real-life example of how structural empowerment can be enhanced through organisational policies implemented by leaders that foster nurses' access to empowering opportunities in a meaningful way. This project demonstrated that access to opportunity can be improved by providing experienced nurses with opportunities to lead and share their experience in senior nurse leader positions, facilitating scheduled time for professional learning and development activities, and strategically taking on projects that develop and enhance nurses' skills. The results of this initiative demonstrate the value of translating theory and research into effective theory-driven evidence-based management practice. Leaders play a crucial role in establishing policies that support empowering work environments, as well as translating those policies from words on paper into action.

The role of nursing leadership is critical in ensuring patient safety and the quality of the work environment for staff. As demonstrated throughout this chapter, leaders have many theoretically based choices when it comes to developing their leadership skills and abilities in a way that will help create work environments that empower nurses to do their jobs effectively. By embracing a relationally focused leadership style, such as authentic or resonant leadership, leaders become more in tune with the abilities, values and needs of themselves and the people they work with, allowing them to exercise emotional intelligence. When leaders are aware of the needs and values of the members of their organisation, they are better equipped to make decisions that enhance access to sources of empowerment that are relevant and valued by these members. On the other hand, leaders who embrace a behaviour-focused leadership style are motivated to develop habits that promote excellence in themselves and others and try to make work meaningful and inspiring to members of the organisation. As a result, they will ensure that nurses have a voice in the decision-making process and have access to the structures that allow them to be their professional best.

There is a wide range of roles and functions in nursing management, ranging from executive level to clinical management (Dignam et al., 2012); both are complex in quite different ways. Nevertheless, it is important that managers and leaders, in whatever capacity they are employed, have adequate educational preparation. Some leadership skills can be learned and there are various strategies for doing so ranging from formal to informal methods of learning and teaching. However, perhaps the most critical skill required is knowing the staff and their skills to ensure sufficient feedback is provided for them to grow and develop (Thoms & Duffield, 2012). Positive work environments do not 'just happen'. The influence of first-line nurse managers in ensuring an environment fosters job satisfaction and satisfaction with nursing cannot be underestimated. Research indicates two factors that are critical are 'a nurse manager or immediate supervisor who is a good manager or leader' and 'a senior nursing administrator who is highly visible and accessible to staff' (Duffield et al., 2009; Duffield, Roche et al., 2011). Organisations looking to restructure in a form that diminishes the power base of these individuals or, worse, seeks to remove these positions from decision making, may well find themselves with greater staff turnover than anticipated. The theory and empirical findings presented in this chapter attest to the importance of empowering front-line nurses to optimise their professional practice and ensure high-quality patient care.

CONCLUSION

Positive leadership practices play a critical role in empowering nurses for effective professional practice and satisfaction with their jobs and career choice by creating worklife conditions that help optimise nurses' abilities to accomplish their work in meaningful ways. Research has shown that structurally empowering workplaces are strongly related to important work attitudes and behaviours that promote both nurses' workplace wellbeing and high-quality patient care. Thus, Kanter's model of structural empowerment provides a theory-driven evidence-based approach to guide leaders in their efforts to optimise nursing practice environments that retain nurses and contribute to the sustainability of the nursing workforce.

REFLECTIVE EXERCISE

1. How do relationally focused and behaviourally focused leadership styles compare in their approach to creating empowering nursing work environments? Which approach would you consider adopting to improve work effectiveness in your role as a nurse manager or leader?

2. Why is leadership a key antecedent to structural empowerment? Can you have one without the other?

3. Consider the key components of Kanter's model. Thinking about your own experiences to date, how would access to these empowerment structures affect your day-to-day work?

4. Nurses in formal leadership positions have often been the focus of research on leadership and empowerment. Although formal leaders are vital to the creation of a healthy, empowering work environment, what do you think is the role of staff nurses in contributing to a workplace that is empowering for nurses and other members of the team? What could you do in your role to enhance structural empowerment for yourself and your colleagues? What barriers might you face?

Recommended Readings

Greco, P., Laschinger, H. K. S., & Wong, C. (2006). Leader empowering behaviours, staff nurse empowerment, and work engagement/burnout. *Canadian Journal of Nursing Leadership, 19*(4), 41–56.

Laschinger, H. K. S. (2008). Effect of empowerment on professional practice environments, work satisfaction, and patient care quality: Further testing the nursing worklife model. *Journal of Nursing Care Quality, 23*, 322–330.

Laschinger, H. K. S., Finegan, J., & Wilk, P. (2011). Situational and dispositional influences on nurses' workplace wellbeing: The role of empowering unit leadership. *Nursing Research, 60*, 124–131.

Laschinger, H., Gilbert, S., Smith, L., & Leslie, K. (2010). Towards a comprehensive theory of nurse/patient empowerment: Applying Kanter's empowerment theory to patient care. *Journal of Nursing Management, 18*, 4–13.

Laschinger, H. K. S., Wong, C., & Grau, A. L. (2013). Authentic leadership, empowerment and burnout: A comparison in new graduates and experienced nurses. *Journal of Nursing Management, 21*, 541–552. doi:10.1111/j.1365-2834.2012.01375.x.

References

Avolio, B. J., & Gardner, W. L. (2005). Authentic leadership development: Getting to the root of positive forms of leadership. *The Leadership Quarterly, 16*(3), 315–338.

Bamford, M., Wong, C. A., & Laschinger, H. (2012). The influence of authentic leadership and areas of worklife on work engagement of registered nurses. *Journal of Nursing Management, 21*(3), 529–540. doi:10.1111/j.1365-2834.2012.01399.x.

Blegen, M. A., Goode, C. J., & Reed, L. (1998). Nurse staffing and patient outcomes. *Nursing Research, 47*(1), 43–50.

Boyatzis, R. E., & McKee, A. (2005). *Resonant leadership: Renewing yourself and connecting with others through mindfulness, hope, and compassion.* Boston, MA: Harvard Business Press.

Cicolini, G., Comparcini, D., & Simonetti, V. (2013). Workplace empowerment and nurses' job satisfaction: A systematic literature review. *Journal of Nursing Management,* Advance online publication. doi:10.1111/jonm.12028.

Conger, J. A., & Kanungo, R. N. (1998). *Charismatic leadership in organizations.* Thousand Oaks, CA: Sage.

Cummings, G. G., Midodzi, W. K., Wong, C. A., & Estabrooks, C. A. (2010). The contribution of hospital nursing leadership styles to 30-day patient mortality. *Nursing Research, 59*(5), 331–339.

Dahinten, V. S., Macphee, M., Hejazi, S., Laschinger, H., Kazanjian, M., McCutcheon, A., et al. (2014). Testing the effects of an empowerment-based leadership development programme: part 2–staff outcomes. *Journal of Nursing Management, 22*(1), 16–28.

Dansereau, F., Graen, G., & Haga, W. (1975). A vertical dyad approach to leadership within formal organizations. *Organizational Behavior and Human Performance, 13*, 46–78.

Davies, A., Wong, C. A., & Laschinger, H. (2011). Nurses' participation in personal knowledge transfer: The role of leader–member exchange (LMX) and structural empowerment. *Journal of Nursing Management, 19*(5), 632–643.

Dignam, D., Duffield, C., Stasa, H., Gray, J., Jackson, D., & Daly, J. (2012). Management and leadership in nursing: An Australian educational perspective. *Journal of Nursing Management, 20*(1), 65–71.

Duffield, C., Baldwin, R., Roche, M., & Weiss, S. (2013). Job enrichment: Creating meaningful career development opportunities for nurses. *Journal of Nursing Management,* Advance online publication. doi:10.1111/jonm.12049.

Duffield, C., Diers, D., O'Brien-Pallas, L., Aisbett, C., Roche, M., King, M., et al. (2011). Nursing staffing, nursing workload, the work environment and patient outcomes. *Applied Nursing Research, 24*, 244–255.

Duffield, C., Roche, M., Blay, N., & Stasa, H. (2011). Nursing unit managers, staff retention and the work environment. *Journal of Clinical Nursing, 20*(1–2), 23–33.

Duffield, C., Roche, M., O'Brien-Pallas, L., Catling-Paull, C., & King, M. (2009). Staff satisfaction and retention and the role of the nursing unit manager. *Journal of the Royal College of Nursing Australia, 16*(1), 11–17.

Force, M. V. (2005). The relationship between effective nurse managers and nursing retention. *Journal of Nursing Administration, 35*(7–8), 336–341.

Goleman, D., Boyatzis, R. E., & McKee, A. (2002). *The new leaders: Transforming the art of leadership into the science of results.* London: Little, Brown.

Greco, P., Laschinger, H. K. S., & Wong, C. (2006). Leader empowering behaviours, staff nurse empowerment, and work engagement/burnout. *Canadian Journal of Nursing Leadership, 19*(4), 41–56.

Houser, J. (2003). A model for evaluating the context of nursing care delivery. *Journal of Nursing Administration, 33*(1), 39–47.

Irvine, D. M., & Evans, M. G. (1995). Job satisfaction and turnover among nurses: Integrating research findings across studies. *Nursing Research, 44*(4), 246–253.

Kanter, R. M. (1977). *Men and women of the corporation*. New York: Basic Books.

Kanter, R. M. (1993). *Men and women of the corporation* (2nd ed.). New York, NY: Basic Books.

Kearin, M., Duffield, C., & Johnston, J. (2007). The impact of restructuring on the nursing workforce. *Australian Journal of Advanced Nursing, 24*(4), 42–46.

Kouzes, J. M., & Posner, B. Z. (1995). *The leadership challenge: How to keep getting extraordinary things done in organisations*. San Francisco: Jossey-Bass.

Krugman, M., & Smith, V. (2003). Charge nurse leadership development and evaluation. *Journal of Nursing Administration, 33*, 284–292.

Lake, E. T. (1998). Advances in understanding and predicting nurse turnover. *Research in the Sociology of Health Care, 15*, 147–172.

Laschinger, H. K. S. (2008). Effect of empowerment on professional practice environments, work satisfaction, and patient care quality: Further testing the nursing worklife model. *Journal of Nursing Care Quality, 23*, 322–330.

Laschinger, H. K. S., Almost, J., Purdy, N., & Kim, J. (2004). Predictors of nurse managers' health in Canadian restructured health care settings. *Canadian Journal of Nursing Leadership, 17*(4), 88–105.

Laschinger, H. K. S., & Fida, R. (2013). A time-lagged analysis of the effect of authentic leadership on workplace bullying, burnout, and occupational turnover intentions. *European Journal of work and Organizational Psychology*, Advance online publication.

Laschinger, H. K. S., Finegan, J., & Wilk, P. (2011). Situational and dispositional influences on nurses' workplace wellbeing: The role of empowering unit leadership. *Nursing Research, 60*, 124–131. doi:10.1097/NNR.0b013e318209782e.

Laschinger, H., Gilbert, S., Smith, L., & Leslie, K. (2010). Towards a comprehensive theory of nurse/patient empowerment: Applying Kanter's empowerment theory to patient care. *Journal of Nursing Management, 18*, 4–13. doi:10.1111/j.1365-2834.2009.01046.x.

Laschinger, H. K. S., & Grau, A. (2012). Creating empowering work environments to promote professional nursing practice. In J. I. Erickson, D. A. Jones, & M. Ditomassi (Eds.), *Fostering nurse-led care: Professional practice for the bedside leader from Massachusetts General Hospital* (pp. 39–63). Indianapolis, IN: Sigma Theta Tau International.

Laschinger, H. K. S., Leiter, M., Day, A., & Gilin, D. (2009). Workplace empowerment, incivility, and burnout: Impact on staff nurse recruitment and retention outcomes. *Journal of Nursing Management, 17*(3), 302–311.

Laschinger, H. K. S., Purdy, N., & Almost, J. (2007). The impact of leader–member exchange quality, empowerment, and core self-evaluation on nurse managers' job satisfaction. *Journal of Nursing Administration, 37*(5), 221–229.

Laschinger, H. K., & Smith, L. M. (2013). The influence of authentic leadership and empowerment on new-graduate nurses' perceptions of interprofessional collaboration. *Journal of Nursing Administration, 43*(1), 24–29.

Laschinger, H. K. S., & Wong, C. (1999). Staff nurse empowerment and collective accountability: Effect on perceived productivity and self-rated work effectiveness. *Nursing Economic$, 17*(6), 308–316.

Laschinger, H. K. S., Wong, C., & Cummings, G. (In press). Resonant leadership and workplace empowerment: The value of positive organizational culture in reducing workplace incivility. *Nursing Economic$*.

Laschinger, H. K. S., Wong, C. A., & Grau, A. L. (2012). Authentic leadership, empowerment and burnout: A comparison in new graduates and experienced nurses. *Journal of Nursing Management, 21*(3), 541–552.

Laschinger, H. K. S., Wong, C., & Grau, A. L. (2013). Authentic leadership, empowerment and burnout: A comparison in new graduates and experienced nurses. *Journal of Nursing Management, 21*(3), 541–552. doi:10.1111/j.1365-2834.2012.01375.x.

Laschinger, H. K. S., Wong, C., Grau, A., Read, E., & Stam, L. (2012). The influence of leadership practices and empowerment on Canadian nurse managers. *Journal of Nursing Management, 20*(7), 877–888. doi:10.1111/j.1365-2834.2011.01307.x.

Laschinger, H. K. S., Wong, C., McMahon, L., & Kaufmann, C. (1999). Leader behavior impact on staff nurse empowerment, job tension, and work effectiveness. *Journal of Nursing Administration, 29*(5), 28–39.

Leiter, M. P., & Laschinger, H. K. S. (2006). Relationships of work and practice environment to professional burnout: Testing a causal model. *Nursing Research, 55*(2), 137–146.

Liden, R. C., & Maslyn, J. M. (1998). Multidimensionality of leader–member exchange: An empirical assessment through scale development. *Journal of Management, 24*(1), 43–72. doi:10.1177/014920639802400105.

Lucas, V., Laschinger, H. K. S., & Wong, C. (2008). The impact of emotional intelligent leadership on staff nurse empowerment: The moderating effect of span of control. *Journal of Nursing Management, 16*(8), 964–973. doi:10.1111/j.1365-2834.2008.00856.x.

MacPhee, M., Skelton-Green, J., Bouthillette, F., & Suryaprakash, N. (2012). An empowerment framework for nursing leadership development: Supporting evidence. *Journal of Advanced Nursing, 68*(1), 159–169.

Manojlovich, M., & Laschinger, H. K. S. (2007). The nursing worklife model: Extending and refining a new theory. *Journal of Nursing Management, 15*(3), 256–263.

Manojlovich, M., & Laschinger, H. K. S. (2008). Application of the nursing worklife model to the ICU setting. *Critical Care Nursing Clinics of North America, 20*(4), 481–487. doi:10.1016/j.ccell.2008.08.004.

McNeese-Smith, D. (1995). Job satisfaction, productivity, and organizational commitment: The result of leadership. *Journal of Nursing Administration, 25*(9), 17–26.

McNeese-Smith, D. (1997). The influence of manager behavior on nurses' job satisfaction, productivity, and commitment. *Journal of Nursing Administration, 27*(9), 47–55.

Meyer, R. M., O'Brien-Pallas, L., Doran, D., Streiner, D., Ferguson-Pare, M., & Duffield, C. (2011). Front-line managers as boundary spanners: Effects of span and time on nurse supervision satisfaction. *Journal of Nursing Management, 19*(5), 611–622.

Nedd, N. (2006). Perceptions of empowerment and intent to stay. *Nursing Economic$, 24*(1), 13.

Ning, S., Zhong, H., Libo, W., & Qiujie, L. (2009). The impact of nurse empowerment on job satisfaction. *Journal of Advanced Nursing, 65*(12), 2642–2648.

Patrick, A., Laschinger, H. K. S., Wong, C., & Finegan, J. (2011). Developing and testing a new measure of staff nurse clinical leadership: The clinical leadership survey. *Journal of Nursing Management, 19*(4), 449–460. doi:10.1111/j.1365-2834.2011.01238.x.

Smith, L., Andrusyszyn, M. A., & Laschinger, H. K. S. (2010). Effects of workplace incivility and empowerment on newly-graduated nurses' organizational commitment. *Journal of Nursing Management, 18*(8), 1004–1015.

Squires, M. A. E., Tourangeau, A. N. N., Laschinger, H. K. S., & Doran, D. (2010). The link between leadership and safety outcomes in hospitals. *Journal of Nursing Management, 18*(8), 914–925.

Thoms, D., & Duffield, C. (2012). Clinical leadership. In E. Chang & J. Daly (Eds.), *Transitions in nursing: Preparing for professional practice* (3rd ed., pp. 225–234). Sydney, Australia: Elsevier Australia.

Tourangeau, A. E., Lemonde, M., Luba, M., Dakers, D., & Alksnis, C. (2003). Evaluation of a leadership development intervention. *Nursing Leadership, 16*(3), 91–104.

Tuckey, M. R., Bakker, A. B., & Dollard, M. F. (2012). Empowering leaders optimize working conditions for engagement: A multilevel study. *Journal of Occupational Health Psychology, 17*(1), 15.

Weberg, D. (2010). Transformational leadership and staff retention: An evidence review with implications for healthcare systems. *Nursing Administration Quarterly, 34*(3), 246–258.

Wing, T., Regan, S., & Laschinger, H. K. S. (in press). The influence of empowerment and incivility on the mental health of new graduate nurses. *Journal of Nursing Management.*

Wong, C. A., & Cummings, G. G. (2009). The influence of authentic leadership behaviors on trust and work outcomes of health care staff. *Journal of Leadership Studies, 3*(2), 6–23. doi:10.1002/jls.20104.

Wong, C. A., & Laschinger, H. K. S. (2012). Authentic leadership, performance, and job satisfaction: The mediating role of empowerment. *Journal of Advanced Nursing, 69*(4), 947–959. doi:10.1111/j.1365-2648.2012.06089.x.

Wong, C. A., Laschinger, H. K. S., & Cummings, G. G. (2010). Authentic leadership and nurses' voice behaviour and perceptions of care quality. *Journal of Nursing Management, 18*(8), 889–900. doi:10.1111/j.1365-2834.2010.01113.x.

Yang, J., Liu, Y., Huang, C., & Zhu, L. (2013). Impact of empowerment on professional practice environments and organizational commitment among nurses: A structural equation approach. *International Journal of Nursing Practice, 19*(S1), 44–55.

Young-Ritchie, C., Laschinger, H. K. S., & Wong, C. (2009). The effects of emotionally intelligent leadership behavior on emergency staff nurses' workplace empowerment and organization commitment. *Canadian Journal of Nursing Leadership, 22*, 70–85.

CHAPTER FOURTEEN

Leadership and health policy

Joanne Travaglia, John Daly, Debra Jackson
& Sandra Speedy

LEARNING OBJECTIVES

At the completion of this chapter, the reader will be able to:

▲ describe attributes and characteristics of policy;
▲ explain the concept of the policy cycle;
▲ delineate the stages of the policy cycle and key challenges in successful policy implementation;
▲ understand the critical role of policy in governance in healthcare at local, national and global levels;
▲ appreciate the power of policy as a tool to enhance nursing's contribution to health system leadership in a multidisciplinary healthcare team context;
▲ understand the role of leaders in influencing, developing, implementing and evaluating health policy.

INTRODUCTION

As discussed in other chapters in this book, numerous international health leadership organisations such as the Institute of Medicine (IOM) in the USA (IOM, 2011) and the World Health Organization (2011, 2013a, 2013b) and others are calling for nursing to more fully exploit its potential for leading change in healthcare systems in partnership with other members of the healthcare team. The World Health Assembly has passed resolutions in the recent past and directed strategy to some extent in efforts to strengthen nursing and midwifery internationally (WHO, 2013a).

Nurses are currently under-represented in senior executive ranks in health service leadership organisations including at higher government level. Historically, the reasons for this are many and varied. Undoubtedly gender politics and traditional professional hierarchies in health education and healthcare have exerted a major impact (see Chapter 4 for more discussion on gender and politics). The profession could also shoulder some responsibility for that situation, as author Suzanne Gordon (2010) has observed, 'nurses tend to emphasize virtue rather than knowledge'. She also calls for nursing to become more assertive and 'activist'.

An active role in system reform is vital if the profession of nursing is to maximise its contribution to healthcare enhancement. The demands on health systems are increasing exponentially. Shifts in demography (as many developed countries like Australia and Japan age rapidly, while other, developing countries, increase their demand for better child and maternal care), illness profiles (including a global increase in non-communicable diseases), workforce ageing and shortages, and the persistence of medical errors, mean that both public and private healthcare providers are seeking better ways to become more effective, efficient, appropriate, equitable and, most of all, viable. Nursing has the potential to play a very significant leadership role along with other health professionals in responding to these challenges.

Increases in patient and system complexity, resource and quality and safety issues have also led to a more systems view in many health system contexts (Schyve, 2009). Indeed, Schyve (2009, p. 1) suggests that 'Rather than thinking of the healthcare organization as a conglomerate of units, think of it as a "system"—a combination of processes, people, and other resources that, working together, achieve an end'. It is here that nurses are finally being recognised as key collaborators in the 'working together process' which involves at its core, theorising ways of achieving future system changes (from bedside to boardroom argues the IOM (2011)) in order to ensure that equitable, sustainable quality healthcare is to be able to be achieved and sustained.

Policy therefore needs to be part of the professional lexicon for all nurses. Purposeful efforts at capacity building to achieve greater levels of knowledge and skill in policy development, implementation and evaluation, among nurses at all levels will be crucial if nursing is to expand its potential to contribute to effective transformation endeavours in healthcare.

WHAT ARE THE ATTRIBUTES AND CHARACTERISTICS OF POLICY?

There have been numerous calls in the international literature for nursing to engage and more fully participate in health policy development and implementation (Gordon, 2010; Hinshaw & Grady, 2011; Mason, Leavitt, & Chaffee, 2014). But what is policy and how does it relate to the work of nurses in general and nursing leadership in particular?

Policy as a concept can mean many things and there is no clear agreement in the literature on a simple or all-encompassing definition (Althaus, Bridgman, & Davis, 2013). The concept is in widespread use in many sectors and institutions in society, particularly in politics and organisational theory. This points to an almost implicit assumption on the part of those who use the term freely, that all who are exposed to it will understand its meaning and implications. Althaus et al. (2013) position policy as a concept, and assert that a 'multitude of meanings is inevitable, since policy is a shorthand description for everything from an analysis of past decisions to the imposition of current political thinking' (p. 6).

The political nature of policies is closely related to their focus. Anderson (2014) talks about public policies as addressing, by their very nature, a problem or a matter of public concern. For Dye (1995) public policy is defined much more simply. Created by governments, policies are, in practice, *whatever they choose to do or not do* and *the difference it makes*. At an even simpler level we can understand policies as those directives or guidelines by which the actions of governments, systems, organisations, teams or individuals are facilitated or constrained.

What is clear, and what we will discuss in the next section, is that policy is value-laden, political, often contested, a potentially powerful tool or instrument of governance, and action oriented, most often in a collective sense (Althaus et al., 2013; Brownson, Chriqui, & Stamatakis, 2009). Policy, according to Colebatch (2009), is a way of creating and maintaining order and predictability, of establishing and mobilising goals within complex circumstances, through the creation and development of linkages. It is also, at the same time, about creating stability and managing change. In this sense policy is less about the decision-making process and more about a process of ongoing societal [and in our case, professional] negotiation (Colebatch, 2009).

Policy attributes

The attributes of policies can be as difficult to pin down as their definition (and, of course, for the same reason). At a very basic level, policies can be either formal (such as policies enacted as laws or regulations) or informal (policies which operate as guidelines). Policies can vary in where and how they are generated, their focus, their type, their direction and their outcomes. We will discuss each briefly in turn.

Policies are generated from a variety of institutions. This is particularly true of policies in the health sector. Health policies are made, implemented and monitored at international (i.e. World Health Organization), national, state and local government levels, as well as by systems, organisations, services, teams and units.

Policies have a variety of foci. They can address: the production (creation, management), distribution and consumption of resources; identity issues (including national and professional identities); and in reflexive mode, how policies themselves are made and who is involved in the process (that is, policies on policy making, such as the inclusion of patients on local health district boards) (Fenna, 2004).

Policies also differ in type. Policies can be distributive, redistributive, constituent, regulatory (Lowi, 1972) or symbolic (Edelman, 1964). Distributive policies (sometimes also known as material policies) shape the way in which resources are allocated across a country, system or organisation. They can determine, for example, what proportion of the national budget is spent on health services, or what amount of a hospital budget goes to paediatrics compared with surgery.

Redistributive policies are a mechanism by which resources are shared across different groups. One example is the Pharmaceutical Benefits Scheme in Australia, which subsidises some medications for some groups. Constituent policies are understood by some to be those policies which direct actions (such as the legislation) required to ensure redistribution occurs, but by others are considered to be about the non-material aspects of redistribution, such as governance.

Regulatory (or self-regulatory as in the case of professional bodies) policies determine what is considered acceptable behaviour by individuals or groups. A good example of regulatory policies are those which are issued by Colleges of Nursing and/ or Midwifery, and which direct expectations of length and type of training, as well as appropriate types of professional, ethical behaviour.

One final category, symbolic policies, are those which have no material resources attached, and which either can have symbolic power or which can be used to shift the focus away from a fully resourced policy. A good example of the former is that the shift to person-centred care does not necessarily affect the type or amount of funding a service or unit receives (although it can) but as a policy it has shaped the behaviour of both clients and clinicians (Epstein, Fiscella, Lesser, & Stange, 2010). An example of the latter is any policy which '... permit[s] elected leaders to show great concern but relieve them of the need to allocate resources' (Schneider & Ingram, 1993, p. 338).

Policies, Palmer and Short (2010) argue, can have different directions. They can be about intentions or objectives—that is, they can be about directing future action (such as the focus of nursing education) or they can be directed at remedying something that has occurred in the past (such as the establishment of the Australian Dust Diseases Board to pay compensation to people exposed to asbestos).

These two examples—nursing education and compensation for an acquired illness—speak to some of the other characteristics of policies. Policies can be substantive; that is, they can address a whole issue or area (for example, higher education). But they can also be procedural; that is, a way of establishing *what actions* need to be taken, by *which individuals,* and according to *what rules.* Hand hygiene policies are also a good example of the latter.

Finally, and equally importantly, policies can have two basic outcomes. These are intended and unintended. One of the key elements of good policy making is the ability to not only plan for intended outcomes but also to assess as many potential unintended outcomes as possible.

THE POLICY CYCLE: HOW IS POLICY MADE?

For Colebatch (2009), policy is an organisational construct that has three dimensions, vertical, horizontal and scene setting. The vertical dimension is where the dominant account of policy is the 'authorised choice', in other words the authority of governments to make policy that they believe will solve problems in an autonomous, goal-oriented and purposive way. The horizontal includes the pattern of structured interaction amongst participants or stakeholders, each with a different understanding of 'the' problem, with conflicting, overlapping, negotiated and compromised interactions rather than the 'decision and order' that seems to operate vertically. Finally, there is the scene-setting dimension, which refers to shared values, ideals and understandings within a policy-making milieu (Colebatch, 2009). But what does this mean in practice? As Colebatch (2009) states:

> *These dimensions are not alternatives: rather, each tends to assume the others. ...*
> *Policy practitioners use both accounts: they recognize the need to try and ensure*
> *that the relevant interests have been involved in framing the policy outcome*
> *(horizontal) before it is presented for official approval (vertical). In their more*
> *reflective moments, they are likely to recognize also that there is another dimension,*
> *where their contribution is less direct: the sphere of shared understandings*
> *and values within which the negotiation and the decision making take place ...*
> *the scene-setting dimension (p. 36).*

The scene-setting dimension also speaks to the other elements of policy making. The process, as we will discuss in the next section, is well understood and documented. But the process does not take place in a vacuum. At the beginning of this chapter we offered several definitions that spoke about policy address problems. But how does something become a social or a health problem? Factors such as politics and the relative power of stakeholders make all the difference and can influence something to be recognised as a problem or concern that needs addressing in/by policy.

The political will of governments to create and enact adequate resource policies is shaped by any number of stakeholders. These can include (amongst others) the public (as in the case with increased gun control), professionals (e.g. health professionals' concern about obesity), researchers (e.g. providing the evidence around smoking) and/or lobby groups (e.g. the fast food industry and support or voluntary groups including those for specific diseases and conditions such as breast cancer).

The relative power of these stakeholders shapes what is on the agenda and what is left off. One of the most important aspects of policy making that needs to be considered is that the lack of a formal policy can itself operate as a policy. Not banning fast food advertising at peak TV watching times for children is effectively a policy that acts to allow children to see such advertisements.

It is important to remember Colebatch's (2009) dimensions as we consider the policy cycle model. The problem with any model or linear (or in this case circular, but with the same limitations) representation is that they tend to present an idealised version of the process.

The policy model represents an idealised process. However, in reality the process is more fluid, more complex and less predictable (Althaus et al., 2013). While reality of the policy process is much closer to Durkheim's notion of the profane (that is, the mundane, the messy and the everyday) than to the 'sacred' model (Durkheim, 1915), the policy cycle does provide us with a basic guide and some useful stepping stones for the process.

The policy cycle

The terms *policy process* and *policy cycle* are used in the literature and they appear to be interchangeable. The process is complex and a range of factors, if not anticipated and managed well, may result in policy failure. Policy development is best approached in a systematic way. The policy process or cycle model is composed of a number of stages that need to be considered to optimise chances of a successful outcome. Althaus et al. (2013) assert that 'good policy should include the basic elements of the cycle. That is, a policy process that does not include everything from problem identification to implementation to evaluation has less chance of success. This will not hold true for every example—some policy issues are so simple that investment in process is redundant. But on balance, and across cumulated experience of policy making, a more thorough policy process is less likely to produce an obvious policy mistake. A policy cycle assists systematic thinking, even if many different types of policy cycle are conceivable' (p. 34).

The policy cycle process

What has come to be known generally as the policy process, or the policy cycle, is more precisely understood at the technical or institutional or rationalist choice model of policy making (Althaus et al., 2013). This model involves a series of steps that are seen to flow logically from one another. The difference between the linear model and the cycle is simply that in cyclical models once the policy is implemented and evaluated, the policy makers go back to the start and reconsider what emerging (in both the political and practical sense) problems may require additional policy.

The rational aspect of this model makes it very attractive to policy makers who are interested in evidence-informed decision or policy making. As in evidence-based clinical practice, evidence-based decision making is centred on the justification of decisions based on the best research evidence. In the shift from an individual-clinical to a population-policy level, the decision-making context becomes more uncertain, variable and complex (Dobrow, Goel, & Upshur, 2004, p. 207). Evidence-based (or evidence-informed decision making) is one attempt to address this uncertainty (Oxman, Lavis, Lewin, & Fretheim, 2009).

There are alternatives to this type of policy-making model. These speak to a less linear and vertical model, incorporating (or at the very least recognising) more of the horizontal negotiation and scene-setting or contextual processes. Some alternatives (there are others) to the rationalist model of policy making include the:

- ▲ *Incrementalist or 'muddling through' model* which argues that it is actually small shifts in what a government or organisation does that create policy and that policy making is essentially a process of such bodies making comparisons between their existing policies and any potential alternatives (Lindblom, 1959).

- ▲ *Garbage can or multiple streams model.* This model recognises the primacy of the elements we discussed in the last section. Proponents of this model say that at any one time there are three independent streams flowing into a policy-making environment—the problems themselves, politics and policy processes (or solutions). Policies are made when the politics of the day allow the policy maker to match the problem and the solution (Cohen, March, & Olsen, 1972; Kingdon, 2010).

- ▲ *Advocacy coalition framework* (Sabatier, 1988). In this model of policy making, coalitions form around specific policy issues. These can include policy makers and analysts, researchers and academics, the public and the media. Policy or policy change happens when a particular coalition (e.g. the anti-smoking lobby) rises to power above other coalitions (e.g. tobacco companies, tobacco growers) and is able to set the policy agenda.

- ▲ *Punctuated equilibrium framework* (Baumgartner & Jones, 1993) argues that policy making is essentially about long periods of small incremental changes (as above) followed by short periods of major policy change.

THE STAGES OF THE POLICY CYCLE AND KEY CHALLENGES IN SUCCESSFUL POLICY IMPLEMENTATION

The policy process essentially involves several key steps. These are presented in Table 14.1.

The attractiveness of this approach to policy making is clear. It is logical, 'do-able' and seemingly consistent with the principles of evidence-based practice. Many of the shortfalls have been identified in the explanation of the steps. It is clear, for example, that good evidence is needed to support the case for a policy intervention (as opposed to any other mechanism for change) for a specific problem (as opposed to multiple other issues), utilising a specific policy (the actual policy intervention chosen).

Table 14.1 Steps and explanation of the policy process

Step	Explanation
1. Identify and define the problem	What is deemed a problem? By whom? How do problems come to the attention of policy makers? How can they be defined? What alternative conceptualisations and perspectives need to be taken into account?
	How will you get agreement from key stakeholders on what the problem is and how it should be addressed? (Hint: engage them at this point.)
a. Establish your goals and objectives	Who is involved in the process of setting goals and objectives?
	How do you know your goals and objectives are achievable?
	How broad or specific do your goals need to be?
2. Identify the evidence	What are your sources of evidence? What will you do if there is little or no evidence?
a. What are the known causes of the problem?	What evidence do you have about the causes of the problem itself, and from which sources? How will you ensure that the voices of the vulnerable are included?
b. What evidence is there for the impact of previous policies, strategies or interventions?	What has been shown to work? To not work? By whom? When? Which scene-setting or contextual factors do you think might have impinged on the impact of previous attempts to address this problem?
c. Why do you think a policy is appropriate?	What alternatives or adjuncts to policy can you employ?
3. Identify your options	What do you think you will do as a result of your policy?
	What features of the community, system or organisation (scene setting) do you need to take into account?
a. What evidence do you have for the appropriateness, effectiveness and impact of your chosen options?	How do you know that your options are sound and are the right response to the problem and its causes?
4. Select the evaluation criterion	How will you know if the policy has met your objectives? How will you know what outcomes (expected and unexpected) and impact (desirable and undesirable, and for whom) it has had? Who needs to be involved in the evaluation? What baseline data do you need to collect before you commence the implementation?
5. Determine known (desirable) outcomes and potential unknown outcomes (both desirable and undesirable)	What are your expected outcomes, and what are your potential outcomes (good and bad)?
	What types of scenarios can you construct and test before implementation?
6. Evaluate the options	How feasible and implementable are your options? How do you know? Who do you need to consult? How will you hear the voices of the vulnerable?

Table 14.1 cont

Step	Explanation
a. What are the costs (resources, politics, power, etc.)?	What will it take to implement your policy? Who will you need to engage in the negotiation process? What politics and power relations will you need to consider, or to bring onside? How will you do this? What alternatives will you have if your policy cannot be fully implemented?
b. Decide on your best option	Based on a) above, what is your best option (intervention) in addressing the problem?
c. Find support	How will you gain the support you need? Who do you need to include in the implementation process? Who do you need to lobby?
7. Implement your chosen option	How will you implement your option(s)? How will you convert your goals and objectives into a specific plan? Who will you engage in the implementation process? How long will this take?
8. Evaluate	According to the criteria established in step 4: How will you disseminate the findings? How will you ensure the continued employment of any successful options? How will you address any negative outcomes?
9. Identify and define the problem	Given what you know now, what is the next problem you need to address?

Hoy and Miskel (2013), writing about educational administration, identify some potential traps in evidence gathering and decision making that can also beset the making and implementation of healthcare policies. These include the:

▲ Anchoring Trap: Giving disproportional weight to initial information.

▲ Comfort Trap: A bias towards alternatives that support the status quo.

▲ Recognition Trap: Tendency to place a higher value on that which is familiar.

▲ Representative Trap: Tendency to see others as representative of the typical stereotype.

▲ Sunk-Cost Trap: Tendency to make decisions that justify previous decisions that are not working.

▲ Framing Trap: Framing of the problem impacts the eventual solution.

▲ Prudence Trap: Tendency to be overcautious when faced with high-stakes decisions.

▲ Memory Trap: Tendency to base predictions on memory of past events, which are often very influenced by both recent and dramatic events.

Implementation is critical to success in policy outcomes, including achievement of a policy's objectives. Sabatier (2007) (of the advocacy coalition model) gives some insights into why policies are difficult to develop and to implement. He argues that:

▲ For any one policy there are hundreds of actors (stakeholders and other) from different agencies, organisations, levels of government, interest groups, academics, legislators and media representatives who are or could be involved in the development and implementation process.

▲ Policy cycles can typically take a decade (and up to 40 years) from the time when a problem is identified through the period when there is enough evidence on its cause and consequences, to when the actual impact of the implemented policy can be assessed.

▲ There is rarely only one policy at work. Whatever the issue, there are often a number of different programs, players and policies all interacting (and at times competing) with each other.

▲ Policy is developed and played out in different arenas. The debates, which shape and direct policies, can take place in Ministries of Health, but they are also shaped by public inquiries, political debates influencing the development of government regulations and interventions and judicial processes.

▲ The policy process can involve deeply held social or religious values (such as those surrounding terminations and euthanasia) and financial interests (including industry).

Policy is being made constantly. Like communication, even when you think you or others are not making policy, you are. Because of the complexity of most policy processes, and the speed at which they can be required by governments, systems and services (as opposed to the speed at which the problem can gestate), nurses need to be more than actively involved, as noted by Gordon (2010) at the beginning of this chapter. They need to take the lead. In the next section we address just that question.

NURSING AND HEALTH POLICY

In healthcare, policy is associated with change and as has been argued in Chapter 4, imposed change is acknowledged as a contributor to some of the work-based adversity issues facing nursing, including retention, burnout and job dissatisfaction (Kowalski et al., 2010). One way that nurses can act against imposed change, and ensure that nursing concerns and interests are considered in the change process, is for nursing to actively contribute to policy change and policy development.

In an earlier chapter of this book we highlight the importance of nurses being politically aware and being able to operate at the level of the political (see Chapter 4). This political insight and confidence is essential if nurses are to contribute to policy development and health reform. It may be that the role of nurses in relation to policy is seen as simply being one of implementing policy. But we argue that nurses are key to health reform, and so have a much more holistic role to play in relation to policy—nurses have roles in all aspects of policy development and implementation—right from recognition of a need for policy (or policy reform), through to contributing to its development and implementation. Further, it is crucial that nurses engage in policy development and implementation beyond the local level and contribute at the regional, national and international levels.

When considering the types of policies discussed earlier—distributive, redistributive, constituent, regulatory and symbolic policies—it is important to consider where nursing involvement might be centred currently, and where there is a need to increase or enhance the nursing contribution.

Nursing leaders in particular have a role to play here—not only a role in contributing to the development of policy themselves, but in two other important areas: 1.) advocating for nursing involvement and inclusion in all levels and types of policy development forums; and 2.) facilitating nurses to develop the skills and confidence needed to participate in policy development and reform.

CONCLUSION

Policy is a crucial and often powerful instrument in governance of healthcare. Choices made in crafting policy for health can have profound implications for healthcare structure, process, resourcing and delivery. Leaders in nursing are well positioned to make important contributions to debate in, and indeed to become significant architects of, health policy. To do so, like other leading health professionals, they require a lexicon, skill set and the confidence to engage in the policy development, implementation and evaluation processes. Health policy can serve as a vehicle for further enabling and expanding nursing's contribution to healthcare in partnership with other health professional policy leaders.

REFLECTIVE EXERCISE

Consider nursing in relation to the types of policies influencing healthcare and delivery.

1. Can you describe examples of nurse involvement in the various forms of policy?
    a. Distributive?
    b. Redistributive?
    c. Constituent?
    d. Regulatory?
    e. Symbolic?
2. How can nursing's involvement in creating and implementing the various types of policy be improved?
3. Conduct an internet search to establish how nursing has contributed to policy development from the local to the international context.

Recommended Readings

Colebatch, H. K. (2009). *Policy: Concepts in the social sciences* (3rd ed.). Berkshire, UK: Open University Press.

Gordon, S. (2010). Nursing and health policy perspectives. *International Nursing Review*, Editorial, 403–404.

Head, B. W. (2008). Three lenses of evidence-based policy. *Australian Journal of Public Administration, 67*(1), 1–11.

Hinshaw, A. S., & Grady, P. (Eds.), (2011). *Shaping health policy through nursing research.* New York: Springer.

Institute of Medicine (2011). *The future of nursing: Leading change, advancing health.* Washington, DC: National Academies Press. Retrieved from <http://www.nap.edu/catalog.php?record_id=12956>.

References

Althaus, C., Bridgman, P., & Davis, G. (Eds.), (2013). *The Australian Policy Handbook* (5th ed.). Sydney: Allen & Unwin.

Anderson, J. E. (2014). *Public policymaking* (8th ed.). Stamford: Cengage Learning.

Baumgartner, F. R., & Jones, B. D. (1993). *Agendas and instability in American politics.* Chicago: University of Chicago Press.

Brownson, R. C., Chriqui, J. F., & Stamatakis, A. (2009). Policy, politics and collective action: Understanding evidence-based public health policy. *Government, Politics & Law, 99*(9), 1576–1583.

Cohen, M., March, J., & Olsen, J. (1972). A garbage can model of organizational choice. *Administrative Science Quarterly, 17,* 1–25.

Colebatch, H. K. (2009). *Policy: Concepts in the social sciences* (3rd ed.). Berkshire, UK: Open University Press.

Dobrow, M. J., Goel, V., & Upshur, R. E. G. (2004). Evidence-based health policy: Context and utilisation. *Social Science & Medicine, 58,* 207–217.

Durkheim, D., & Swain, J. W. (1915). *The elementary forms of the religious life.* London: Allen & Unwin.

Dye, T. R. (1995). *Understanding public policy* (8th ed.). Englewood Cliffs, N.J.: Prentice Hall.

Edelman, M. (1964). *The symbolic uses of politics.* Urbana: University of Illinois Press.

Epstein, R. M., Fiscella, K., Lesser, C. S., & Stange, K. C. (2010). Why the nation needs a policy push on patient-centered health care. *Health Affairs, 29*(8), 1489–1495.

Fenna, A. (2004). *Australian public policy* (2nd ed.). Frenchs Forest: Pearson.

Gordon, S. (2010). Nursing and health policy perspectives. *International Nursing Review,* Editorial, 403–404.

Hinshaw, A. S., & Grady, P. (Eds.), (2011). *Shaping health policy through nursing research.* New York: Springer.

Hoy, W., & Miskel, C. (2013). *Educational administration: Theory, research, and practice* (9th ed.). New York: McGraw-Hill.

Institute of Medicine (2011). *The future of nursing: Leading change, advancing health.* Washington, DC: National Academies Press. Retrieved from <http://www.nap.edu/catalog.php?record_id=12956>.

Kingdon, J. W. (2010). *Agendas, alternatives, and public policies* (2nd ed.). Pearson: Essex.

Kowalski, C., Ommen, O., Driller, E., Ernstmann, N., Wirtz, M. A., Kohler, T., et al. (2010). Burnout in nurses—the relationship between social capital in hospitals and emotional exhaustion. *Journal of Clinical Nursing, 19*(11–12), 1654–1663.

Lindblom, C. E. (1959). The science of "muddling through". *Public Administration Review, 19,* 79–88.

Lowi, T. J. (1972). Four systems of policy, politics, and choice. *Public Administration Review, 33*(3), 298–310.

Mason, D. J., Leavitt, J. K., & Chaffee, M. W. (Eds.), (2014). *Policy and politics in nursing and healthcare.* St Louis: Elsevier Saunders.

Oxman, A. D., Lavis, J. N., Lewin, S., & Fretheim, A. (2009). SUPPORT Tools for evidence-informed health Policymaking (STP) 1: What is evidence-informed policymaking? *Health Research Policy and Systems, 7*(Suppl. 1), S1.

Palmer, G. R., & Short, S. D. (2010). *Health care and public policy: An Australian analysis* (4th ed.). South Yarra: Palgrave MacMillan.

Sabatier, P. (1988). An advocacy coalition framework of policy change and the role of policy-oriented learning therein. *Policy Sciences, 21*(2–3), 129–168.

Sabatier, P. A. (2007). *Theories of the policy process.* Colorado: Westview Press.

Schneider, A. L., & Ingram, H. (1993). Social construction of target populations: Implications for politics and policy. *American Journal of Political Science Review, 87*(2), 334–346.

Schyve, P. M. (2009). *Leadership in healthcare organizations: A guide to Joint Commission leadership standards*. San Diego: The Governance Institute.

World Health Organization (2011). *Strategic directions for strengthening nursing and midwifery*. Geneva: WHO.

World Health Organization (2013a). *WHO nursing and midwifery progress report 2008–2012*. Geneva: WHO.

World Health Organization (2013b). *Interprofessional collaborative practice in primary health care: Nursing and midwifery perspectives*. Geneva: WHO.

CHAPTER FIFTEEN

Developing and sustaining self

Marion Broome & Jason Gilbert

Through imagination we can envision the worlds within us.
— **Stephen Covey (FranklinCovey Co. Used with permission)**

LEARNING OBJECTIVES

At the completion of this chapter, the reader will be able to:

▲ describe the developmental trajectory of a nurse leader;

▲ discuss the responsibility of each emerging leader to engage in self-assessment and reflection as critical professional development activities;

▲ evaluate two existing leadership assessment tools for their purpose, theoretical foundation, relevance and usefulness to nurse leaders;

▲ describe how one evaluates the reliability and validity of a leadership assessment tool;

▲ select and complete a leadership inventory tool to examine one's own areas of strength as a leader;

▲ describe the role mentors play in a leader's development and journey;

▲ identify three strategies nurse leaders use to nurture their own continued growth based on their self- and others' assessment to sustain their ability to lead others in challenging times.

KEY WORDS

Development, leadership assessment, nurturing growth as a leader

INTRODUCTION

The successful development of an effective nurse leader depends on a variety of experiences and opportunities created by others, as well as the individual themself (McBride, 2011). In this chapter we will focus on how the individual can take advantage of opportunities that will challenge them to enlarge their perspective about an issue confronting them, shape how they approach solving problems and how they inspire and lead others. These growth opportunities will present themselves on a regular basis throughout a career but the individual must recognise and embrace them, be open to seeking advice and counsel from coaches and mentors, reflect on their own growth, take risks and commit to reflection and lifelong learning. In this chapter we will describe how leadership qualities evolve over time during a career. We will discuss numerous approaches to assessing one's own strengths and weaknesses as a leader, how to evaluate the various tools commonly used, how to best utilise the feedback from the use of standardised tools and shape one's own growth curve. Mentorship as a form of growth enhancement and support will be explored as well as the way leaders need to seek out a sense of balance to sustain their ability to lead. Finally we will explore various dimensions of sustainment of self during the leadership journey.

ASSESSMENT OF LEADERSHIP POTENTIAL

Listening and reflection: learning about self as leader

Many nurse leaders who look back on their careers retrospectively will share that their own perception of 'self as leader' lagged behind the perceptions of others in their environment (Taylor, Wang, & Zhan, 2012). Many seasoned leaders can identify times when others whom they worked for and with, encouraged them to take on more responsibility or praised them for doing a good job of leading a team through a challenging implementation of a plan. These observations of others often resulted in a change in self-perception of the emerging leader's strengths. Alternatively, in a predominantly female profession, there are pragmatic realities related to stereotyping, bias and prejudice about women as leaders that every emerging leader in nursing will face at some point in a career. The research literature has documented the pervasive phenomenon that women leaders have faced when others do not recognise their strength, or see those characteristics as being 'too soft'. Yet these people skills that women excel at are now recognised in many sectors of business as very crucial to building teams, inspiring others, engaging followers, etc. (Ibarra, Ely, & Kolb, 2013; McEldowney, Bobrowski, & Gramberg, 2009). The observations of others about one's strengths, success with setting and accomplishing goals, reflection about how one handled a difficult team assignment and brought it to completion, all help young leaders to begin to believe in their own strength and unique characteristics that stand out from others (Hughes & Beatty, 2005).

One reason the emerging leader has difficulty seeing how well they managed a situation and demonstrated leadership behaviours is they are often caught up in the emotional aspects of the challenging situation. 'Trying on' leadership behaviours (e.g. setting a vision for a team goal; managing conflict on a team) for the first few times often feels awkward. But as others in the environment, especially well-regarded leaders in the organisation, comment on how well those behaviours manifested themselves, the emerging leader begins to slowly integrate those perceptions into their own self-image, and are more likely to apply those behaviours in another situation. In my own [Broome's] career, as I moved into a new career phase, I felt very awkward—sometimes even like an imposter (Heinrich, Hurst, Leigh, & Oberleitner, 2009). I often questioned my actions and decisions when conceptualising new initiatives and

Table 15.1 Reflections for emerging leaders

Question	Reflection
How do I know others think of me as a leader?	When you work with others, do they listen to how you frame the problem? Do you find others asking you what you think should be a solution?
How well do I listen to what others are saying? Do I change my mind about something when others provide evidence and rationale for a decision?	Do you find yourself thinking about what you will say next when someone is speaking?

developing goals implementation strategies. Fortunately, I was a hard worker, focused and liked working with people. But although I set goals for myself, I was very hesitant to set goals for and lead teams of people. It was only when I heard others share how well organised an initiative was, how creative my approach was, how much they learned, or how much they enjoyed seeing a 'young nurse' leading other faculty from across campus to meet a specific project goal, that I began to see myself as a leader. And the more specific their feedback was about what I did well the more likely I was to repeat it and experiment with that style when working with other people. Hughes and Beatty (2009) discuss the criticality of learning through experience in the development of a leader and how emerging leaders must seek out challenging experiences to stretch themselves. The questions in Table 15.1 can be used to reflect on a recent experience that has helped you shape your leadership 'strengths'.

Assessing leadership potential using structured assessment tools

The assessment of one's leadership potential is one of the first, and regular, steps any leader should engage in. As was mentioned earlier, regular and objective assessment is critical as so many emerging, and even seasoned, leaders often do not see their strengths as an influencer and vision 'holder' in the way that others see them (Rath, 2007). Unfortunately, some leadership workshops do not include a self-assessment component, leaving emerging leaders to try and emulate or 'try on' one leadership strategy after another. The use of structured assessment tools allows one to use the items, questions and scores to compare strengths in certain areas with others and view competences thought to be important for a self-identified leader.

There are a number of tools available to assess leadership characteristics and style. There are many self-assessment tools that measure overall leadership behaviours and qualities, such as setting a vision, inspiring others, etc. In addition, these tools will assess and provide information about specific competences, such as conflict management, ability to initiate change or team-building skills. Ideally, leadership assessment tools are usually based on or linked to a theoretical model of leadership. The theoretical model will describe what the key variables (factors) are in leadership. The model also helps to understand what we think the relationships between the various leadership concepts or components are and make it possible to predict if, for example, we do 'this', 'that' will happen. For instance, what might be the relationship between the ability to manage conflict and the ability to build and maintain teams.

A theoretical foundation is an important distinction among leadership assessment tools. If a measure is not based on a theoretical model that describes the overall leadership framework, it will be more difficult for an individual to see where they 'fit' within the overall leadership journey and what they can expect during the leadership journey.

ASSESSMENT TOOLS FOR LEADERSHIP

There are a plethora of leadership models and frameworks, assessment tools and tool kits one can use to guide a self-assessment. Table 15.2 includes several examples of approaches that can be used by emerging and seasoned leaders in a variety of settings and across their leadership journey. These include the assessment of leadership strengths, clinical leadership, transformational leadership strategies, etc. These are just selected examples and the reader is encouraged to explore the literature and leadership training sites before selecting one or two. In the next section one leadership model, The Leadership Challenge Model, is used to illustrate how one might use a framework and assessment tool to gain insight into one's own potential as a leader.

Selecting the most appropriate leadership assessment tool

There are three important characteristics of any assessment scale that one should look at before choosing the most appropriate for use. These include a) reliability; b) validity; and c) feasibility. Reliability is defined as how consistently an assessment tool measures the same person's attributes over time—assuming nothing has changed about the individual's knowledge and skills. There are a numbers of ways tool developers determine this (Litwin, 1995), and most credible tools have this information available on their websites. Validity is a property of an assessment tool that reflects its ability to measure what it says it is measuring. For instance, different items on an assessment tool should distinguish between transactional leadership behaviours and those reflecting transformative actions.

ILLUSTRATIVE EXAMPLE OF A LEADERSHIP MODEL
The Leadership Challenge Model

The Kouzes and Posner model is one leadership model (Kouzes & Posner, 2007) that describes five major leadership practices thought to be important: 1) Model the Way, 2) Inspire a Shared Vision, 3) Challenge the Process, 4) Enable Others to Act and 5) Encourage the Heart. The Leadership Performance Inventory (LPI) is available for emerging leaders to complete and compare their scores on each component.

Selected behaviours associated with each exemplary practice can be found in Table 15.3. To assess your leadership style, reflect on selected behaviours in the right column and describe, according to your own assessment, to what degree you believe it is characteristic of you.

Respondents are asked to think about their typical response in an actual work setting and indicate whether they perform the behaviour, for example, fairly often, seldom, etc. Each response is given a point from 1 to 10 (never, seldom, always) and then the item's responses summed for each of the five subscales.

When I [Broome] completed the LPI the first time, I was struck by 1) how well the scores in each component actually reflected my actual experience and comfort with certain practices vs. others and 2) how two of the scores were very high (Inspire a vision and Model the way) and two very low (Enable others to act and Encourage the heart). This assessment gave me pause and I spent a great deal of time talking with trusted colleagues and reflecting about the individual items on these subscales,

Table 15.2 Selected examples of leadership assessment tools

Leadership assessment tool	Conceptual components (subscales)	Items	References/order
Leadership Practices Inventory (Kouzes & Posner, 2007)	Model the way Inspire a vision Challenge the process Enable others to act Encourage the heart	30 items/5 subscales/10-point response format	www.leadershipchallenge.com
Multifactor Leadership Questionnaire (MLQ-Form 5x) (Bass & Avolio, 2004)	Idealised influence Inspirational motivation Intellectual stimulation Individual consideration Contingent reward Active and passive management Laissez-faire	45 items/3 factors: Transformational/ Transactional/ Avoidant-Passive	www.mindgarden.com
Clinical Leadership Competency Framework: Self-assessment tool (National Health Service, 2012)	Demonstrating personal qualities Working with others Managing services Improving services Setting direction		www.leadershipacademy.nhs.uk
StrengthsFinder 2.0 (Rath, 2007)	Thirty-four themes and ideas for action include Relator; Ideation; Futuristic, etc. Based on one's core that is calculated online and an individual report is produced that provides a description of your top five strengths and specific suggestions for how to maximise your strengths and minimise any weaknesses.	Assessment tool accessed by code found at end of book by Tom Rath. The assessment takes about 30 minutes.	http://sf2.strengthsfinder .com/research

Table 15.3 Selected items for the Leadership Practices Inventory (LPI)

Leadership component	Selected behaviour
Model the Way	I set a personal example of what I expect from others
Inspire a Shared Vision	I describe a compelling vision of what our future could be like
Challenge the Process	I experiment and take risks even when there is a chance of failure
Enable Others to Act	I support the decisions that others make on their own
Encourage the Heart	I make it a point to let others know about my confidence in their abilities

www.leadershipchallenge.com

what I did well, what behaviours I felt comfortable with and what people who worked with me expected from someone in my position. I then focused on adopting several of the behaviours on the subscales with low scores and 'trying them out' until I felt more genuine and comfortable. In my experience, that worked well to help me 'learn' those behaviours and examine how they worked with others. Did others seem to respond positively to what I was saying and doing? Were there others in my organisation who responded less positively? Was I able to influence the latter group over time to achieve our common goals? I found that the more I enacted some of those behaviours, the more I received positive feedback from others I worked with, which made it easier to enact that behaviour again. Three years later I took the LPI again. My previous high scores remained highest of the five subscales, but I was able to move the scores on two of the five in a more positive direction, while the fifth stayed the same.

The Clinical Leadership Competency Framework

The National Health Service of the United Kingdom has developed a Clinical Leadership Competency Framework for clinicians working to 'deliver quality service' to patients and families (NHS, 2012). Strong engaging leaders are critical to ensuring patients receive the highest-quality, safest care possible. The purpose of that framework is to assist clinical leaders in an assessment of their own ability to lead others. Clinical leadership in health and care services is about delivering high-quality services to patients by 1) demonstrating personal qualities, 2) working with others, 3) managing services, 4) improving services and 5) setting direction (NHS, 2012). In demonstrating personal qualities, the emphasis is on self-management and self-development. There are questions and pragmatic strategies aligned with each component of the competency framework. This toolkit provides very helpful ways to think about competencies needed in each area and differentiates those competencies by level of leader–student, practitioner and expert practitioner. One unique aspect of this leadership model is the integration of expectations for leaders around patient safety and quality of care.

Assessing one's leadership

Several key principles are important to consider when completing and reviewing your answers (i.e. score) with another individual—a coach, sponsor or supervisor or colleague. In terms of process, it is always a good idea to identify someone you respect in terms of their leadership abilities to review the scores and help with the interpretation. This person will almost always share that the first time they completed an assessment tool they, too, focused on those areas they didn't score as highly on (e.g. 'Model the Way'). It is best to take a balanced view of your scores, think about areas you have strong skills in and talk with that individual about ways you might strengthen the areas you found to be less strong, assuming you think it is important to strengthen them. Leaders vary in their strengths and in most organisations the ideal leadership team is composed of individuals who complement each other but also have some common leadership qualities, including the ability to see self as an executive leader, ability to think conceptually, integrity and empathy (Wageman, Nunes, Burruss, & Hackman, 2008).

I found it helpful as I was reflecting on my scores on the Multifactor Leadership Questionnaire (Table 15.2, Bass & Avolio, 2004) to envision how use of some of those strategies in a recent situation might have changed the outcome, given neither I nor those involved were satisfied with the outcome.

This 'critical incident technique' (Chell, 2004) is used to help learners think through a challenging process that they have recent and deep knowledge about. This technique enables the emerging leader to recount an experience and explicate what was important to them in defining the situation. It makes it possible for the learner to imagine hypothetical outcomes that could have resulted and might be worth applying in the next situation.

THE ROLE OF MENTOR IN THE LEADERSHIP JOURNEY

Engaging with a mentor can be a very profound experience that accelerates self-development and growth. The mentor–protégé relationship can be defined as a 'developmental relationship between a more experienced or skilled mentor and a less experienced protégé whereby both mentor and protégé benefit from the relationship' (Kim, 2007, p. 187). This relationship is generally comprised of three functions: career support, psychosocial support and role modelling (Kim, 2007). Career support includes sponsorship, in which the mentor serves as a champion for the protégé. Career support also includes coaching, advising and involvement in challenging assignments, as well as protection of the protégé (McBride, 2011). The mentor is careful and calculated with exposure and visibility of the protégé to other key individuals who may be influential in the long-term development of the protégé's career (Kim, 2007). The psychosocial support function includes acceptance, confirmation and counselling (Kim, 2007). Necessary elements of this function include the mentor being available to the protégé, active listening, asking clarifying questions, having the ability to give and receive difficult feedback in a supportive way, and celebrating achievements (McBride, 2011). Finally, the role-modelling function provides the protégé with a frame of reference for appropriate behaviour and values through interaction with and observation of the mentor (Kim, 2007).

MENTOR AND PROTÉGÉ CHARACTERISTICS

Both the mentor and the protégé bring different experiences, viewpoints and personalities to their relationship. The mentor–protégé dyad may be created through a formal and structured mentoring program designed to pair more experienced experts with novice learners or through informal natural development in which two individuals are drawn to each other and negotiate the terms of the relationship independently (McCloughen, O'Brien, & Jackson, 2009). Whether brought together formally or informally, there are characteristics of both the mentor and protégé that greatly influence the efficacy of the relationship.

Characteristics of successful mentors include strong self-esteem, optimism and effective communication skills. The mentor should also be highly knowledgeable in the content the protégé wishes to learn, possess the ability to navigate organisational politics, and be interested in new challenges. The mentor should also be altruistic and genuinely interested in developing the career of the protégé (McCloughen et al., 2009). In addition, many successful mentors possess a visionary transformational leadership style in which they are motivated to help others develop to their fullest potential and facilitate the protégé's goals (Middlebrooks & Haberkorn, 2009). The mentor must also be available to the protégé, provide unconditional support, honest feedback and challenging assignments (Kim, 2007; McCloughen et al., 2009).

Successful protégés must have self-management capabilities and be committed to learning (Kim, 2007). Protégés should also be motivated to reach professional goals, be accepting of constructive feedback, be committed and passionate about their career and profession, possess effective communication skills, have the potential to succeed, take initiative for development and have the ability to act responsibly and independently (McCloughen et al., 2009). Since the end goal of this relationship is to have the protégé become independently competent, it is important that the protégé should take an active participatory role in the relationship. Through active participation in the development of learning goals, the protégé learns to become more self-reliant (Fischler & Zachary, 2009).

CHARACTERISTICS OF PRODUCTIVE MENTOR–PROTÉGÉ RELATIONSHIPS

There are characteristics of productive mentor–protégé relationships that enhance the functionality and positive outcomes of the exchange. The nature of the relationship is a voluntary exchange in which there must be shared trust and guidance (Talley, 2008). The focus of this relationship should be on professional growth and development of both the protégé and the mentor. The mentor–protégé relationship differs from other social relationships and should not be confused with a friendship. Although personal in nature, respectful boundaries should be observed and usually develop out of integrity, mutual trust and mutual respect (Kim, 2007; McCloughen et al., 2009). Creating a safe environment with mutual goals, unconditional support and respectful boundaries is important as the mentor and protégé will engage in dialogue that will likely include self-disclosure. Wanberg, Welsh, and Kammeyer-Mueller (2007) found that higher levels of disclosure on the part of the protégé increased the satisfaction with and efficacy of the relationship. Self-disclosure can be a risk to both members of the dyad if mutual trust and respect is violated and these boundaries should be negotiated and respected.

Godshalk and Sosik (2003) found that mentor–protégé relationships are more productive when the conceptual model of learning goal orientation (LGO) is utilised. Successful LGO characteristics are those in which both members of the dyad are focused on the desire to enhance development through skill acquisition, mastery of new and challenging situations and competency improvement (Kim, 2007). The nature of this relationship is fluid in nature and learning goals should be negotiated over time (Talley, 2008). The relationship may take many forms dependent on the availability of a mentor and the learning and developmental needs of the protégé (Kim, 2007). It is also noted that a mentor does not necessarily need to be from the same profession provided that they have the expertise in the content that the protégé desires to learn in the context of the relationship (McCloughen et al., 2009).

Another important characteristic of the mentor–protégé relationship is that of reciprocal teaching. This teaching method has positive effects on both parties in this dyad. The protégé receives the benefit of exposure to new concepts and increased self-reliance, while the mentor receives the benefit of mastery of concepts through teaching, guidance and adjustment of current mentor competence (Middlebrooks & Haberkorn, 2009). A key to this reciprocal teaching characteristic is effective two-way communication in which both parties engage in active listening and open dialogue.

Finally, another key characteristic of a productive mentor–protégé relationship is the development of psychological capital. Four foundational elements of the development of psychological capital that provide the foundation of future leadership activities are self-efficacy, hope, optimism and resiliency (Middlebrooks & Haberkorn, 2009). Over time, the protégé becomes less reliant on the guidance provided by the mentor, thus increasing their self-efficacy (Kim, 2007). The mentor, in entering into the relationship, receives confirmation of personal efficacy and is able to verify knowledge through mentoring activities (Middlebrooks & Haberkorn, 2009). Hope and optimism is fostered in this dyad through clarifying roles and expectations, and achieving goals in a positive manner. Through this engagement, both parties in this dyad may experience an increase in hope through interaction and achievement. While both the mentor and the protégé need to have a sense of optimism for this to be successful, the mentor's ability to be optimistic has a greater effect on the success of this relationship (Middlebrooks & Haberkorn, 2009). Resilience is built through the experience of challenges and failures throughout the course of the relationship. Mentors must assist protégés to face adversity by rolemodelling persistence and achievement despite failures and setbacks (Middlebrooks & Haberkorn, 2009).

STAGES OF THE MENTOR–PROTÉGÉ RELATIONSHIP

Many authors have described the development of the mentor–protégé relationship as it is formed and developed. Like many relationships, there is typically a beginning, a middle and an end, which are marked by different transitional events throughout the career. One common conceptual model delineates four distinct phases of the mentor–protégé relationship as a) initiation, b) cultivation, c) separation, and d) redefinition (Fielden, Davidson, & Sutherland, 2009; Kram, 1983; McCloughen et al., 2009). Each phase along with its associated behaviours is found in Table 15.4.

OUTCOMES OF THE MENTOR–PROTÉGÉ RELATIONSHIP

There are many positive outcomes achieved through the development and cultivation of a productive mentor–protégé relationship. These outcomes, presented in Table 15.5, outline the expected outcomes experienced not only by the protégé, but also by the mentor and the organisation (Ensher & Murphy, 2011; Fielden et al., 2009; Kim, 2007; Wanberg et al., 2007).

PERSONAL REFLECTIONS ON BECOMING BOTH A PROTÉGÉ AND A MENTOR

I [the second author, Gilbert] have had many opportunities to relate to a mentor throughout the course of my career. Beginning as an undergrad student, I sought out

Table 15.4 Stages of the mentor–protégé relationship

Relationship phase	Relationship functions and behaviours
Initiation phase	Mentor and protégé come together either through mutual respect and attraction or formal process Dyad establishes boundaries and terms of relationship Negotiation of learning goals Dyad learns about each other through dialogue and self-disclosure
Cultivation phase	Exposure to new knowledge Completion of challenging assignments and negotiated developmental goals Sponsorship of protégé by mentor through exposure to larger professional network Protégé grows in self-esteem, confidence, independence and competence
Separation phase	Mentor and protégé separate emotionally and geographically through independence of protégé
Redefinition phase	New relationship boundaries are established May include occasional coaching or support Shift to more collegial relationship

Table 15.5 Outcomes of the mentor–protégé relationship

Entity	Possible outcomes
Protégé	Increased compensation Quick promotion Increased career mobility Increased socialisation into organisational roles Improved leadership skills Increased job and career satisfaction
Mentor	Satisfaction in assisting protégé obtain career goals Increased knowledge and insight into leadership practice Continued personal leadership development Renewed sense of organisational commitment
Organisation	Increased productivity Increased ability to recruit and retain talent Decreased turnover Enhanced motivation Improved communication Enhanced succession planning and talent development Increased work environment stability

a faculty mentor who became a trusted advisor throughout my undergraduate career and transition to clinical practice. Entering into practice, another mentor oversaw the advancement of my skills and exposure to new protocols and projects. Upon entering into my first management position and through the transition to the director level, I had yet another trusted mentor who saw in me more possibility than I saw in myself. Engagement with these mentors throughout the course of my career has accelerated my growth and advancement. They are the reason I have continued progressive education, sought out new opportunities outside of my comfort zone and was afforded the opportunity to grow and develop. I am forever indebted to these trusted advisors for helping me to achieve educational and leadership goals while enduring unforeseen setbacks along the trajectory. Equally important has been the relationships developed with those I have been fortunate enough to mentor over my career. Once mastery of one level of leadership was attained, I was able to enhance my skill by guiding others on their leadership journey. Being both a protégé and a mentor has enhanced my leadership practice and has made the journey much more rich and satisfying.

SUSTAINMENT OF SELF DURING LEADERSHIP CHALLENGES AND CHANGE

It is a rare leader that finds the journey without bumps, detours and sometimes seemingly abrupt changes in how one is perceived by others. The challenges to one's leadership vision or execution usually follow a period of time in which the leader may have not timed a new initiative well, didn't fully communicate the impending change, or plan for implementation and consider all the ramifications for everyone involved. It is easy to be a leader and feel good about one's leadership when things function smoothly, praise flows freely from those one works with and change is evolving at a more normal speed. Under those circumstances most leaders are renewed and recharged at regular intervals and look forward to watching new and exciting initiatives unfold. However, that exact scenario is unlikely to present itself very often if one is working in a complex, dynamic work environment.

It is much more difficult to refresh and recharge when change becomes chaos, even for a short period of time, when execution of a planned-for change is fraught with uncertainty and anxiety on the part of those involved. Very quickly a chorus of unhappiness fills the organisation and it is easy for the leader to sink into self-pity and even despair, feeling all of the organisation's difficulties are his/her responsibility alone.

The traditional expectation that a 'good' leader has endless enthusiasm and energy, optimism and hope is not realistic in today's work world. Leaders of complex organisations, which most are, must find ways of doing more for themselves to maintain hope (McBride, 2011) and generosity of spirit while working with others.

Physical energy is also an important part of leadership and a leader today will find it very easy to continue to work well past their reserves on dispatching 'one more email', coaching one more employee, answering one more phone call from a distressed staff member, etc. As a contemporary advertisement points out 'a body in motion stays in motion'—but it is the kind of motion that is critical to ensure that one is renewed and refreshed.

Resilient leaders use a variety of strategies to renew and refresh. Some find they must maintain a regular schedule of physical activity (walking, rowing, badminton, etc.) to reduce stress and devote time to themselves to keep from feeling tired all the

---

Box 15.1 Evidence-based strategies for renewal and sustainment for nurse leaders

What activity outside of work do I enjoy the most? Which gives me the most satisfaction, renewal?

Have I spent less time on that activity in the last three months than before? Than I want to?

How do I make time for that activity?

Are there new strategies I could incorporate (i.e. meditation, mindfulness) in my week that would add to any sense of inner peace I might strive for during unrelenting change?

---

time. Others have a hobby or a vocation that, while taking several hours from their schedule each week, serves as a way to meet needs they have for interaction with others outside of work, learn new ideas, and/or serve others. Other leaders make time for meditation each day, finding that after 30 minutes of inward reflection and quietude they return more awakened, refreshed and serene and ready to face the day's challenges. Others find that time spent with their children, spouse, partner or friends rejuvenates their sense of balance and inner peace.

One might ask what a leader gets out of pursuing these activities. It could be expected that leaders who take time for themselves, and engage in activities outside of work and with others in the community would make better decisions, respond less reactively to challenges and be more creative in generating solutions to problems. Each emerging (and seasoned) leader must make time to reflect, rest and renew their spirit and inner sense of peace and serenity. To do less is not only unfair to the individual leader but also to those in the workplace and in the home. Box 15.1 includes some questions a leader can use to guide their self-assessment related to sustainment and renewal as a leader.

CONCLUSION

Developing and sustaining oneself during the course of a leadership trajectory is an important and necessary component of success. Even though talent and determination are helpful, the ability to reflect on one's actions and learn through experience is vital to grow and develop into a competent and respected leader. There are a variety of leadership models and tools with which one can gauge current performance and develop self-improvement strategies. Engaging with a mentor at every level of the leadership journey can be conducive to self-growth and acceleration of leadership competency. Contemporary leadership practice requires navigation through complex systems with ever-increasing financial and regulatory pressure in both clinical and academic settings. Learning to lead during times of change, taking risk and accepting new challenges with optimism is important in developing as a nurse leader. Balance between professional, personal and scholarly aspirations and obligations can be difficult to achieve, and it is necessary for the leader to recharge and find inner peace through engagement in fulfilling work and leisure activities.

CASE STUDY

Elizabeth is a 28-year-old clinical nurse specialist who was identified by her Vice-President of Nursing as having 'leadership potential' and wanted her to attend a leadership workshop. However, Elizabeth did not view herself as a leader. She knew she was very organised, liked working with teams of people to solve problems in patient care, was able to meet deadlines and stay on task, and always picked up others' work on a team when someone ran into some difficulty meeting their obligations. She was skilled at interpreting what outcomes 'administration' wanted and could reframe for others some change that was impending and get them to see the positive side of the change—to see how they or their patients might benefit.

Elizabeth liked being with other people at work, and was well respected by her peers as an expert clinician who mentors, encourages others, challenges unsafe or low-quality care in the organisation and serves as a role model to direct care nurses.

If you were the nurse manager in Elizabeth's setting, or previous faculty advisor, and she came to you to ask advice, what would you encourage her to do as a next step in her leadership journey? How would you follow up with Elizabeth to best support her as she continues to develop?

REFLECTIVE EXERCISE

1. How do you find the time to engage in reflective practices related to your own leadership?
2. How do you spot emerging leaders? What kinds of support are most appropriate to encourage leadership development?
3. How do you know what 'feeds your soul' as a leader and gets the rest of the job done well?
4. How do you choose a mentor?
5. How do you find energy and engage in self-sustainment practices?

Recommended Readings

Bolman, L. G., & Deal, T. E. (2008). *Reframing Organizations: Artistry, choice, and leadership* (4th ed.). San Francisco: Jossey-Bass.

Ford, J. D., & Ford, L. W. (2009). *The four conversations: Daily communication that gets results.* San Francisco, CA: Berrett-Koehler Publishers.

George, B. (2010). *True north: Discover your authentic leadership* (Vol. 143). San Francisco: John Wiley & Sons.

Gifford, W. A., Davies, B. L., Graham, I. D., Tourangeau, A., Woodend, A. K., & Lefebre, N. (2013). Developing leadership capacity for guideline use: A pilot cluster randomized control trial. *Worldviews on evidence-based nursing: Linking evidence to action, 10*(1), 51–65.

Kellerman, B. (2012). *The end of leadership*. New York, NY: HarperCollins.

Northouse, P. (2013). *Leadership: Theory and practice* (6th ed.). Los Angeles: Sage.

References

Bass, B., & Avolio, B. (2004). *Multifactor leadership questionnaire manual and sampler set* (3rd ed.). Menlo Park, CA: Mind Garden.

Chell, E. (2004). Critical incident technique. In C. Cassell & G. Symon (Eds.), *Essential guide to qualitative methods in organizational research*. London: Sage.

Ensher, E. A., & Murphy, S. E. (2011). The mentoring relationship challenges scale: The impact of mentoring stage, type, and gender. *Journal of Vocational Behavior, 79*(1), 253–266. doi. <http://dx.doi.org/10.1016/j.jvb.2010.11.008>.

Fielden, S. L., Davidson, M. J., & Sutherland, V. J. (2009). Innovations in coaching and mentoring: Implications for nurse leadership development. *Health Services Management Research, 22*(2), 92–99. doi:10.1258/hsmr.2008.008021.

Fischler, L. A., & Zachary, L. J. (2009). Shifting gears: The mentee in the driver's seat. *Adult Learning, 20*(1/2), 5.

Godshalk, V. M., & Sosik, J. J. (2003). Aiming for career success: The role of learning goal orientation in mentoring relationships. *Journal of Vocational Behavior, 63*(3), 417–437. doi. <http://dx.doi.org/10.1016/S0001-8791(02)00038-6>.

Heinrich, K., Hurst, H., Leigh, G., & Oberleitner, M. (2009). The teacher scholar project: How to help faculty groups develop scholarly skills. *Nursing Education Perspectives, 30*(3), 181–186.

Hughes, R., & Beatty, K. (2005). *Becoming a strategic leader*. San Francisco: Jossey-Bass.

Ibarra, H., Ely, R., & Kolb, D. (2013). Women rising: The unseen barriers. *Harvard Business Review*, September, 61–66.

Kim, S. (2007). Learning goal orientation, formal mentoring, and leadership competence in HRD: A conceptual model. *Journal of European Industrial Training, 31*(3), 181–194.

Kouzes, J., & Posner, B. (2007). *The leadership challenge*. San Francisco: John Wiley & Sons.

Kram, K. E. (1983). Phases of the mentor relationship. *Academy of Management Journal, 26*(4), 608–625. doi:10.2307/255910.

Litwin, M. (1995). *How to measure survey reliability and validity*. Thousand Oaks, CA: Sage.

McBride, A. (2011). *The growth and development of nurse leaders*. New York: Springer Publishing Co.

McCloughen, A., O'Brien, L., & Jackson, D. (2009). Esteemed connection: Creating a mentoring relationship for nurse leadership. *Nursing Inquiry, 16*(4), 326–336. doi:10.1111/j.1440-1800. 2009.00451.x.

McEldowney, R., Bobrowski, P., & Gramberg, A. (2009). Factors affecting the next generation of women leaders: Mapping the challenges, antecedents and consequences of effective leadership. *Journal of Leadership Studies, 3*(2), 24–30.

Middlebrooks, A. E., & Haberkorn, J. T. (2009). Implicit leader development: The mentor role as prefatory leadership context. *Journal of Leadership Studies, 2*(4), 7–22.

National Health Service (NHS) (2012). *LeAD Leadership Framework Academy*. Retrieved from <www.leadershipacademy.nhs.uk>.

Rath, T. (2007). *StrengthsFinder 2.0*. New York: Gallup Press.

Talley, V. H. (2008). Mentoring: The courage to cultivate new leaders. *AANA Journal, 76*(5), 331–334.

Taylor, S., Wang, M., & Zhan, Y. (2012). Going beyond self-other rating comparison to measure leader self-awareness. *Journal of Leadership Studies, 6*(2), 6–31.

Wageman, R., Nunes, D., Burruss, J., & Hackman, J. R. (2008). *Senior leadership teams*. Cambridge, MA: Harvard Business School Press.

Wanberg, C. R., Welsh, E. T., & Kammeyer-Mueller, J. (2007). Protégé and mentor self-disclosure: Levels and outcomes within formal mentoring dyads in a corporate context. *Journal of Vocational Behavior, 70*(2), 398–412. doi:10.1016/j.jvb.2007.01.002.

CHAPTER SIXTEEN

Interprofessional education (IPE): Learning together to practise collaboratively

John H. V. Gilbert

LEARNING OBJECTIVES

At the completion of this chapter, the reader will have gained an understanding of the challenges associated with nursing leadership of interprofessional learning as applied to collaborative patient-centred care. The chapter will present discussions about:

▲ the healthcare system—why interprofessional (IP) learning is difficult;

▲ the importance of interprofessional education (IPE) and interprofessional practice;

▲ interprofessional education in practice (IPP): re-thinking collaboration;

▲ moving IPE and IPP into healthcare—how leaders in nursing can plan and build a program of IPE and interprofessional care (IPC).

KEY WORDS

Interprofessional education, interprofessional practice, interprofessional care

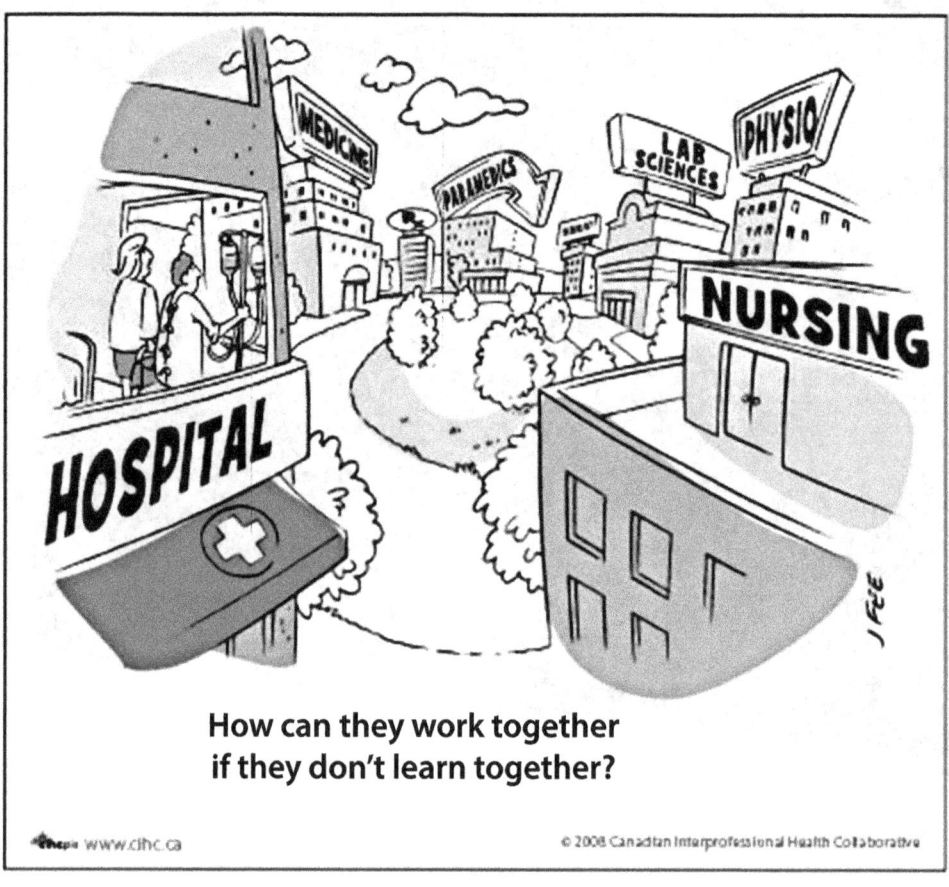

How can they work together
if they don't learn together?

www.cihc.ca   © 2008 Canadian Interprofessional Health Collaborative

INTRODUCTION: THE HEALTHCARE SYSTEM—WHY IP LEARNING IS DIFFICULT

Health professional education is a long and interesting process. It has taken place over the past 100 years in carefully built silos (Gilbert, 2008).

The silo approach to education has led to confusion and many interpretations about healthcare practice. Is it about getting and staying fit and well? Is it about healthcare providers? Is it about body parts and diseases? The complexity of interaction between wellness, illness and providers has been compounded by the siloed education of health professionals (Margalit et al., 2009).

The healthcare workforce is composed of many different professions and many different health occupations of which nursing comprises the greatest number. It is a large and complex mass of people that includes not only regulated professions but also cleaners, desk clerks, technicians, community workers and many others who are frequently unseen in the continuum of care. It's the most highly educated workforce in the world. Yet, when it comes to working as an interprofessional team, it is frequently dysfunctional. Leaders in nursing have great potential to address this dysfunction, and, with leaders in other health professions, lead system change (Gilbert, 2005a).

It is the health system's belief that of course it works as a team. Yet global studies demonstrate the frequent occurrence of events that are adverse for patients because of poor team skills.

These adverse events frequently occur because of the inability of healthcare workers to talk coherently with each other in a common language.

During the past 15 years there has been considerable impetus for healthcare reform. The Institute of Medicine (USA) 1999/2001 reports, which consider health professions' education, illustrated major concerns with quality and safety. As a result, healthcare has seen the gradual incorporation of models from, for example, group dynamics, aviation, crew resource management and LEAN management into policy and practice. Coincidentally, and driven by intense work in Canada, the UK and the USA, the development of sound adult learning principles (andragogy) for IPE have begun to emerge.

It is now clear that interprofessional team-based practice and care have positive impacts, not only for patient care but also in the development of healthy workplaces, human resource planning and a better understanding of chronic disease management. How is IP education related to IP practice, and why is it important? Can health professional education be transformed through inspired nursing leadership to bring health equity?

THE IMPORTANCE OF IP EDUCATION AND PRACTICE

Since 1969, there have been many attempts to introduce interprofessional (IP) concepts in educational programs and a number of recommendations concerning what students should learn, together with how they should learn it (see, for example, WHO, 2010). Professional nursing associations in many countries have been at the forefront of these attempts. The movement towards interprofessional education and learning for collaborative patient-centred practice has included many well-intentioned and, in a few cases, highly successful experiments—funded by governments (e.g. National Health Service, UK; Health Canada, and the Health Resources and Services Administration (HRSA, USA)), non-governmental organisations (e.g. World Health Organization), and foundations (e.g. Macy Foundation, USA). However, despite the fact that there have been numerous attempts to develop IPE programs, building and sustaining even the most moderate program has proven to be difficult.

Interprofessional education (IPE) has been defined as 'Occasions when two or more professions learn from and about each other to improve collaboration and the quality of care' (Centre for the Advancement of Interprofessional Education (CAIPE), 2002). Much that has been written about IPE and the IP team has concentrated on two or at most three professions, primarily medicine, nursing and pharmacy. Educational programs described in the literature tend to focus on activities involving students, practitioners or both. Very little has been written about the structural changes that need to be made within universities, colleges and the healthcare industry such that IPE becomes a joint responsibility across a number of jurisdictions that may then effectively influence institutional practice.

Any educational program for collaboration should provide conceptual opportunities to test assumptions that, at the very least, provide data on the relationships among different professional groups as expressed in the values and beliefs held by their practitioners. The data would include, for example, assessment of the knowledge and skills needed to collaborate and work in teams; delineation of the roles and responsibilities of health and human service professionals in a team; that is, what those professionals actually do in their work lives; and evaluation of the benefits of IPE and collaborative care to patients or clients, to the practice of a profession and to an individual's professional growth.

Institutional structures do not necessarily support collaboration in either the education or the health sectors. Over the years, significant discussion has taken place about barriers to effective IPE programs, and how to address these barriers. There is a broad consensus on the difficulties of scheduling courses, meeting professional requirements, recognising faculty involved in IPE for promotion and tenure and cost implications. Gilbert (2005b) has examined these and other barriers that have prevented (and continue to prevent) the emergence of a culture of interprofessionalism within both the post-secondary education sector and the healthcare industry. Individuals and institutions working to implement IPE, whether in academia or practice, face a number of structural challenges such as:

▲ developing reward structures for faculty who are often not compensated for teaching IP courses (i.e. tenure track excludes IPE);

▲ university/college/institute funding is generally allocated by faculty or department, and excludes IP or co-led programs;

▲ health professionals have limited opportunities and time to focus on IP activities within their organisation (i.e. hospital, health authority, private practice);

▲ many managers and administrators are faced with lack of support when attempting to introduce IPE as a new concept within their organisation;

▲ the healthcare system is driven by the 'issue of the day' with education receiving less attention than clinical areas in terms of budget, human resources allocation, etc.

IPE is often seen as an add-on or 'non-essential' program, and as a result it is frequently a lower priority.

In teaching health professionals, the patient's voice is often lost in the discussion. Indeed, sometimes healthcare sounds as though it is all about healthcare professionals. The patient becomes the object and not the subject of attention. Teaching devolves into a lot of talking about (or at) the patient, but not much talking with the patient.

Leaders in nursing education have to continually and continuously focus attention on the fact that practice is about the patient. The patient should always be the subject of professional attention not the object of some professional goal. Patient-centred care is not about moving a football, it is about caring for a person.

Because of professional silos, there is much duplication of learning—which finds its way into practice. Valuable time, effort and energy are lost when healthcare providers repeat, for strictly professional reasons, the same procedures as their colleagues. The ways in which scopes of practice are developed by each profession present the system with this problem of reduplication.

One major problem of health professional education is that each profession trains its practitioners in different languages. Each profession has a secret code. I call it 'acronish'. All professions develop their own acronyms, and it is clear that frequently one profession does not understand the acronyms used by another profession (see Appendix 1A for a class exercise). It is not surprising that adverse events (errors of practice) occur when language used among health professionals has many attributes of the Tower of Babel. Professionals think that they are using the same language, but frequently the language each profession thinks it understands leads to different conclusions. Close to 80% of the healthcare workforce is female. Yet education has paid little heed to gender differences in language.

Complaints addressed to the health systems administrators are all too frequently attributed to the language problem of poor information transfer. The probability of an honest answer to the question 'Does this piece of clothing make me look fat?' depends on the person you ask—your partner, your parent or your closest friend. We have lots of analogues in healthcare of this kind of information fear of who is asking and answering a question. Much of the interaction in collaborative teams is about confusion in information transfer. Imagine the potential to get things wrong at discharge handoff. At that crucial time healthcare professionals could give incorrect information, or they could omit information or they could simply mangle information. If the team is confused, no wonder patients are confused and that adverse events occur.

If confused and confusing language is not enough to trip up team care, think about the environments in which care is provided—or in which teaching is conducted. It is no wonder that at times the system appears discombobulated. Finding a way through the mazes called 'acute care settings' can seriously interfere with good teaching and practice. Those who have experienced the system know it is good and it is bad and are usually articulate in talking about the good and the bad (see Appendix 1B).

Each discipline on a university, college or institute campus loves to own its space. Think of all the simulation labs being built on the private territory of Faculties x, y or z, which will only ever be used by that faculty, and no other. Can we expect health professionals to work together if they don't learn together? What are the many ways in which leaders in nursing could draw in other health professionals to learning around simulation?

It is recognised that there are no simple solutions to these problems. We suffer from 100 years of silo building, and almost as many years of professional regulation and legislation (see Gilbert, 2008). Change will take time, patience and resources.

Next, consider role clarification. Tied up in scopes of practice, dictated by accreditation and sanctified by legislation, is it any wonder that we see constant iterations of a theme: 'That body part (or that disease) belongs to us. Not to you.' We are inching towards IP practice, but still have a long way to go. So simple solutions cannot be expected. But at least logic can be applied to these problems. Their extent can be assessed and evaluated. Clear plans for change can be developed. Outcomes and impacts can be measured. Attention of this nature is owed to future students, and certainly to patients.

This major movement to IP education and practice will take collaborative nursing leadership—from nurses in post-secondary education, the health sector, professional associations, unions and government and, of course, in their interactions with the health professionals. Health professional education can surely be partly removed from silos to produce graduates who enter practice skilled in collaboration, and with enough knowledge to work together in any kind of healthcare team. With respect to IPE, the future leadership goals of nursing education are: To teach students in nursing to collaborate more effectively and efficiently with other health professionals. This will mean less time protecting turf, ceding pieces of scopes of practice and moving out of silos.

How might this goal be achieved by re-thinking collaboration between nursing and other health professions in everyday practice?

INTERPROFESSIONAL EDUCATION IN PRACTICE (IPP): RE-THINKING COLLABORATION

Around the world, instructional programs in universities, colleges and institutes prepare individuals to practise as licensed professionals and assistants in identified healthcare professions, many of which are regulated and controlled by a variety of complex mechanisms, such as: government legislation, professional associations, facility and educational program accreditation and union membership.

When considering the reality of how patients receive health services, this complexity is further compounded by the large number of health and human service occupations that are not regulated (e.g. home care assistants). To reduce the possibility of disconnection between regulated and unregulated health occupations, it is imperative that IPE be embedded in health and education systems in a manner that helps students and providers to understand each other's competencies and roles. This interconnection can be established through, for example, IPE interventions, which occur when two or more professions learn interactively to improve collaboration and the quality of care; interprofessional practice (IPP) interventions, which are activities or procedures incorporated into regular practice to improve collaboration and the quality of care; and interprofessional organisational (IPO) interventions, which are changes at the organisational level (e.g. space, staffing, policy) to enhance collaboration and the quality of care (Hall & Weaver, 2001).

As noted above, IPE occurs when two or more professions learn with, from and about each other to improve collaboration and the quality of care. IP collaborative practice is closely linked to this definition since it is envisioned as an environment that facilitates communication and decision making, which enables the separate and shared knowledge and skills of different care providers to work together to influence the care provided through changed attitudes and behaviours (after Way, Jones, & Busing, 2000; Kirkpatrick, 1967).

There are, of course, innumerable examples of what constitutes IP collaborative practice settings: acute care—ER, OR; community health clinics—diabetes; extended care, home nursing care; mental health centres; rehabilitation services and social services of many descriptions.

What does IP collaborative practice try to achieve? Its central purposes are to simplify access to other professionals; enhance communication among professionals; promote IP learning; promote evidence-based practice; and allow full scope of practice to be realised.

As noted earlier there are, however, structural barriers to effective IP collaborative practice, which include university, college and institute campuses where frequently curricula are structured entirely around and within individual professional faculties and schools with little discussion about common interfaces around common clinical problems. Effective nursing leadership can do much to overcome these barriers by, for example, bringing faculties together around case-based learning. Despite their critical role in practice (clinical) education, community agencies (e.g. hospitals, health centres, etc.) are not conceptualised as learning environments and, when they are, are inadequately resourced to provide exemplary teaching and learning opportunities. Too often community agencies are viewed strictly as service providers rather than partners in the continuum of learning for preparation to practise, and then for continued learning. As health and human service professions developed during the twentieth century, many statutes were put in place to recognise the distinct difference between professions, which then unfortunately through mechanisms such as licensing and certification, inhibited the impetus to collaborative practice. Finally, the health and human service professions themselves, through their professional associations, set in place the accreditation of educational programs which had no remit to work with other professional accrediting programs to embrace IP education, learning and practice.

In addition to structural barriers to effective IP collaborative practice, there are personal and interpersonal barriers. All professionals, often for very good reasons, dislike uncertainty and are fearful of change. As professions have developed they have built both intra- and interprofessional rivalries and misunderstandings. Because of the way in which health and human services professionals are educated and compensated, there are power, income and status differentials, which can cause anger and hostility. There are, of course, differing conceptual approaches and models of healthcare depending on professional training and in almost all professions a lack of education and training about collaborative teamwork. Finally, there are different and competing organisational priorities both within and between academic and training programs, and healthcare provider organisations, which can lead to a form of undesirable tribal behaviour.

Despite the many barriers to IP collaboration, it is being recognised that there are facilitators that can be invoked to build environments in which effective IP collaboration can be developed as the model for patient-centred practice. These facilitators include a clear and coherent understanding of an institution's shared values and goals, and a clear statement of the institution's objectives. These need to be underpinned and reinforced by clearly defined tasks, procedures and protocols. All members of the provider community need to understand and respect their complementary roles. To achieve this goal there needs to be regular and effective communication in order to build mutual respect and trust and to develop a commitment to collaboration in practice. Ultimately, it is recognised that to sustain these facilitators there needs to be regular review and reflection on progress and informed feedback on performance.

It has become clear that there is a set of abilities needed in order to promote effective IP collaborative practice; these include the ability to network effectively, to communicate and problem solve clearly, to manage confidentiality, to cooperate reflectively, to negotiate honestly, to handle conflict appropriately, and to plan realistically and follow through on that planning. An effective collaborator is a facilitator, an assessor, an evaluator and a communicator.

How then can IPE and IPP be moved into the healthcare system?

MOVING IPE AND IPP INTO HEALTHCARE—HOW TO PLAN AND BUILD A PROGRAM OF IPE AND INTERPROFESSIONAL CARE (IPC)

One of the major issues facing healthcare systems and healthcare professionals is the amount of duplication in service that has resulted from the development of scopes (codes) of practice. Clearly, each health professional needs to be competent in a number of different aspects of patient care related directly to her/his profession. But it is also clear that because, for example, diagnosis follows similar paths regardless of profession, there will be overlap. For example, every health professional needs to know the name and age of a patient, particularly in the absence of a chart or electronic record, and each health professional will need to ask similar questions about current health status. The reiteration of these questions across practitioners is illustrated in the cartoon. The task of moving IPE and IPP into healthcare has, of necessity, to take individual professional knowledge and skills into account, while at the same time reducing reduplication of processes. It is imperative to plan and build a program of IP practice and care that grows out of discipline-specific professional education and extends along the continuum from classroom to practice settings to the larger community of the patient/client.

Planning a program brings us into contact with the problem of terminology, which it is essential that all participants in a program understand and agree upon. A number of terms have been used to describe the interaction between health and human service programs (HHSPs) as they grapple with the problems and complexities

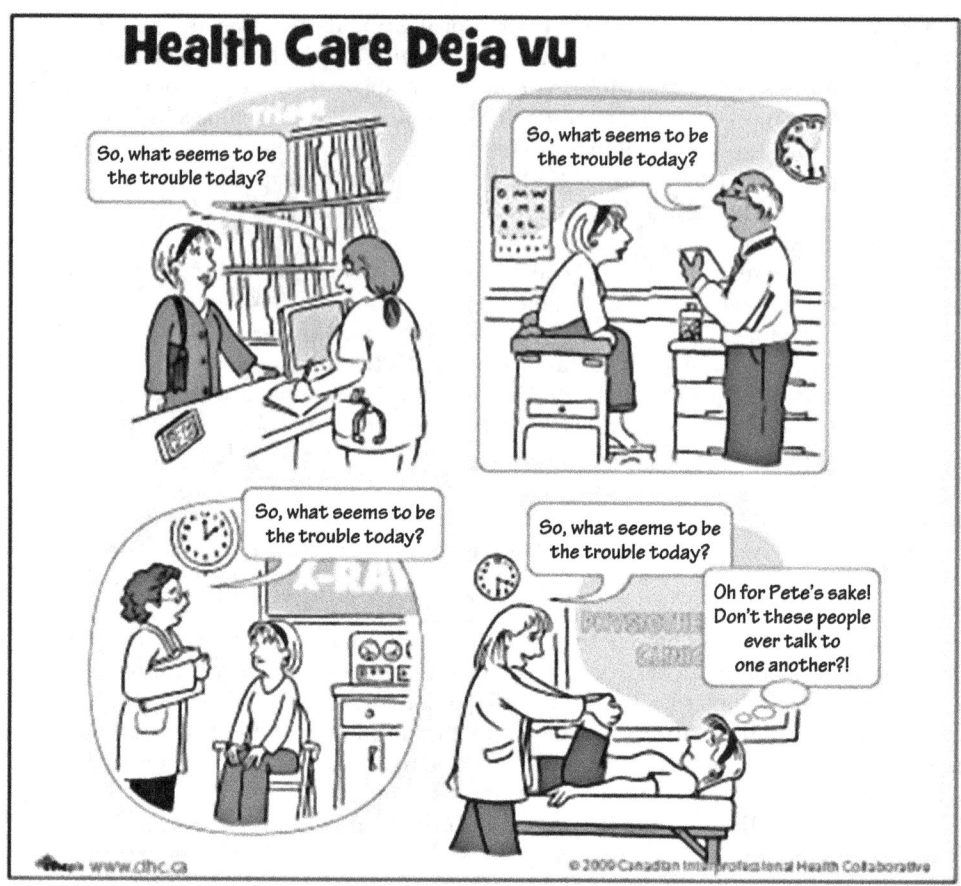

of working together, to maximise their various competencies and reduce reduplication. The term 'interprofessional' is preferred to either multi-professional—which infers work in parallel, or interdisciplinary—a term reserved for discipline-based interactions, since interdisciplinary activity can be practised by any two academics, within any one academic department.

In developing a concept of IPE, it is important to recognise today's understanding of two major concepts: the determinants of health and the parameters of population health. Together these concepts ultimately drive health and human service delivery. Nursing leaders play an important role in bringing health professionals together around these concepts.

When we examine the curricula of diverse health and human service educational programs, many questions are raised as we attempt to understand how such curricula are influenced (or not) by the relationship between the determinants of health and population health, with respect to their effectiveness and efficiency, and application to practice. In the past 10 years we have come to recognise the close links between determinants and safety, and between safety and what in the airline industry is termed 'crew resource management (CRM)' (Gordon, Mendenhall, & O'Connor, 2012).

This series of complex interactions between determinants, population health and safety have moved the discussion about IPE/IPP to a number of questions. How do we educate students to understand the philosophical differences between universal programs; for example, public health issues, targeted programs, such as those that aim at specific populations, and clinical programs that are concerned with a broad range of health issues but within a specific domain? Each of these programs is closely linked to determinants, population health and safety and each requires a clear understanding of how professionals can work together to deliver them as informed IP teams.

Within universities, colleges and institutes, and health service agencies, which may offer a wide range of health and human service programs, grappling with how to encourage those different health and human service programs to collectively and collaboratively understand each other's academic and professional missions, and how to take steps to integrate certain aspects of teaching and learning, can each be approached by asking a number of related questions.

1. How do those various agencies together build a collaborative, civic community by developing such understanding—a community that takes social responsibility for healthcare in the broadest sense envisioned by the World Health Organization (WHO)?

    … there is a health baseline below which no individuals in any country should find themselves: all people in all countries should have a level of health that will permit them to work productively and to participate actively in the social life of the community in which they live (WHO, 2010).

2. How do those various agencies take professional education out of professional practice boxes to ensure that graduates truly understand the effects of a broad IP spectrum of healthcare practices, and how to integrate their learning into such practices?

3. How do those various agencies integrate policy matters—in both education and health—with evidence from scientific inquiry so that such evidence informs IP collaborative practice in a coherent, congruent and timely fashion?

4. How do those various agencies integrate IPE with the health goals espoused in the large number of consultation documents produced by various levels of government in literally every country in the world?

Nursing leaders can facilitate the serious attempts needed to move IPE and IPP into healthcare by participating in collaborative discussions with other health professionals that both understand and answer these and other complex questions. Planning and building a program of IPE and interprofessional care (IPC) must be able to cross professional boundaries, while at the same time respecting and maintaining the integrity of professional programs to educate and train the next generation of excellent practitioners. Planning should also recognise the personal experiences of healthcare professionals (see Appendix 1B for a group exercise on this topic).

All participants recognise, and agree, that the education of health and human service professionals is incredibly complex. There are, for example, over 90 designated health professions in Canada, and similar numbers in other high-income countries. These professions are regulated and controlled by a variety of mechanisms through, for example, government bodies, professional associations, facility accreditation and union agreements.

The intersect of the large number of universities, colleges and institutes with these governing bodies and regulations makes the IPE of practitioners imperative. This education should be focused on helping them understand each other's competencies and roles in the system, prior to graduation into practice. It is far easier to train for

IPC than it is to change to IPC when in practice (Blue, Mitcham, Smith, Raymond, & Greenberg, 2010).

What arenas exist for IP work? Who should be engaged in this for it to work? There are at least four ways of viewing the arenas and participants in IP education and practice and in which nursing leaders can be prime movers.

1. We can look at IPE and practice from the perspective of service providers. Those service providers work at the forefront of care and report to managers, directors, and chief executive officers in their various agencies, as they perform services called for in their job descriptions. Front-line practitioners are vital partners in IPE and IPC.

2. We can look at IPE from the point of view of faculty members in the wide variety of educational institutions. Those faculty members must meet internal expectations of academic excellence; that is, teaching and research, depending on the institution, whilst at the same time ensuring that their educational institutions meet requirements of external accrediting, licensing and other agencies.

3. We might look at IPE from the point of view of the client/patient/citizen—the purchaser or user of the services of the professions we educate. We have evidence from an extensive body of work that the client/patient/citizen responds favourably to care when served by an IP team that has a true understanding of the role of the team in patient care. Clients/patients are becoming central players in changing educational and service institutions.

4. We might examine IPE from the point of view of governments—federal, local and municipal—who all work under the constraints of their tax bases. Governments have a strong interest in ensuring that service is delivered in timely, appropriate and economically reasonable ways that meet their programmatic needs.

As noted by Gilbert (2005b, 2008) it is somewhat perverse that in a number of ways, each of these four players has developed barriers to IP cooperation.

An example of these barriers to IPE can be found within just one of these players—the university.

All members of university programs that train health and human service professionals recognise the enormously important role of community agencies in IPE. It is clear, however, that only by understanding the barriers to IPE in educational institutions will it be possible to formulate strategies for working around barriers to interprofessional practice (IPP) community agencies.

Barriers to IPE as opposed to IPP have their roots in the development of universities. Despite any difference in their origins, however, universities by and large have inherited historically similar faculty and departmental structures.

In universities, faculty structures are modelled on departments with reward systems that usually place greater emphasis on disciplinary, as opposed to interdisciplinary, scholarship and teaching. This disciplinary emphasis usually means that faculty members who wish to engage in IP or interdisciplinary activities do so at some peril, since their promotion, tenure and merit adjustments are predicated on service to a single department or discipline.

In addition, most professional programs are subject to accreditation, and professional accrediting authorities make demands of departments about what should or should not be included in curricula. Frequently, accrediting bodies pay lip service to IPE, usually because it is so poorly understood.

It has been said that: 'Changing a college curriculum is like moving a graveyard— you never know how many friends the dead have until you try to move them.' (Variously attributed to either Calvin Coolidge or Woodrow Wilson.)

And then, of course, there is external licensing legislation. Again, licensing requirements are frequently written with very little (or no) recognition of the role of IPE.

How then might we overcome these barriers to IPE encountered in our universities?

Health and human service community agencies have proven to be models for teamwork, although this teamwork is not necessarily interprofessional. Community agencies tend towards programmatic service delivery; for example, to entities such as diabetes clinics, rehabilitation centres, cardiac clinics and clinical entities for other chronic diseases.

Programmatic service delivery implies a flattening of organisational structures such that within service organisations, departments of X, Y and Z no longer exist but have been replaced by teams of professionals in these specific programs. There are also many very well-documented examples of excellent community-level activities run by human service agencies; for example, mental health. All of these many and diverse programs offer a wide range of IPE opportunities which are directly related to IP practice and care.

It is ironic that programmatic approaches to care in the provider community have heightened awareness to the fact that although disciplinary health professional education programs produce competent practice-ready graduates, those graduates are all too frequently not job ready.

It is now understood that 'not job ready' means new graduates are unable to work in these new programmatic team settings without a considerable amount of additional education by employers, to bring graduates into the organisation's program structure. At the same time, however, this additional education by employers is mostly about focusing on the specific knowledge and skills needed by that institution, rather than driven by a desire to develop IP practice and care.

How then might an institution begin to plan for IPE?

1. Most important is to identify people who have a clear interest in IPE and IPC. To begin this may only be a small team of three or more health professionals, which must include nursing. It is equally important that these 'champions' have access to all levels of administration. They should include clinical faculty and managers for clinical placements. They should represent a cross-section of disciplinary interests and skills and be capable of teaching IP competencies. The small team should certainly include a patient/client who has been engaged as a teacher and understands the importance of team-based care and, from the start, students should be part of the planning—in countries where IPE has begun to thrive, students have been major interlocutors for its importance in their professional education (see, for example, http://www.cihc.ca/nahssa).

2. The team should explore conceptual ideas for curricular formats: a) How to mount big, multi-disciplinary courses using lectures and demonstrations, which are foundational to IPE; for example, Population Health, Determinants of Health, Bases of Teamwork; b) How to develop small, team-teaching, team-learning IP courses using problem-based, case-based and scenario-based learning for topics such as issues in primary healthcare and chronic disease management; for example, HIV Aids, Disability and Justice, Palliative Care, using a variety of methods for presenting such courses including: collaborative

learning, egalitarian learning, group-directed learning, experiential learning or reflective learning.

3. It is now recognised that the principles of adult learning should drive IPE.

4. Scheduling of IP learning offers many opportunities to be very flexible; that is, a 'course' can be one day (for example, seminars); it may be one week (for example, workshops); it may be one month (for example, intensive courses); or it might be one year (for example, a typical full course).

5. Focus on practice (clinical) education sites, and resolve some critical issues related to placements, so that they are truly interprofessional. Focus on developing curricula with Practice (clinical) Educators, who are key players and must understand principles of evaluation of IPE, how the knowledge gained from learning 'with, from and about' is attained, and that sharing, disseminating and communicating lessons as they are learned is a fundamental part of sustaining such programs. We have to recognise that IP collaboration is not learned by osmosis, nor in a classroom—it is learned by working with patients and with professional colleagues.

6. The team must understand that institutions (both educational and health) must clearly acknowledge the roles and responsibilities of participating faculty/clinicians, and therefore that appropriate rewards must be offered to faculty (both campus and clinical) for participating in the new challenges that IPE and IPP bring.

7. Set out foci for preparing individuals for IP collaborative practice; that is, following the work of Kirkpatrick (1967), establish the bases of knowledge; show how to acquire new skills; ensure that learning changes attitudes; work to change inappropriate behaviours and develop perceptions that pave the way for collaborative practice: between professions, within and between organisations, and with patients/clients, their caregivers and communities.

There is of course much more to be said (for example, what constitutes the theoretical basis for IPE and what testable hypotheses does such theory present?). We only have a few of the necessary answers and need much more research evidence. We know from global experiences with conferences that centre on IPE; for example, All Together Better Health (see http://www.atbh7.pitt.edu) and Collaborating Across Borders (see http://cabiv.ca), that it is possible to 'collaborate across professional boundaries' by ensuring that IPE forms a solid part of the education of health and human service professionals (Thistlethwaite, 2012).

CONCLUSION

Ultimately, every health and human service program must recognise that IPE forms a vital and permanent part of the curriculum. IPE is not an add-on—not dumbing down—and not multiskilling. IPE must become a necessary part of educating health and human service professionals. Every graduating student should justifiably claim that they have met and worked with other aspiring health professionals before entering the workforce. Today each profession has tended to forget that it is only one of many that are serving patients. Moving the culture of healthcare in small steps to ensure that patients are not compromised by lack of understanding and communication about shared roles and responsibilities among health professionals must be a goal. It is imperative that knowledge of IP care is enshrined in accreditation and licensure, and that health professionals entering practice collaborate for the better health of patients. The health workforce is claimed to be the most highly educated in modern societies. But that education too often runs along parallel tracks that never meet. To improve the effectiveness of—and the 'value for money' from—that educational investment, we shall have to develop innovative ways of education and training. And those ways will need to recognise the vast range of similarities among the multiplicity of professional preparations, rather than emphasising the differences. The necessary changes will require continued patience and perseverance.

REFLECTIVE EXERCISE

As a nurse leader, what strategies would you bring to address the following questions in a group of fellow health professionals from related disciplines?

1. What is the relationship between interprofessional education (IPE), patient safety and quality of care?
2. What kinds of research are necessary to examine the links between IPE and improved clinical practice and outcomes?
3. How would you build an IP curriculum for a chronic disease, such as diabetes?
4. What factors would you use to facilitate the growth of IPE and IPC at your institution?
5. How would you evaluate the outcomes, and impacts, of an IPE curriculum?

Recommended Readings

Lait, J., Suter, E., Arthur, N., & Deutschlander, S. (2011). Interprofessional mentoring: Enhancing students' clinical learning. *Nurse Education in Practice, 11*(3), 211–213.

Laschinger, H. K. S., & Smith, L. M. (2013). The influence of authentic leadership and empowerment on new-graduate nurses' perceptions of interprofessional collaboration. *The Journal of Nursing Administration, 43*(1), 24–29.

Miers, M., & Pollard, K. (2009). The role of nurses in interprofessional health and social care teams. *Nursing Management, 15*(9), 30–35.

Schwartz, L., Wright, D., & Lavoie-Tremblay, M. (2011). New nurses' experience of their role within interprofessional health care teams in mental health. *Archives of Psychiatric Nursing, 25*(3), 153–163.

WHO (2010). Framework for action on interprofessional education & collaborative practice. Retrieved from <http://www.who.int/hrh/resources/framework_action/en/>.

References

Blue, A. V., Mitcham, M., Smith, T., Raymond, J., & Greenberg, R. (2010). Changing the future of health professions: Embedding interprofessional education within an academic health center. *Academic Medicine, 85,* 1290–1295.

Centre for Advancement in Interprofessional Education (CAIPE) (2002). Interprofessional education—a definition. Retrieved from <http://www.caipe.org.uk/>.

Gilbert, J. H. V. (2005a). Interprofessional education for collaborative patient-centered practice. *Journal Nursing Leadership, 18*(2), 32–37.

Gilbert, J. H. V. (2005b). Interprofessional learning and higher education structural barriers. *Journal of Interprofessional Care,* (Suppl. 1), 87–106.

Gilbert, J. H. V. (2008). Abraham Flexner and the roots of interprofessional education. *Journal of Continuing Education in the Health Professions, 28*(S1).

Gordon, S., Mendenhall, P., & O'Connor, B. B. (2012). *Beyond the checklist: What else health care can learn from aviation teamwork and safety.* Ithaca: Cornell University Press.

Hall, P., & Weaver, L. (2001). Interdisciplinary education and teamwork: A long and winding road. *Medical Education, 35,* 867–875.

Institute of Medicine (IOM) (1999). *To err is human: Building a safer health care system.* Washington, D.C.: National Academy Press.

Institute of Medicine (IOM) (2001). *Crossing the quality chasm: A new health system for the 21st century.* Washington, D.C.: National Academy Press.

Kirkpatrick, D. L. (1967). Evaluation of training. In R. Craig & L. Bittel (Eds.), *Training and development handbook.* New York: McGraw Hill.

Margalit, R., Thompson, S., Visovsky, C., Geske, J., Collier, D., Birk, T., et al. (2009). From professional silos to interprofessional education: Campus-wide focus on quality of care. *Quality Management in Health Care, 18*(3), 165–173.

Thistlethwaite, J. (2012). Interprofessional education: A review of context, learning and the research agenda. *Medical Education, 46,* 58–70.

Way, D., Jones, L., & Busing, N. (2000). *Implementation strategies: Collaboration in primary care—family doctors and nurse practitioners delivering shared care.* Toronto, Canada: Ontario College of Family Physicians.

WHO (2010). Framework for action on interprofessional education & collaborative practice. Retrieved from <http://www.who.int/hrh/resources/framework_action/en/>.

APPENDIX 1

A. The Acronish Exercise © John Gilbert

Object: To show how the secret languages of professions might impact care.
Time: 30 minutes.
Format: Groups of 8/9 different health professionals with one large sheet of paper and pens.

Part 1. Five minutes per group: One person keeps the group on time

Each member of the group writes as many acronyms that s/he uses in daily care. Writers must not say the words of the acronym aloud as they write them—this is very important. It does not matter if there are duplicates.

Part 2. Two minutes per person

▲ Each member of the group chooses ONE acronym.

▲ Her/his task is to spell out the words, then to describe how the acronym is used in patient care.

▲ Every member of the group is responsible for keeping every speaker to time!

▲ So, at the end of the two minutes, the person to the left of the speaker says 'Time'!

Part 3. Seven minutes per group

Each member of the group gets 30 seconds to say if the one acronym she or he chose helps or hinders IP collaboration. 'I think it helps/hinders because ...'

Use the same timekeeping rules as for Part 2.

B: The Personal Experience Exercise © John Gilbert

Object: To reflect on aspects of team-based care.

Time: One hour.

Format: Groups of up to six participants from different health professions.

Individual task: Think about a situation that you have been involved in OR heard about that fits into one of the following two scenarios:

▲ Tell a story about the BEST experience you have had in an acute care or chronic care situation you experienced—especially one that involved interprofessionally working closely together. Describe the situation with as much detail as you can. How did interprofessional care (IPC) contribute to the positives of the situation? Did you have a role in the success? If so, what?

▲ Tell a story about an acute care or chronic care situation that was ABSOLUTELY THE WORST you have experienced. What went wrong? Describe the situation with as much detail as you can. As you think about the situation, what could have changed? How might (improved) IPC contribute to improving the situation?

Take about three minutes to make some notes privately. Then you will share your story within your table group, with each person having about three minutes to tell his/her story.

Ask the group to assign a discussion leader and timekeeper.

'Imagine it is five years from now. Your institution has a well-functioning interprofessional education (IPE) program that is grounded in a collaborative care model.'

▲ What does the IPE program look like?

▲ How did it get created?

▲ What obstacles were overcome as it was created?

▲ What is most successful about it, and how do you know (what are the measurable indicators)?

Then in groups of three people (a combination of guests and fellows) from your table, share what you are imagining for the future of IPE at your institution.

Directions: Within your group of three, discuss and prepare to report on the most promising ideas that you heard in your three-way dialogue.

CHAPTER SEVENTEEN

Leadership and the role of professional organisations

Rosemary Bryant & Debra Thoms

LEARNING OBJECTIVES

At the conclusion of this chapter, the reader will be able to:

▲ describe professional organisations;
▲ understand the roles of professional organisations and how success is seen;
▲ discuss challenges for professional organisations;
▲ describe how professional organisations provide leadership;
▲ describe how professional organisations contribute to the development of leadership within individuals.

KEY WORDS

Professional organisations, leadership, membership, advocacy, networking, mentoring

INTRODUCTION

This chapter explores the role that professional organisations play within the nursing profession. We will provide an overview of the different types of organisations that identify as professional organisations and the challenges that such organisations face. The role and contribution that such organisations make to the broader nursing profession both nationally and internationally will be considered. In particular the focus will be on how these organisations provide leadership for and to the profession and also enable individuals to develop leadership capabilities.

PROFESSIONAL NURSING ORGANISATIONS

It is in the nature of human beings to want to come together with like-minded people to network, share and problem solve. The coming together of people with similar interests provides a focus and avenue to pursue common objectives. The first international health professional organisation was established in 1899 in the United Kingdom. This was the International Council of Nurses (ICN), an organisation that continues to be extant. Its original charter was signed by individual nurses from the United Kingdom, the USA and Germany. Its goals to this day are to bring nurses together, influence health policy, advance the socio-economic welfare of nurses and advance the profession of nurses. The membership of ICN is made up of national nursing organisations from around the world. Within these member associations there are different types of professional nursing organisations (ICN, 2014).

In the early part of the last century, nursing organisations were established in many countries including the United Kingdom, Canada, China and Australia. In the case of Australia, organisations were established on a state-to-state basis, some of which were branches of the Royal British Nurses Association. In more recent decades there has been a move to more nationally based organisations in Australia. This has been seen in the harmonisation of the New South Wales Nurses Association (now NSW Nurses and Midwives Association—NSWNMA) with the Australian Nursing Federation (now Australian Nursing and Midwifery Federation) and the unification of The Royal College of Nursing, Australia and The College of Nursing to form the Australian College of Nursing (ACN) (NSWNMA, 2014; ACN, 2014).

The motivation behind the founding of these organisations can largely be seen to fall into two main underpinning areas: the promotion of professional standards of nursing and advocacy for nurses' working conditions. Since that time, it has been observed that nursing bodies have in most countries split into three familiar types of organisation—professional, industrial and regulatory, although at times these may be combined within one organisation. In Canada at the provincial level, for example, the nursing association is also the regulator.

Being a member of a profession is seen by many as bringing with it some special obligations that non-professionals are not subject to—this is because of the social contract that is seen to exist between the professions and society (Welchman & Greiner, 2005). Welchman and Greiner (2005) outlined what these special obligations are:

▲ individually to provide competent, beneficent, just and confidential care;

▲ collectively:

   ✛ self-regulation—to maintain a satisfactory level of quality in education and professional practice;

   ✛ conduct research and develop new skills, knowledge and techniques to improve;

✛ identify and try to redress obstacles to fair and open access to all—advocacy.

The authors argue that it is difficult for individuals to do all three of these on their own and that it is through professional associations that the responsibilities of quality control, research and advocacy are met. Through their involvement with professional organisations individuals can then meet their obligations as professionals. Individuals also need to provide the information and assist the professional organisation in discharging these responsibilities as they cannot perform their function without the active engagement of its members. In recent years in a number of countries it has become more common for advocacy to be seen as an individual responsibility (Welchman & Greiner, 2005, p. 297). Many of the issues that confront the profession cannot be argued by individuals alone and it is through the collective voice of a professional organisation that change can be achieved. The move of nursing education into the higher education sector in Australia in the 1980s represents this collective advocacy for the profession and the community. The lead-up to the change saw a number of key professional nursing organisations working together to achieve a common goal.

The organisations

These organisations have a focus on what are described as professional nursing issues and do not generally participate in regulatory or industrial matters except to provide a professional perspective. The mission of professional nursing associations centres on the promotion of nursing standards for the benefit of the public. For example, the objects of the Australian College of Nursing are 'to cultivate and maintain the highest principles of nursing and healthcare'. The American Nurses Association (ANA) says that it is 'dedicated to ensuring that an adequate supply of highly skilled and well-educated nurses is available, and. ... is committed to meeting the needs of nurses as well as healthcare consumers. The ANA advances the nursing profession by fostering high standards of nursing practice, promoting the economic and general welfare of nurses in the workplace, projecting a positive and realistic view of nursing, and by lobbying the Congress and regulatory agencies on healthcare issues affecting nurses and the general public' (ANA, 2013). Royal College of Nursing (UK) aims to develop and educate nurses professionally, build professional networks to represent the interests of nursing and the nursing profession, influence government bodies and policy makers and promote the value of nurses in all their diversity (RCN, 2013). The objects of Canadian Nurses Association as defined in the Letters Patent (2013 revision) are:

▲ to advance nursing excellence and positive health outcomes in the public interest;

▲ to promote profession-led regulation in the public interest;

▲ to act in the public interest for Canadian nursing and nurses, providing national and international leadership in nursing and health; and

▲ to advocate in the public interest for a publicly funded, not-for-profit health system.

As can be seen, the organisations cited all have similar aims but they employ different strategies to achieve these. Nevertheless, their main functions encompass policy analysis and implementation, research, advocacy in its many forms, development of clinical and other standards and, of course, membership services.

Industrial and professional

It is not unusual to find that organisations represent themselves as both an industrial and professional association. The Royal College of Nursing in the UK states it 'represents nurses and nursing, promotes excellence in practice and shapes health policies' (RCN, 2013). It also is the key organisation that undertakes industrial bargaining. Within Australia, the Australian Nursing and Midwifery Federation is registered as an industrial and professional association. While engaging in professional activities these organisations are often known more for their industrial activities than for their professional although they do actively engage in areas such as standards development and policy commentary. The American Nurses Association as an alternative example works predominantly at the national level and is seen to have a stronger focus on professional activities with state-based nursing associations undertaking wage bargaining and other industrial activities. One of the challenges that can present for organisations that are both industrial and professional is the balance between the two perspectives and managing the occasions where a professional perspective may not be entirely congruent with the industrial perspective. Some members may be more interested in the industrial issues and others the professional (and some both), which may influence their expectations of the organisation. Tensions concerning resource allocation to these respective activities can also occur.

Regulatory organisations

In those countries with a clear regulatory framework leading to registration of nurses and midwives there are examples of professional associations that also undertake regulatory functions. In countries such as Australia, New Zealand and the United Kingdom, the regulatory organisation or Nursing/Midwifery Board is a separate organisation that has a very specific role. The regulatory role that some organisations have will not be considered in this chapter.

Specialty nursing organisations

Some nursing organisations exist for a specific purpose such as representing a specialty of nursing or a geographic section of the nursing community. These tend to be focused more on professional activities specific to the specialty areas of practice such as standards and competency development, working with what is often a larger industrial professional association for industrial issues. Some of these have international affiliations; for example, critical care nurses. Membership of a specialty group may be in addition to membership of a more generic nursing organisation or nursing union.

The advantage of specialty organisations is that they are well placed to develop the requisite standards and other professional documents such as guidelines and competencies. The disadvantage is the consequence of their size. Often they may be led entirely by volunteers whose effectiveness is often dependent on the time and energy they have to devote to the business at hand. Over time, some of these groups opt to become a section of a larger more general nursing organisation where they have access to professional media and policy development personnel. In these situations it is critical that the unique nature of their goals and objectives is maintained within the larger organisation. Reluctance to surrender independence is often cited as the reason why smaller specialist groups are maintained, even when they are struggling to survive.

ROLES OF PROFESSIONAL ORGANISATIONS

Nurses who join a professional organisation will find themselves with opportunities to be exposed to a broader view of nursing and health. Through active engagement it is possible to meet with other nurses with similar interests to network, discuss and explore areas of mutual interest. This may be focused locally, nationally or even internationally.

Opportunities provided by such organisations enable nurses to contribute to the broader nursing agenda through critical review, debate and contribution to organisational responses on nursing and health matters. By meeting and networking with nurses beyond your own organisation you can gain wider understanding of nursing, health and associated issues. Most professional organisations provide opportunities for continuing professional development through relevant education. Within some organisations there can also be opportunities to participate in nursing projects internationally providing an opportunity to not only grow as an individual but to contribute positively to the global nursing effort to improve healthcare.

Policy development and advocacy

In all professional nursing organisations, advocacy—for their members, for the community or for the profession—plays a central role. Policy development is the vehicle that underpins advocacy and is therefore a significant part of any nursing organisation. The leadership of the governing body and chief executive is critical to the success of advocacy activities as it is they who represent the organisation externally and drive the direction internally. Many nursing organisations will be involved in addressing policy issues on behalf of their members. Recent research has identified that nursing organisations address a variety of policy issues including: professional or practice issues, targeted health issues or populations, social determinants of health, equity or public policy in general. The researchers found that over half were for issues such as scope of practice, prescribing rights, education requirements and workplace issues such as nursing shortages (MacDonald, Edward, Davies, & Marck, 2012, p. 34).

Success for the organisation can also be achieved through alliances and working together, often on a specific issue. This may take the form of nursing and midwifery groups advocating on a common issue in a fixed time frame or a broader alliance, which may be longer term, such as in a Memorandum of Understanding. Creating alliances with consumer groups sends a powerful message to decision makers as significant synergies can be achieved through such alliances. Alignments with groups representing other health professionals can be powerful as well—again, usually for a specific purpose. Leadership and political acumen are critical to the success of these forays as there may be areas where the aims of other organisations are diametrically opposed to those of the nursing organisation. Avoidance of sensitive issues and respectful discourse are essential. Leadership is required to keep these alliances focused on the target at hand.

Policy and advocacy interests will also be impacted by whether the professional organisation operates at a national or state/provincial level. At the local or state level it is often easier to have more targeted responses, while at the national or even international level the strategies to be employed may be numerous and varied in order to represent the nursing perspective (MacDonald et al., 2012, p. 37).

Advocacy by nurses as individuals can be difficult to achieve success in when acting alone—by working with and through professional organisations the potential for achieving desired outcomes is enhanced. The collective position expressed through professional organisations will be able to bring issues to the fore more successfully than an individual could (Mahlin, 2010).

Practice and research

Nursing organisations will be engaged in contributing to debate on practice standards but also in promoting the use of evidence in practice. Through the provision of continuing professional development activities and also by the development of standards, professional organisations can contribute to the professional standing of nursing and midwifery. Standards work by professional organisations can range from the development of papers and guidelines to competency development and credentialling or certifying levels of practice. Some of these are focused on clinical practice but may also be centred on areas such as management and leadership. As an example, the American Organisation of Nurse Executives (www.aone.org) has a program of work that provides education and certification of nurse managers, nurse leaders and nurse executives. In Australia, the Australian College of Mental Health Nurses offers a credentialling program for nurses working in mental health (www.acmhn.org) that focuses more on the clinical practice of nurses in mental health.

MEMBERSHIP

The success of any nursing organisation (apart from the regulator) is dependent on a strong and active membership base. The most obvious reason for this is that membership fees are the drivers of activity and determine the extent to which the organisation can engage in its essential activities. An active membership also assists in driving policy development and achievement of the goals of the organisation. Achieving a strong membership base is primarily the responsibility of the chief executive but in reality all members have a role in ensuring that their colleagues participate in their professional organisation. To a degree success follows success as the more influential the organisation is, the more attractive it becomes for prospective members. The leadership of the president and chief executive is crucial to membership engagement. Conversely, members will vote with their feet if they feel that the organisation is not advocating successfully on their behalf or representing their views. As mentioned earlier the active engagement of members is critical for the success of an organisation but also for the achievement of desired outcomes for the profession.

CHALLENGES

Any organisation representing a profession has its own unique culture that has developed over many years. It can have entrenched views about the profession or about how the organisation should operate. In the case of nursing professional organisations, the board or governing council are generally elected from the membership of the organisation. This may mean that those who stand for office possess limited requisite skills to function in a governance position. They may see election to these positions in their organisations as prestigious and a step that will enhance their stature. Moreover, not many nurses are exposed to the world of health politics and they are therefore often not experienced in this regard. While such an appointment may be advantageous for their own professional development, their organisation itself may not benefit. The sum effect of this situation is that the paid secretariat officers, especially the chief executive, need to be competent political operators and skilled at guiding the board. Education for elected officials, particularly concerning their ethical and legal activities and responsibilities, is vital. Of equal importance is the need for elected members to understand the role of the board as either a board of management or a board of governance. This will underpin the relationship between the paid staff and the board and the functions that each undertake. It will also impact on the relationship with the broader members as the expectations of the board members need to be clear in terms of their strategic and operational responsibilities.

One of the drawbacks experienced by many nursing organisations is the heavy reliance often placed on the small number of those in leadership positions. In reality this is most often the executive officer or chief executive and possibly the president. While individuals are often dynamic in their leadership, the organisations often falter once the individual resigns or retires. This is particularly the case when the organisation is led by an entirely voluntary leadership team.

In larger nursing organisations that have paid secretariats, the performance and expertise of the chief executive officer are critical. This is not dissimilar to the situation in any not-for-profit enterprise. In the case of the president and governing body being weak, the organisation can quickly lose its relative political advantage as well as its profits. Once again this illustrates the dependence of such organisations on individuals. Strong and capable individuals serving on governing bodies are frequently the only mitigating factor in these situations.

It can also be argued that the number of nursing organisations can impact on the collective voice of nursing as a profession. As noted above, the capacity to collaborate between these various specialty groups can be limited at times as these groups often will be focused on issues related to the specialty only and not on issues beyond the specialty, but which can have an impact on nursing overall (MacDonald et al., 2012, p. 36).

For many nurses the decision to join a professional organisation can be difficult. Consideration of issues that are important to you as an individual can assist in making that decision by comparing what you seek with the aims and objectives of the relevant organisation. Membership of professional organisations can also be costly and is a continuing challenge for many. The understanding of members of how to effectively engage and the role the organisation has in ensuring this happens is continuing to challenge as the profile of the profession changes.

Professional associations themselves need to have clarity around their own functions and how they exercise these; for example, if an organisation is both professional and industrial it may need at times to balance the agendas between the two aspects, which may not meet with the approval of all members.

Members are often very diverse and achieving consensus on major issues can be time-consuming and costly. Large organisations will need to have clear processes in place to engage with members with all understanding that there may, at times, be individuals that hold a different view to the one ultimately put out by the organisation.

LEADERSHIP

Growing nurses as leaders

Nurses who are involved with professional organisations have opportunities to grow and develop their own leadership skills and capabilities. This will vary depending on the level of involvement of the individual and the types of opportunities that are presented to them. Stein (2001) in her work, identified three types of informal learning that can occur through membership of a professional organisation. These were mentoring, coaching and networking. While many of these activities were not undertaken in a formal way, often being ad hoc, the outcomes able to be identified indicated that mentoring, coaching and networking did occur. These relationships can offer practical advice on issues that are being confronted, career guidance and an opportunity to connect with colleagues beyond their usual groups. It was evident that members had developed increased self-confidence, which translated into communication and willingness to try new things; others sought new jobs or education opportunities. What was seen as particularly important was that the participants in Stein's study felt that they had 'grown'. They reported being able to see the nuances that exist within many situations and no longer saw things as black or white—they saw themselves as professionals who could make important contributions to the profession (Stein, 2001; Walsh & Borkowski, 2006).

Professional organisations can assist those in their early career to connect with later career and more experienced professionals. As those members who mentor others develop the individual, they are also developing broader leadership. These relationships serve not only as a way to pass on knowledge to the next generation but challenge and support the later career nurses to continue to grow and develop in their own practice as well as the profession more broadly.

Networks take time to develop but do provide access to complementary resources that may not be available in the workplace (Walsh & Borkowski, 2006). These networks may provide additional information and can also be a source of support to an individual. Activities such as information exchange, access to resources and the promotional opportunities that can occur have been called 'instrumental functions' of these networks (Walsh & Borkowski, 2006, p. 367). Professional organisations provide a mechanism to find colleagues with similar interests and opportunities to work together to mutual benefit. As an individual's career develops, the availability of such networks can become even more important as a source of not only information but support and guidance.

Professional nursing organisations also provide more structured educationally based leadership development for members and nurses more broadly. The ACN Emerging Nurse Leader Program identifies early career nurses and provides some formal activities to grow in leadership and other informal activities more directly driven by the participants themselves. ICN has the Global Nursing Leadership Initiative, which provides exposure for individuals to an internationally developed program. As already mentioned, the AONE has made a considerable investment in the provision of leadership development programs in the United States of America.

Individuals will also identify opportunities to develop leadership skills and capabilities through active engagement in local leadership activities, taking on a position perhaps locally, initially, and then perhaps state/province and then nationally. Taking on a position as a committee chair or holding a formal position within the membership structures can develop leadership skills (Guerrieri, 2010). For nurses who aspire to leadership roles, being a member of a professional nursing organisation and interacting and networking with colleagues from different areas of practice and employment can assist to understand the variety of ways that individuals approach their lives and their work and what holds groups together. It can also help to grow an understanding of things such as integrity, advocacy and teamwork, which are all important when exercising leadership (Guerrieri, 2010). Workplaces have changed greatly over the years and the demands of work have impacted on the socialisation that occurs in the workplace, sometimes leaving individual nurses feeling quite isolated. Membership of a professional organisation can provide a sense of belonging and help to reduce the risk of burnout. Sharing of issues with other colleagues as well as hearing of the new and innovative approaches that some may be taking can provide encouragement to continue or to try new approaches (Guerrieri, 2010).

SUCCESS

The markers of success of professional nursing organisations are many and again rely heavily on the expertise of the leader or leaders. Successful organisations are, above all, relevant to their stakeholders both external and internal. External stakeholders include governments, chief government nurses, education providers, other nursing and health professional organisations and consumers. Internal stakeholders are the members and staff of the organisation. Loss of relevance can spell the demise of the organisation much in the same way that insolvency can. A good leader is attuned to this possibility and acts to ameliorate it quickly.

Other markers include sound financial management and investment; an active and representative membership base; good relationships with stakeholders; stable and competent staff; a governing body that is engaged and politically adept; and strong and able leadership.

CONCLUSION

Professional organisations provide more than the opportunity to network with like-minded colleagues. Used effectively they can bring about advancement for both the individual and the profession. Understanding the aims and objectives of an organisation can help you to decide whether or not you may wish to join. Many offer opportunities to grow and develop leadership skills and to contribute to policy debate on major health issues.

REFLECTIVE EXERCISE

1. Consider your current career stage, goals and path:
   a. Have you considered joining a professional association?
   b. Are many of your colleagues members of a professional association?
   c. Does your organisation promote any professional memberships?
   d. Are you primarily interested in industrial issues or professional issues or both?
   e. Do you wish to be actively involved?

   This exercise will help you to identify your current situation with respect to professional associations and think about which one may be of most benefit to you if you were to join.

2. Reflect on your own membership of nursing professional associations:
   a. Do you have a clear understanding of their objectives?
   b. Do these meet with what you wish to gain from being a member?
   c. In your view, to what extent does your professional organisation meet its objectives?
   d. Are you active in your membership; that is, do you participate in the activities of the organisation or are you a passive recipient of information and material?

   This exercise will help you to identify how well you are using your professional organisation membership to develop your own career.

3. Reflect on your awareness of international nursing organisations such as the International Council of Nurses.

    a. Do you know who the member organisation is for your country?

    b. Are you aware of the activities of the international organisation?

    c. Do you know how to access information on the organisation's activities; for example, its website, local contact organisation?

    This exercise will increase your awareness of international nursing organisations.

4. Reflect on your need for leadership development:

    a. Does your professional organisation provide leadership development programs?

    b. What are the critical elements of a leadership development program in your view?

    This exercise will help you reflect on your role and plans for development of your career.

Recommended Readings

Frank, K. (2005). Benefits of professional nursing organization membership. *AORN Journal, 82*(1), 13–14.

Holleman, G., Eliens, A., van Vliet, M., & van Achterberg, T. (2006). Promotion of evidence-based practice by professional nursing associations: Literature review. *Journal of Advanced Nursing, 53*(6), 702–709.

Zabel, D. (2009). The mentoring role of professional associations. *Journal of Business and Finance Librarianship, 13*(3), 349–361.

References

American Nurses Association (ANA) (2013). *Statement of Purpose*. Retrieved 3 December 2013 from <http://nursingworld.org/FunctionalMenuCategories/AboutANA/ANAsStatementofPurpose.html>.

Australian College of Nursing (ACN) (2014). Retrieved 24 March 2014 from <http://www.acn.edu.au/about>.

Canadian Nurses Association (2013). *Letters patent*. Retrieved from <http://www.cna-aiic.ca/sitecore%20modules/web/˜/media/cna/files/en/cna_letters_patent_bylaws_june2013.pdf#search=%22letterspatent%22>.

Guerrieri, R. (2010). Learn, grow and bloom by joining a professional association. *Nursing*, May, 47–48.

International Council of Nurses (ICN) (2014). Retrieved 24 March 2014 from <http://www.icn.ch/about-icn/about-icn/>.

MacDonald, J. A., Edwards, N., Davies, B., & Marck, P. (2012). Priority setting and policy advocacy by nursing associations: A scoping review and implications using a socio-ecological whole systems lens. *Health Policy, 107*, 31–43.

Mahlin, M. (2010). Individual patient advocacy, collective responsibility and activism within professional nursing organisations. *Nursing Ethics, 17*(2), 247–254.

New South Wales Nurses and Midwives Association (NSWNMA). (2014). Retrieved 24 March 2014 from <http://www.nswnma.asn.au/about-us/history/>.

Royal College of Nursing (RCN) (2013). *Our Mission and Strategic Plan*. Retrieved 3 December 2013 from <http://www.rcn.org.uk/aboutus/our_mission_and_strategic_plan>.

Stein, A. M. (2001). Learning and change among leaders of a professional nursing association. *Holistic Nursing Practice, 16*(1), 5–15.

Walsh, A. M., & Borkowski, S. C. (2006). Professional associations in the health industry: Factors affecting female executive participation. *Women in Management Review, 21*(5), 366–375.

Welchman, J., & Greiner, G. G. (2005). Patient advocacy and professional associations: Individual and collective responsibilities. *Nursing Ethics, 12*(3), 296–304.

CHAPTER EIGHTEEN

Leading nursing in the Academy

Kathleen Potempa & Philip Furspan

LEARNING OBJECTIVES

At the completion of this chapter, the reader will be able to:
▲ explore barriers to change in the Academy;
▲ examine challenges and opportunities facing higher education in the US and globally;
▲ examine the challenges of healthcare for higher education;
▲ define the characteristics of successful leaders in the Academy;
▲ provide insight into the innovative requirements of leadership.

KEY WORDS

Higher education, nursing education, leadership, policy, technology

INTRODUCTION

Type Leadership into the Amazon electronic search engine and more than 100,000 books across disciplines and contexts will be returned. What makes the topic of such universal interest? When a problem exists, regardless of business or social sector, often the need for leadership is invoked. When a difficult process of change is managed in business, leadership skill is the focus of accolade. Leadership is seldom captured in a static definition or singular context.

Leadership in this chapter will be explored in the context of higher education and nursing. Because nursing education rests in two institutional contexts, higher education and healthcare, the challenges and opportunities for leaders within these two sectors in modern society will be discussed.

THE CONUNDRUM OF THE ACADEMY

The 'Academy', as higher education is often referred to, has a centuries-old history that has evolved from an elite education for the clergy and aristocracy, to what is now a fundamental expectation of many (Kerr, 2001). While the Academy has evolved, many traditions of today are rooted in the ancient beginnings. For example, systems of hierarchy related to academic achievement as illustrated by the promotion process through academic ranks; 'faculty governance' that distributes leadership across a body of the professoriate such that decisions are highly dependent on consensus; and, resistance to change that comes from long-standing traditions among a stable group of tenured faculty (Brubacher & Rudy, 1997).

While the traditions within the Academy remain visible, the institutions of the Academy have evolved within the context of changing societies. In the United States (US), for example, many contemporary external pressures are challenging the Academy, including the need for greater access, demand for lower cost, and the push for higher degree completion rates (Crow, 2010). What was once considered an 'elite' opportunity governed by the standards of faculty, the college degree is evolving as a 'right' for access to jobs, long-term economic success and social mobility. As the demand for higher education rises around the world (Schofer & Meyer, 2005), the pressures on the modern Academy to be relevant to diverse populations, accessible regardless of geographic location, and affordable in cost have never been greater (Adams, 2011).

Government and private sector leaders are applying pressure to higher education leaders demanding changes in the Academy. While the 'hallowed halls' of the Academy have matured over the last centuries to now be the research and knowledge engines of the world, the modern world expects even more. Like many mature institutions, the very characteristics that fostered its success in the past are the same characteristics impeding change into the future. The traditions of faculty governance, scholarship/research as the 'elite' mission area, and cautious approach to change make the modern university less resilient in responding to a rapidly changing world. It is unlikely that the forms and rules that served an isolated, homogeneous university in the past will be effective in the modern complex, multicultural and globally oriented university. Thus, it is imperative that the Academy strives for nimble ways to adapt and thrive in new and rapidly changing environments. Change at this level will require the active involvement and direction of the leaders in higher education.

Leaders in higher education now face the imperative to innovate 'academic structures, practices, and operations' in order to meet contemporary challenges. This is nothing less than complete transformation or 'institutional turnaround' with all of the accompanying culture change required to achieve such magnitude of change (Crow, 2010). As Kezar opines, '... the future of higher education rests on creating a new set of leaders across campuses who embrace new concepts and abilities of leadership' (Kezar & Carducci, 2009).

PRESSURES AND OPPORTUNITIES FOR THE ACADEMY

Institutions of higher education rest within countries experiencing sweeping changes related to globalisation, the rise of new economic epicentres around the world, unprecedented technological capability, and political volatility and philosophical swings that affect education policy. Whereas these challenges exert pressures on the Academy, they present opportunities as well.

Globalisation and internationalisation of universities

Once, the concept of the Academy as an ivory tower distant from the concerns of the world had a certain validity. However, the increasing ease and rapidity of travel and communication over the past decades have accelerated the internationalisation of universities. At first, admission to the 'elite' universities of countries such as the United States, the United Kingdom, Canada and Australia was sought only by the wealthy or citizens with high social standing of less economically advantaged countries as a pathway for advanced degrees and a cosmopolitan experience (De Witt, 2009). Later, as the advantages of this educational pathway became more prominent, foreign governments began to sponsor their citizens to study abroad through scholarships and stipends. 'Elite' universities of the high-resourced countries became centres of diversity of language, cultures, religions and philosophies demonstrated in the student body, faculty and courses of study.

As internationalisation has evolved in higher education, many universities around the world now not only accept but encourage foreign citizens to study at their campuses (Marginson, 2007). Two factors have contributed to this rapid evolution: the availability of technology to increase access and communication; and the capacity of some universities to compete favourably on the cost of tuition and the expenses of living abroad (Altbach, 2013). As the cost of tuition and living increases in the high-resourced countries such as the US, the availability of good universities in other countries as alternatives is an ever-growing reality. Thus globalisation, while initially only a force for the internationalisation of elite universities in the world, now promulgates competition among universities around the world for the very best students. Most pronounced is the competition for students prepared for study in the STEM fields (science, technology, engineering and medicine). Technology is rapidly increasing the capacity of elite universities such as the Massachusetts Institute of Technology, Stanford University, the University of Michigan, for example, to put courses online that reach thousands, if not hundreds of thousands of participants worldwide (Flynn, 2013). Course content, once only available on campus, is now available for use by citizens and faculty alike around the world. Some universities have put whole curriculums online for free use. While the elite universities reap the benefit of this generosity through increasing applications for their degree programs, universities slow to enter the global arena are falling behind.

According to a survey study by the American Council on Education, 'internationalization is not a high priority on most college campuses' (Green, Luu, & Burris, 2008). For example, the survey revealed that 'Less than 40% of institutions made specific reference to international or global education in their mission statements ...' Although not necessarily a factor in the slippage of US market share of all international students during the past decade (Douglass & Edelstein, 2009) it should be of concern to leaders in the Academy. For nursing schools in the US, the non-US resident enrolment at all levels (baccalaureate, master's and doctoral) more than doubled between 2002 and 2007; however, the subsequent five-year period saw a 16% decline in enrolment, mostly in the baccalaureate category (AACN, 2013). Universities in the US, UK, Canada and Australia, for example, prepared many of the world leaders in nursing and deans of colleges of nursing around the world. As these leaders establish new schools of nursing, more students are able to meet their education goals through domestic opportunities.

The influence of technology

While mimeographs, overhead projectors, filmstrips, etc. were the technological main-stays of higher education pedagogy for several decades, a recent sea change has been brought about by the development of the personal computer, the high-speed internet and the smartphone. For the first time in history students need not be physically present to hear a lecture, ask questions, take an exam, hand in homework, etc. One response of the Academy to these technological innovations has been a steadily increasing availability of online classes in both public and private institutions as well as the development of for-profit universities that offer a large proportion of their classes online. An outgrowth of these classes, MOOCs (massive open online courses), featuring unlimited participation and open access via the internet, have proliferated and drawn much interest and scrutiny in the past couple of years (Flynn, 2013). Although many elite universities have begun to embrace MOOCs it is still not clear how courses enrolling up to hundreds of thousands of students worldwide for free will fit in the tradition-bound, slow-to-change Academy. Although it is unlikely that MOOCs and how to use them are a pressing concern for leadership in nursing educa-tion they must deal with other technological innovations such as advanced patient mannequins, the digital clinics of Second Life and, as recently reported in the *New York Times*, the use of apps on handheld devices to store and access information, such as drug interactions, that once had to be memorised.

The rising cost of higher education

Throughout much of history access to higher education has been perceived as a privi-lege reserved for the aristocratic, the well-born and the wealthy. In colonial times less than 1% of the population was enrolled in college (Cremin, 1970). The century fol-lowing the signing of the Declaration of Independence saw huge growth in the number of institutions awarding bachelor's degrees; 500 by 1870 (Handlin & Handlin, 1970). In 2009, about 7% of a much larger US population was enrolled in an institu-tion of higher learning. In 2012, the US Census Bureau reported that, for the first time, more than 30% of American adults held bachelor's degrees (Perez-Pena, 2012). Despite reaching this milestone, the US lags behind many other developed countries, especially in the youngest cohort studied, those 25–34 years of age (OECD, 2011). In fact, the rate for this youngest cohort is identical to that of the oldest cohort, age 55–64 years, indicating no improvement in the percentage of the population with bachelor's degrees in more than 30 years. The reasons for this poor showing are complex but can in large part be attributed to two factors: the skyrocketing cost of post-secondary education and an anaemic graduation rate. In the past 30 years, tuition, fees and room and board costs at both public and private four-year schools have more than doubled (in 2013 dollars). And, perhaps relatedly, six-year graduation rates have hovered at little more than 50% for the last decade or more (Knapp, Kelly-Reid, & Ginder, 2011). This state of affairs is likely to worsen as the US Census Bureau recently released statistics revealing that college enrolment in the fall of 2012 dropped by nearly half a million compared with a year earlier (Census Bureau, 2013). Although enrolment in entry-level baccalaureate nursing programs in the US has increased every year since 2001 (AACN, 2011), the attainment of the goal set forth by the Institute of Medicine (IOM) of a nursing workforce wherein 80% hold a bachelor's degree or higher by 2020 is still uncertain (IOM, 2011). The main impediment to this goal remains a shortage of nursing school faculty (AACN, 2011). From 2002–2010, almost 300,000 qualified applicants were turned away from schools of nursing (AACN, 2011). The shortage of qualified faculty and resources are cited as the reasons for this situation (AACN, 2011). These are challenges that leaders in nursing education must tackle if we are to meet the demands of the evolving healthcare landscape.

In 2008, the 34 countries of the Organization for Economic Co-operation and Development (OECD) spent an average of 1.9% of combined GDP from both public and private sources on tertiary education (OECD, 2011). Although the full extent of the effect of the global recession on that average is not yet known, in the US, educational appropriations for higher education in 2012 had decreased by more than 23% (SHEEO, 2012).

Cost pressures for higher education in the midst of global changes in the economic forces and related political responses will undoubtedly continue well into the twenty-first century. These economic and political forces are a further challenge to nursing education, which is already affected by faculty shortages. Leaders in nursing education must find transformative means to be efficient, not only within their own institutions but potentially across institutions as faculty are a rare national, if not international, resource.

Innovation and the Academy

With the onset of MOOCs, campus-based online or 'blended technology'-driven courses, international competition for students and rising costs pressuring universities, the challenge of Crow (2010) to transform 'academic structures, practices and operations' now seems insufficient to address these challenges. Universities are indeed grappling with their mission (Keohane, 2013). This is especially true for colleges and universities that are primarily residential or have high value for the in-person experience of students.

The role of the university in research and knowledge generation is also being challenged as search engines, reference material and library capabilities, often unique to major research universities, are available to the public online. 'Think Tank' organisations, foundations and private corporations are taking up major efforts in either supporting research or performing research. Knowledge generation is no longer the essence of a university alone. As well, research costs are escalating and universities are re-evaluating their 'core mission' in order to survive, if not thrive, for their academic purpose.

The tally of challenges facing leaders in the Academy today, including soaring costs, anaemic degree completion rates, disruptive technological innovations, and, for nursing, a lack of faculty, are perceived by many as a daunting crisis in higher education. However, as President Kennedy once remarked, 'When written in Chinese, the word "crisis" is composed of two characters. One represents danger and the other represents opportunity' (Puymbroeck, 2004). In response to the recent global financial crisis, but equally applicable here, Crow recommended that institutions embrace change and complexity (Crow, 2010). He goes on to suggest that when 'confronted by the entirely new environment' in which they must operate they 'should seek to establish *institutional cultures of innovation'* [his emphasis]. The challenges of cost and degree completion rates will require innovation in almost all aspects of the university, mission, operations and source of funding (Crow, 2010).

In some cases the challenge and the opportunity are flip sides of the same coin; for example, MOOCs. A fundamental question is whether expertise and course content are the singular essence of the 'academic course' brought by faculty, whether in person or online? Or, is education much more—reflecting not only content driven by expert faculty, but the dynamic experience and interaction of students, faculty and the flexible content evolving, in real time, with this interaction.

For nursing education leaders the challenge of faculty shortages can be met with several opportunities. One is provided by the Patient Protection and Affordable Care Act (ACA) 'which reauthorizes and strengthens the nursing programs funded by the Health Resources and Services Administration (HRSA)—the primary source of federal funding for nursing education' (Wakefield, 2010). A third opportunity arising from faculty shortages is to create active learning environments that use electronic methods to provide content, while direct interaction is saved for faculty–student activity in clinical settings, research settings and other extracurricular events (Luo, Ng'ambi, & Hanss, 2010).

THE CHALLENGES OF HEALTHCARE FOR HIGHER EDUCATION

Healthcare in the US nearly doubled in per capita cost between 2000 and 2011 (CMS. gov, 2013). However, despite spending much more per capita in dollars and as a percentage of GDP, the US ranked near the bottom (46th) in healthcare efficiency of the 48 countries studied (Bloomberg.com, 2013) and 37th in health outcomes worldwide (WHO, 2000). This inefficiency and broken-value proposition have contributed to a national health picture that is one of the most dismal among high-income countries. In a 2013 study of 17 affluent countries by the NIH, the US had the highest or near-highest prevalence of infant mortality, heart and lung disease, STDs, adolescent pregnancies, injuries and disability (NRC/IOM, 2013). Other issues resulting from this are manifold. The high cost of healthcare and the millions of uninsured means that many people delay seeking treatment and when they do so it is often in emergency rooms, the high cost of which is passed on to the insured through higher insurance premiums (Burt, McCaig, & Rechtsteiner, 2007; Hadley, 2007). The fragmented nature of the US healthcare system has made coordination of patient care problematic, including long waits for diagnostic tests and loss or misplacement of test results (Harris-Interactive, 2007). Access and treatment disparities for ethnic minorities in the US are well documented with the result of 'more chronic diseases, higher mortality, and poorer health outcomes than individuals classified as white' (Tuckson, 2004). These healthcare issues are some of the more pressing ones to be addressed by and, at least partly, rectified by the ACA. The important role of nurses in the accomplishment of many of the provisions of the ACA is evinced by the provisions in the act designed to address training and shortages of nurses at all levels: baccalaureate, master's and doctoral (Wakefield, 2010). To address the latter, the ACA lifts the cap on funding for the Advanced Education Nursing Traineeship and the Nurse Anesthetist Traineeship programs. The ACA also has provisions to provide low-interest loans and partial loan cancellation for nursing students from disadvantaged backgrounds and underrepresented groups. To address the shortage of nursing faculty, there is now more money available for the Nurse Faculty Loan Program, which provides loans for master's and doctoral students interested in becoming teachers. Because the nation not only needs more but also better-educated nurses, the Nurse Education, Practice, and Retention program will address the quality of nursing care. The need to know and do more has grown rapidly as nurses have been asked to fill primary care roles, help manage chronic illnesses, keep up with and use new and complex technologies and information management systems, and collaborate with other healthcare professionals in the coordination of patient care. For these reasons, one of the key messages of the IOM report on the Future of Nursing is that 'nurses should achieve higher levels of education and training through an improved education system that promotes seamless academic progression' (IOM, 2011). Not only do nurses need to know and do more, they must do so with fewer resources and less help as they bear the brunt of the increasing emphasis on cost-cutting and increased productivity at all levels of healthcare (Grandfield, 1992). Rather than passively accept these sub-optimal working conditions, the IOM has called upon nurses to take an active leadership role in the transformation of the US healthcare system by serving as 'leaders in the design, implementation, and evaluation of, as well as advocacy for, the ongoing reforms to the system that will be needed' (IOM, 2011).

LEADERSHIP IN THE NEW ERA

There are many parallels in the challenges of higher education and healthcare in societies that want more for lower cost, international shortages of nurses and the knowledge explosion. No longer is the requirement to be a strong academic in the sense of scholarly prominence, publications and affiliations with prestigious professional organisations the singular hallmark of leadership preparation in the Academy. Leaders of nursing in the Academy today are expected to be chief financial officers, chief executive officers, and 'dean' of faculty. Expected to have business-like acumen, the qualities necessary to lead in the current era are unlike those of previous generations of leaders.

A recent study by Witt/Kieffer compared the qualities of leaders in higher education to those of business and found that leaders from these different environments 'show very similar personality profiles when assessed characteristics are viewed as a whole' (Witt/Kiefer, 2013). However, when looked at individually, several of the characteristics and values did differ between the two groups; in particular, the values of 'Mischievous', 'Aesthetics', 'Altruistic' and 'Commerce'. The report concludes that:

> These differences deserve particular consideration and attention when higher education leaders are asked to adapt to new market conditions or strategic directions, or conversely, when executives from the private sector are asked to step into academic leadership roles (Witt/Kieffer, 2013).

The results of these studies bode well for the contemporary challenges facing higher education/nursing leadership. Current leaders need not be replaced to respond to the difficulties of leading in these challenging and changing times. Instead, there is an imperative to acquire the skills appropriate to the challenges facing higher education/nursing at this time.

As noted at the beginning of this chapter, there is no dearth of resources for the nurse leader in education or healthcare who is intent on improving and adding to their leadership skill set. One of the seminal works in this area (Kouzes & Posner, 1995) elucidates five fundamental principles that the authors claim are universally found in effective leaders: '1) They challenge the process; 2) They inspire a shared vision; 3) They enable others to act; 4) They set an example, and 5) They encourage the heart.' Going beyond these principles in the case of nurse leaders, McNamara

(2009) asserts, based on the findings of a study by Antrobus and Kitson (Antrobus & Kitson, 1999), that:

> ... *nursing knowledge derived from nursing practice is the basis of the identity and legitimacy of all nursing leaders, regardless of whether they operated primarily in the clinical, organisational, political or academic domains. Nursing knowledge from practice for leadership combines an understanding of the philosophical bases of nursing, including the ethics and ideology of caring, with a firm grasp of the wider external and internal factors that might compromise nursing values and promote or inhibit developments in nursing practice.*

The role of innovation as a core opportunity in this current era cannot be over-emphasised. Supporting innovation is a particular skill, as a leader weighs the investments in maintaining the current programs while also investing in the capital necessary to inspire and resource projects that can lead to new innovation. Creating a culture that is open to change requires collaborative capacities, teamwork and willingness to manage chaos that can come from implementation. Implementing change by its nature can never be fully planned because by definition the new processes are untested. Thus, administrative leaders in particular, need to inspire resilience on the part of faculty and students.

The passage of the ACA has presented an unprecedented challenge to the nurse leaders in both education and practice who must prepare nurses, both new and experienced, for their integral role in the enactment and success of many of its provisions. Nurse leaders are responding to this challenge in innovative ways. The past decade has seen the development and implementation of practice-academic partnerships (Beal, 2012) designed 'to keep schools of nursing entwined with what is evolving clinically and to keep clinical nurses closely involved with trends and issues in contemporary nursing education' (Donaldson & Fralic, 2000). In 2010, the same year the ACA was passed into law, this innovative approach to 'advance nursing practice and improve the quality of care' was endorsed by two top US nursing organisations, the American Association of Colleges of Nursing (AACN) and the American Organization of Nurse Executives (AONE), with the issuance of guiding principles, and an interactive toolkit, for developing and sustaining academic-practice partnerships (AACN, 2010).

Although we have concentrated on what we know best, nursing education and healthcare in the United States, we are cognisant that many, and more, of the issues and concerns we have discussed are problems worldwide (Nardi & Gyurko, 2013). In 2005, an innovative response to these global challenges manifested itself in the formation of the Global Alliance for Nursing Education and Scholarship (GANES) (Daly, Macleod Clark, Lancaster, Orchard, & Bednash, 2008). This organisation, comprising national associations of Nursing Deans and Schools of Nursing, strives to 'offer information, support and advice to health care policy makers and nurse educators across the world'. GANES has positioned itself as a resource that nursing education leaders around the world can turn to for information and assistance with which to address shared problems such as the shortage of nurses and the lack of academically qualified faculty needed to teach in schools of nursing (Nardi & Gyurko, 2013).

As this new era of changing educational paradigms and healthcare systems progresses, nursing leadership in the Academy would do well to reflect on these questions:

Am I open to and do I encourage innovation in nursing pedagogy, research and service?

Am I informed about the changes occurring in healthcare that may necessitate changes in the way nurses are educated?

Am I communicating my vision and priorities effectively?

Do I continuously engage in my own leadership development?

Do I encourage others to develop leadership skills relevant to the changing social context of universities?

CONCLUSION

Leadership quality, capacity, capability and innovation in nursing education will be even more crucial to ongoing strategic development of the discipline of nursing in higher education in the future. The 'academy' in nursing faces many challenges that cut across the higher education sector internationally. These challenges include, among others, increased scrutiny and accountability demands by governments and other funders for prudent use of resources, resource constraints and fiscal austerity, changing societal expectations and consumer demands and rapid transformation in educational delivery driven largely by innovation in technology.

Leadership in this complex, continually changing context will be enhanced by nimble, flexible, well-informed, politically intelligent, economically efficient and transformative approaches. Skill development and continual skill renewal appropriate to the challenges facing nursing will also be crucial to success.

Recommended Readings

Altbach, P. G. (2013). Globalization and forces for change in higher education. In *The International Imperative in Higher Education* (pp. 7–10). Rotterdam, The Netherlands: Sense Publishers.

Crow, M. M. (2010). Toward institutional innovation in America's colleges and universities. *Trusteeship, 18*(3), 8–13.

IOM (2011). *The future of nursing: Leading change, advancing health.* Washington, DC: National Academies Press.

Kezar, A. J., & Carducci, R. (2009). Revolutionizing leadership development: Lessons from research and theory. In A. J. Kezar (Ed.), *Rethinking leadership in a complex, multicutural, and global environment.* Sterling, VA: Stylus Publishing.

Kouzes, J. M., & Posner, B. Z. (1995). *The leadership challenge: How to keep getting extraordinary things done in organizations.* San Francisco: Jossey-Bass.

References

AACN (2010). Academic-practice partnerships. Retrieved 26 November 2013 from <http://www.aacn.nche.edu/leading-initiatives/academic-practice-partnerships>.

AACN (2011). *Shaping the future of nursing education and practice: 2011 Annual Report.* Washington, DC: American Association of Colleges of Nursing.

AACN (2013). *Research and Data Services.* Washington, DC: American Association of Colleges of Nursing.

Adams, J. (2011). Oppportunities and obstacles: The imperative of global citizenship. In D. Brenneman & P. Yakoboski (Eds.), *Smart Leadership for Higher Education in Difficult Times* (pp. 115–127). Northampton, MA: Edward Elgar Publishing.

Altbach, P. G. (2013). Globalization and forces for change in higher education. In *The International Imperative in Higher Education* (pp. 7–10). Rotterdam, The Netherlands: Sense Publishers.

Antrobus, S., & Kitson, A. (1999). Nursing leadership: Influencing and shaping health policy and nursing practice. *Journal of Advanced Nursing, 29*(3), 746–753.

Beal, J. A. (2012). Academic-service partnerships in nursing: An integrative review. *Nursing Research and Practice*, 9, doi:10.1155/2012/501564. Retrieved from <http://dx.doi.org/10.1155/2012/501564>.

Bloomberg.com (2013). Bloomberg visual data: Most efficient health care: Countries. Retrieved from <http://www.bloomberg.com/visual-data/best-and-worst/most-efficient-health-care-countries>.

Brubacher, J. S., & Rudy, W. (1997). *Higher education in transition: A history of American colleges and universities*. New Brunswick, NJ: Transaction Publishers.

Burt, C. W., McCaig, L. F., & Rechtsteiner, E. A. (2007). *Ambulatory medical care utilization estimates for 2005*. Hyattsville, MD: US Department of Health & Human Services, Centers for Disease Control and Prevention, National Center for Health Statistics.

Census Bureau, US (2013). *After a recent upswing, college enrollment declines, Census Bureau reports*. Retrieved from <http://www.census.gov/newsroom/releases/archives/education/cb13-153.html>.

CMS.gov (2013). National health expenditure data: Historical. *National Health Expenditure Accounts*. Retrieved from <http://www.cms.gov/Research-Statistics-Data-and-Systems/Statistics-Trends-and-Reports/NationalHealthExpendData/NationalHealthAccountsHistorical.html>.

Cremin, L. A. (1970). *American education: The colonial experience, 1607–1783* (Vol. 2). New York: Harper & Row.

Crow, M. M. (2010). Toward institutional innovation in America's colleges and universities. *Trusteeship*, *18*(3), 8–13.

Daly, J., Macleod Clark, D., Lancaster, J., Orchard, C., & Bednash, G. (2008). The global alliance for nursing education and scholarship: Delivering a vision for nursing education. *International Journal of Nursing Studies*, *45*(8), 1115–1117.

De Witt, H. (2009). *Internationalization of higher education in the United States of America and Europe*. Charlotte, NC: Information Age Publishing.

Donaldson, S. K., & Fralic, M. F. (2000). Forging today's practice-academic link: A new era for nursing leadership. *Nursing Administration Quarterly*, *25*(1), 95–101.

Douglass, J. A., & Edelstein, R. (2009). The global competition for talent: The rapidly changing market for international students and the need for a strategic approach in the US. *Research and Occasional Papers Series*. Retrieved from <http://escholarship.org/uc/item/0qw462x1>.

Flynn, J. T. (2013). MOOCs: Disruptive innovation and the future of higher education. *Christian Education Journal*, *10*(1), 149+.

Grandfield, S. (1992). Do more with less: Strategies for improving productivity in community health nursing. *The Health Care Manager*, *11*(1), 37–42.

Green, M. F., Luu, D. T., & Burris, B. (2008). *Mapping internationalization on US campuses: 2008 edition*. Washington, DC: American Council on Education.

Hadley, J. (2007). Insurance coverage, medical care use, and short-term health changes following an unintentional injury or the onset of a chronic condition. *JAMA: The Journal of the American Medical Association*, *297*(10), 1073–1084.

Handlin, O., & Handlin, M. (1970). *The American college and American culture: Socialization as a function of higher education*. New York: McGraw-Hill.

Harris-Interactive (2007). Uncoordinated care: A survey of physician and patient experience. Retrieved from <http://www.chcf.org/publications/2007/09/uncoordinated-care-a-survey-of-physician-and-patient-experience>.

IOM (2011). *The future of nursing: Leading change, advancing health*. Washington, DC: National Academies Press.

Keohane, N. O. (2013). Higher education in the twenty-first century: Innovation, adaptation, preservation. *PS, Political Science & Politics*, *46*(1), 102–105.

Kerr, C. (2001). *The uses of the university*. Cambridge, MA: Harvard University Press.

Kezar, A. J., & Carducci, R. (2009). Revolutionizing leadership development: Lessons from research and theory. In A. J. Kezar (Ed.), *Rethinking Leadership in a Complex, Multicultural, and Global Environment* (pp. 1–38). Sterling, VA: Stylus Publishing.

Knapp, L. G., Kelly-Reid, J. E., & Ginder, S. A. (2011). *Enrollment in postsecondary institutions, fall 2009; graduation rates, 2003 & 2006 cohorts; and financial statistics, fiscal year 2009*. Washington, DC: NCES, IES, US Department of Education.

Kouzes, J. M., & Posner, B. Z. (1995). *The leadership challenge: How to keep getting extraordinary things done in organizations*. San Francisco: Jossey-Bass.

Luo, A., Ng'ambi, D., & Hanss, T. (2010). *Towards building a productive, scalable and sustainable collaboration model for open educational resources*. Paper presented at the Proceedings of the 16th ACM international conference on Supporting group work.

Marginson, S. (2007). Global position and position taking: The case of Australia. *Journal of Studies in International Education, 11*(1), 5–32.

McNamara, M. S. (2009). Academic leadership in nursing: Legitimating the discipline in contested spaces. *Journal of Nursing Management, 17*(4), 484–493.

Nardi, D. A., & Gyurko, C. C. (2013). The global nursing faculty shortage: Status and solutions for change. *Journal of Nursing Scholarship, 45*(3), 317–326.

NRC/IOM (2013). *US health in international perspective: Shorter lives, poorer health*. Washington, DC: National Academies Press.

OECD (2011). Education at a Glance 2011: OECD Indicators. Retrieved from <http://www.oecd .org/education/school/educationataglance2011oecdindicators.htm>.

Perez-Pena, R. (2012). U.S. Bachelor Degree Rate Passes Milestone. *New York Times*. Retrieved from <http://www.nytimes.com/2012/02/24/education/census-finds-bachelors-degrees-at -record-level.html>.

Puymbroeck, M. (2004). When written in Chinese, the word 'crisis' is composed of two characters. One represents danger, and the other represents opportunity. John F. Kennedy. *Therapeutic Recreation Journal, 38*(4), 394.

Schofer, E., & Meyer, J. W. (2005). The worldwide expansion of higher education in the twentieth century. *American Sociological Review, 70*(6), 898–920.

SHEEO (2012). *State higher education finance FY 2012*. State Higher Education Executive Officers.

Tuckson, R. (2004). *Understanding health disparities*. Columbus, OH: Health Policy Institute of Ohio.

Wakefield, M. K. (2010). Nurses and the Affordable Care Act. *AJN The American Journal of Nursing, 110*(9), 11. doi:10.1097/1001.NAJ.0000388242.0000306365.0000388244f.

Witt/Kiefer (2013). How college and university leaders compare with corporate executives. *Leadership traits and success in higher education*. Retrieved from <http://www.wittkieffer .com/file/thought-leadership/practice/Leadership%20Traits%20and%20Success%20in%20 Higher%20Education_a%20Witt%20Kieffer%20Study_final.pdf>.

World Health Organization (WHO) (2000). *The world health report 2000: Health systems: Improving performance*. Geneva: WHO.

CHAPTER NINETEEN

Avoiding derailment: Leadership strategies for identity, reputation and legacy management

Daniel Pesut

LEARNING OBJECTIVES

At the completion of this chapter, the reader will be able to:

▲ explain the concept of leadership derailment;
▲ contrast differences between identity and reputation;
▲ identify and define behaviours that derail leaders;
▲ describe the value of shadow work for personal and professional leadership success;
▲ create a personal strategy for self-management of potential leadership derailers;
▲ reflect on the importance of creating and crafting a leadership legacy.

KEY WORDS

Leadership, derailment, identity, reputation management, shadow work, legacy

INTRODUCTION

Do you know someone who initially showed great promise in their academic, clinical or administrative career and along the way became sidetracked or derailed? Perhaps they were not promoted, or did not gain the confidence of people in the organisation they were leading? Maybe they developed a reputation for being a difficult or challenging personality? Perhaps they had a reputation for being a 'taker' rather than a 'giver' or 'matcher' (Grant, 2013)? While advancing themselves personally maybe they failed to pay attention or seek out feedback from others? Perhaps they received feedback and chose to ignore or disregard it. Or maybe they did engage some type of 360-degree feedback process and worked with a coach to craft a personal and professional development plan that helped them manage and work through their challenges with insight, understanding, appreciation and success.

The purpose of this chapter is to describe and discuss the concept of leadership derailment, and connect the concept to issues of identity, reputation and legacy management. Derailment takes place when people who are perceived as having high potential in an organisation plateau at a lower level than expected, are demoted or leave the organisation voluntarily or involuntarily (Lombardo & McCauley, 1988).

The chapter begins with a discussion about the contrasts between identity and reputation. Positive and negative behaviours that support effective leadership are described. Both the 'light' and the 'dark' side of leadership are explained. The dark sides of leadership are those conscious or unconscious behavioural characteristics that get in the way of leadership success and professional advancement. People who lead with intention and integrity seek out feedback from the environment and embrace knowledge about themselves and work through issues of identity, belonging, projection and introjection (Smith & Berg, 1997). The courage to work through issues of derailers often results in more effective reputation management and the creation of a positive leadership legacy. Successful leaders who are conscious and awake rather than unconscious and closed, engage in the inner work and the deep change that is required for mastery of an effective leadership skill set (Quinn, 1996).

LEADERSHIP MASTERY: INNER WORK FOR OUTER SERVICE

Throughout my years as a clinician, consultant, educator and coach, I have had a keen interest in learning about an individual's strengths and talents. I believe that knowing one's strengths is a prerequisite to understanding how best to lead and influence in any context. Helping people master the knowledge, skills and abilities of leadership is a personal and professional mission (Pesut, 2001, 2007, 2013). Leadership requires mastery of one's self, mastery of communication, mastery of relationships and mastery of multiple ways of being, thinking and feeling, doing and influencing in order to transform problems into desired outcomes. Personal mastery also requires attention to inner work and the management of one's psychological projections or shadows. An aspect of the inner work required of every nurse is personal reflection and self-management of those behaviours and characteristics that may negatively affect their relationships with others, patients, families, co-workers, colleagues and most importantly their own professional goals and aspirations.

Becoming more conscious of one's thoughts, feelings, beliefs and projections is an invitation for personal growth and professional development related to leading and influencing (Sullivan, 2013; Patterson, Grenny, Maxfield, McMillan, & Switzler, 2008). Inner work, attending to issues of archetypes, symbols and shadow is one way to help people understand the complexities of intra- and interpersonal dynamics and personal healing (Pesut, 2001, 2007). A variety of tools and resources support learning and reflection and the requisite inner work required to develop personal leadership insights. This chapter provides some references and suggested activities that support elements of knowing, being and doing for nurses who want to explore and expand their personal and professional leadership skill set. Knowledge derived from thoughtful reflection of one's purpose, strengths and values, and understanding the inside, bright side (golden shadows) and dark side (dark shadows) of one's leadership behaviours leads to successful self-management of one's reputation and contributes to the experiences and stories people are likely to tell about leaders. Legacies are passed on in the stories people tell (Kouzes & Posner, 2006). It is important to consider the future self that you want to create based on your values, beliefs and achievements.

IDENTITY AND REPUTATION

Marshall Goldsmith and Mark Reiter (2009) note that leaders need to be vigilant about four aspects of productive joyful living. The first is **Identity** which answers the question—who do you think you are? The second is **Achievement**, which answers the question—what have you done lately? The third is **Reputation management**, which answers the question—who do people think you are? And the fourth is **Acceptance** which poses the question—when can you let go? Perhaps the most complex of the four aspects is the issue of identity. Goldsmith and Reiter suggest each person has at least four identities based on a combination of self and other perceptions as well as past experiences and future aspirations. For example, did you grow up with scripting of some sort from your parents about who you would become, or what you would do in terms of a career? This is one's *prescribed* identity. As you gained experience and people came to know and experience you, other kinds of scripting or attributions likely came your way as people suggested what you would be good at or what role and/or career would suit you based on their experiences with you over time. This is one's *reflected* identity. After reflecting on what others suggested and related to you, combined with your personal aspirations, perhaps you developed a *remembered* identity. Finally, one weighs the opinions and suggestions of parents, friends and colleagues, considers one's personal thoughts, feelings and beliefs and values and then negotiates who they want to be. A fourth identity emerges as we craft a future for ourselves based on our experience and who we want to be. This is a *created* identity and it is our created identity that gives us the most joy and meaning as it enables us to fully be who we are based on our values, beliefs, strengths, destiny, calling and character (Secretan, 2010).

Identity is a first person or 'actor's view' of one's values, beliefs, character, strengths, aspirations, hopes, dreams and goals. As Robert Hogan (2007) and Hogan and Hogan (2002) assert, identity is not easy to measure and often is not reflected in behaviours. In contrast, Hogan and others believe the reputation is an 'observer's view' of an individual and can be described and measured in terms of characteristics. Characteristics reflect how a person's behaviour can be evaluated by others over time as a result of interactions and experiences with that person. Hogan (2011) and his team believe that characteristics can be used to predict behaviour and performance and they suggest there is an inside, light side and dark side to a person's leadership skill set.

The inside of leadership is best described as a person's key values and drivers—the activities that a person enjoys that give meaning and value to the life they want to live. There are a number of commercial assessments available that help people learn about key strengths, values and motivations. As a coach and educator, I encourage people to learn about and know their top five signature strengths. Rath and Conchie (2008) have fine-tuned a strengths' assessment that helps people discern their strengths and relate the strengths they possess to the needs followers have; namely, trust, compassion, hope and stability. Knowing one's strengths helps to make sense of the types of activities and strategies one can use to build trust, compassion, stability and hope among a followership. In addition to strengths, another important source of information that helps clarify the inside of leadership is a values inventory.

The Values in Action (VIA) Survey (www.viasurvey.org) assesses 24 character strengths (Values in Action Institute). The strengths are grouped by the virtue categories of wisdom, courage, humility, justice, temperance or transcendence. Knowledge of character strengths and learning edges promotes insight, action and development (Peterson & Seligman, 2004). One of the values of taking the strengths and character strengths assessments is the results help to clarify identity and provide people with a vocabulary they can use to describe who they are and what they do best. As one comes to appreciate the nuances of strengths and character, one can be clearer about values and beliefs as well as skills and talents that support a personal and professional sense of identity in light of leadership challenges. Knowing one's strengths and values provides insights into one's motivations. Hogan (2011) defines the inside of leadership in terms of 10 dimensions: aesthetics, affiliation, altruism, commerce, hedonism, power, recognition, science, security and tradition.

The bright sides of leadership according to Hogan (2011) are the positive aspects of leadership; for example, the degree to which a person is calm and self-accepting, confident and competitive, sociable, interpersonally sensitive, conscientious and prudent, creative and interested in problem solving and open to learning. Such leaders are often intelligent and insightful, sensible and responsible, honest, sincere, positive and optimistic, active and productive, respectful, kind, courteous, inclusive, tolerant, forgiving, caring, hopeful and inspiring. Leaders who activate and embody the bright side of leadership often have very positive reputations and esteemed legacies.

In contrast, the dark sides of leadership are those behavioural characteristics and risk factors that if unmanaged or unchecked can support the development of a negative reputation and be the source of leadership derailment. For example, enabling people rather than being more assertive or forceful or focusing on operations when a strategic orientation is called for may get leaders into trouble. Other dark-side characteristics include excitability, scepticism, cautiousness, being too reserved, boldness, mischievousness and being too colourful, imaginative or dutiful (Hogan, 2011). When people are stressed or tired, they may act out tendencies that are counterproductive to their leadership efforts. Such counterproductive efforts may overuse strengths and prevent the development of leadership versatility (Kaplan & Kaiser, 2013). Taken to extremes and going unchecked, the negative behaviours associated with the dark side of leadership can result in a negative reputation which can derail a leader and contribute to an undesirable legacy.

LEADERSHIP DERAILMENT

The word 'derailment' conjures up images of a train wreck. And so it is an apt metaphor for describing what can happen to a leader who loses a job or who does not get promoted because of an inability to manage their behaviour and relationships with others. There is a growing body of literature about the concept of derailment and leadership success and/or failure. There are many reasons that a leader may derail. Table 19.1 lists many potential derailing behaviours and characteristics gleaned from the literature (Burke, 2006; Dotlich & Cairo, 2003; George & Sims, 2007; Hogan, 2007; Kovach, 1989; Leslie & Van Velsor, 1996; Lombardo & McCauley, 1988; Maccoby, 2003; McCartney, 2006; Sutton, 2007).

Table 19.1 Potential derailing characteristics and behaviours of leaders

Aloofness: Pattern of disengagement and disconnection

Arrogance: Belief they are right and everyone else is wrong

Callousness: Uncaring, unkind, ignoring the needs of others

Corruption: Lies, cheats, steals, places self-interest first

Eager to please: Wants to win any popularity contest

Eccentricity: Belief that it is fun to be different just for the sake of it

Excessive caution: Fails to make decisive decisions

Evil: Does psychological or physical harm to others

Glory seekers: Motivated by seeking world's acclaim

Habitual distrust: Focuses on the negatives

Imposters: Lacks self-awareness and self-esteem

Incompetent: Lacks will or skill to create effective action and positive change

Insular: Ignores the needs and welfare of those outside the group

Intemperate: Lacking in self-control

Loners: Fails to build personal support structures

Melodrama: Always grabs the centre of attention

Mischievousness: Believes rules are only suggestions

Passive resistance: Silence is misinterpreted as agreement

Perfectionism: Gets the little things right while the big things go wrong

Rationalisers: Deviates from their values

Rigid: Stiff, unyielding, unable or unwilling to adapt to the new

Shooting stars: Lacks grounding in an integrated balanced life

Volatility: Mood shifts are sudden and unpredictable

SHADOW WORK AS A LEADERSHIP PRACTICE

Hogan and Hogan (2002) note the development of social political intelligence is an essential leadership skill. Sociopolitical intelligence includes the skills to: accurately read interpersonal cues; accurately communicate intended meanings; have the ability to convey trustworthiness; build and maintain relationships with others and, finally, be a rewarding person to work with. An aspect of sociopolitical intelligence is being honest with oneself regarding one's bright and dark sides of leadership and one's shadows and projections. Until recently, shadow work was a key practice in therapeutic circles. David Richo writes, 'The shadow is the archetype of the unconscious that represents the feared, denied, and unaddressed, forbidden and excluded parts of ourselves' (1991, p. 93). The negative shadow relates to those things we are unconscious of in ourselves that we disown and consequently recognise and condemn in others. Positive shadows are those things that we admire and perhaps envy in others that in fact are our own good qualities that we disavow in ourselves.

One of the most challenging things I have come to realise is how my dislike, discomfort, criticism or outrage and anger with someone is really more about me than the person who is the object of my feelings—either positive or negative. I have come to realise through personal shadow work that what I most dislike or admire in someone is really an aspect of myself that I dislike or admire. William Miller (1981) proposes this exercise as one way to tap into one's shadow. Think of someone you dislike. List all the qualities you do not like in that person. Perhaps it is control, ego-centrism, arrogance, defensiveness, sarcasm, clinging behaviour, dependency. These identified qualities are the seeds for shadow work. What we dislike in others, often are qualities we ourselves possess and may not even be aware that we possess! Nega-tive qualities are called dark shadows. The same dynamic of noting positive qualities in others may reveal our golden shadows. What we admire in others are, in fact, qualities that we possess in ourselves. The less one engages in shadow work, the more likely one is open to derailment, disregards reputation management and fails to con-sider legacy issues. Understanding personal shadows is one way to master the leader-ship skill set to manage derailment and safeguard reputation disturbances in one's professional career.

Shadow work is a leadership practice that involves intense honesty and reflection and inner work, dedicated to integration of personal and professional hopes, fears and desires (Richo, 1991). William Miller writes, '... only he who is substantially con-scious of the light should journey into his darkness. For the darkness will convict him and seek to destroy him and only the light can save him. Therefore we seek more light, more goodness, more moral strength and stamina when we make friends with our shadow. For that we must do, no matter what' (Miller, 1981, p. 142). Shadow work is one way to maximise leadership success, foster a positive reputation and create a lasting positive legacy.

William Miller (1981) offers five strategies to gain shadow insights: 1) soliciting feedback from others as to how they perceive us; 2) uncovering the content of our projections; 3) examining our behaviour and exploring what is really occurring when we are perceived other than we intend to be perceived; 4) considering our humour and identifications; and 5) studying our dreams, daydreams and fantasies.

Dotlich and Cairo (2003) offer leaders three specific coaching techniques that help leaders use inner and outer resources to fight failure. First, they suggest an adversity analysis. Adversity analysis involves reflection on the five biggest failures in one's leadership life. Once these failures have been identified, leaders are invited to reflect on what behaviours in those circumstances did not serve them well? What would one's worst critics say about how they acted? Is there a theme or pattern to the behaviour and do any of the derailers fit this pattern?

Second they suggest a direct report evaluation (Dotlich & Cairo, 2003, pp. 144–145) that involves posing the following questions to one's direct reports:

How can I be a better leader?

What do I do that makes you nuts?

How do I force you to work around me rather than with me?

When you get together to complain about me what do you complain about?

When I am under stress, what do I do that you think is counterproductive?

Third, they suggest one find a confidant and share with that person some of the derailers noted in Table 19.1 and invite them to help discuss, monitor and challenge the leaders about these vulnerabilities and how they might manage them in order to prevent derailment and leadership failure.

Additional practices that support shadow work include surfacing competing commitments and assumptions that support one's immunity to change. For example, Robert Kegan and Lisa Lahey (2001, 2009) provide strategies and techniques to uncover hidden assumptions and competing commitments that individuals or groups may hold that promote an immunity to change. Working through these assumptions in a systematic way supports insights and the development of strategies for behaviour change and personal mastery.

The 3-2-1 Shadow Process is an integral life practice (Wilber, Patton, Leonard, & Morelli, 2008) that helps a person engage in working through any intra- or interpersonal disturbances in the environment, positive or negative. It involves unpacking and exploring several perspectives in order to gain insight, understanding and personal ownership of issues. Exploring issues from a third-person perspective, second-person perspective and then first-person perspective enables an individual to appreciate and understand the dynamics of the shadow process. More specifically, the 3 in the 3-2-1 process is observing and noticing the positive or negative disturbance that you experience with someone. From this perspective individuals are encouraged to describe the disturbance in as much detail as possible—keeping the description in the third person (he, him, she, her, they, their, it, its). Next, in the 2-phase of the 3-2-1 process, individuals are invited to start a dialogue with the disturbance. Engaging in a dialogue with the person, situation or image, and posing questions—who or what are you? What do you want from me? What do you need to tell me?—gives a second-person perspective relating to the disturbance. The intention is to gain as much information as possible from this inner dialogue. Finally, the 1 of the 3-2-1 process is relating knowledge and information gained from the observation and dialogue with the issue to a first-person insight—how is it that the disturbance you have witnessed and related to is an aspect or part of one's own way of being? Acknowledging that an interpersonal disturbance is a part of self (dark or golden shadow), the 3-2-1 Shadow Integral Life Practice is a strategy to face, talk to and be the shadow that is projected towards others and learn from the process how best to self-manage the thoughts, feelings and beliefs and behaviours that may lead to leadership derailment. Positive management of shadow issues results in the generativity of a legacy.

THE GENERATIVITY OF A LEGACY

John Kotre (1999) notes that a deep satisfaction can come when a life is lived with generativity in mind—a sure knowledge that one's life has 'counted'. A generative leader is someone who creates and fosters creativity wherever they go. Generative leaders encourage cooperative strategies among agents in a system with the intention of building new capabilities that address previously unknown opportunities (Hazy, 2008). Generative leaders are solution focused, outcome oriented and excel at framing and reframing. Generative leaders challenge the people in systems in which they work to think in new ways and produce creative solutions to intractable problems. Generative leaders ask the question: 'What do I want to create for myself and the people I care about?' Generative leaders are accountable and consistently ask the question: 'How am I responsible for what is happening to me?', 'How can I positively influence the outcomes I want to see in this situation?' Generative leaders are purpose-driven individuals who have spent time clarifying their highest goal, as they confront and manage their shadows, in service to their followers. Generative leaders are clear about who they are, what they believe and work towards, developing the capabilities and skill sets to accomplish what they desire in the environments in which they find themselves. Generative leaders embrace shadow work and in so doing build positive reputations that lead to positive legacies (Yount, 2007).

Kouzes and Posner (2006) note successful leaders want to make a difference in the world and do so through service and sacrifice to a greater good. Successful leaders pursue their aspirations with courage and conviction and along the way pay attention

Table 19.2 Reputation—legacy management reflections

Have you made the impact you wanted to in your career?

What is your reputation among peers, colleagues, supervisees and/or other leaders?

How do you manage the difficult people in your life and/or organisation? Are you one of those difficult people?

Are you aware of behaviours that may lead to derailment? How do you currently manage those behaviours and characteristics?

What do you do now to manage and gather information about your reputation?

Do you have a trusted confidant or coach who can provide you with honest direct feedback?

Have you ever taken a leadership assessment or been involved in a 360-degree feedback exercise? If so, how did you respond to the results? What difference did the feedback make for you?

What is more important to you in your nursing career—the results you achieve or how you achieve them?

Will nursing and other health profession colleagues remember you as someone who made a difference in their lives?

When you are gone what 'mark' will you leave on the organisations in which you have worked?

How, specifically, will you know that your identity and reputation has contributed to the legacy that you imagined you would leave?

Will the values you instilled and live by endure long after you have left the organisation in which you are working?

Have you put into place a system that enables others to have a sense of clarity, knowledge and information that each needs to be effective?

How have you contributed to helping others understand the value and importance of identity, reputation and legacy management?

---

to loving critics. They write, 'Legacies are not the result of wishful thinking. They are the results of determined doing. The legacy you leave is the life you lead. We live our lives daily. We leave our legacy daily. The people you see, the decisions you make, and the actions you take—they are what tell your story' (Kouzes & Posner, 2006, p. 180). How well leaders manage their shadow issues and model the bright side of leadership has an impact and effect on their reputation and the stories people will tell about their leadership into the future. What stories will people tell about you in the future? What are the legacies that you as a leader want to promote? Living a life with generativity in mind leads one to ponder on the nature of a personal and professional leadership legacy. Reflect on the questions listed in Table 19.2 and consider your answers in light of your future legacy aspirations.

CONCLUSION

The purpose of this chapter was to describe and discuss the concepts and issues associated with leadership derailment, reputation and legacy management. Differences between identity from an actor's point of view and reputation from an observer's point of view were discussed. Types of behaviours that illustrate the positive and negative aspects of leadership have been identified. The concept and process of shadow work was introduced as a self-management strategy leaders can engage as a means of working through difficult intrapersonal or interpersonal dynamics in organisations and professional relationships. Working through dark and golden shadow issues supports the growth and development of leaders and assists in positive reputation management. Several strategies and techniques to engage in shadow work were described and discussed. Leaders need to think about the impact and difference they want to make in a profession, career or organisation, attention to the legacy they want to leave, influences and effects of the decisions they make, the relationships they foster and the impact that they want to have in terms of their highest goal and greater aspirations. Proactive self-management of potential derailing behaviour can keep leaders on track with positive reputations and significant legacy contributions.

REFLECTIVE EXERCISE

1. Determine your strengths and values. Complete the StrengthsFinders survey (Rath, T. & Conchie, B. (2008). *Strengths based leadership: Great leaders, teams and why people follow.* New York, NY: Gallup Press).

2. Complete the Values Inventory of Strengths Assessment: http://www.viasurvey.org/. See how your top values dovetail and support your leadership strengths.

3. Listen to this audio program about the 3-2-1 Shadow Process: http://www.youtube.com/watch?v=x64razil_4I

4. Start a book club and read George, B. & Sims, P. (2007). *True North.* John Wiley & Sons, NY, and use the online resources to explore more of the *True North* concepts http://www.truenorthleaders.com/

5. Write yourself a Sage Letter. Imagine that you are 70 years old looking back on your career. Write a letter to your younger self and explain the lessons you learned, the reputation you developed and the legacy that you created during your working years. Or consider writing a letter to the future self you aspire to become. Explore this resource: http://www.futureme.org/what

Recommended Readings

3-2-1 Shadow Process (n.d.) Retrieved 3 November 2013 from <http://integrallife.com/member/topher-hunt/blog/3-2-1-shadow-process-example>.

Egan, G. (1994). *Working the shadow side: A guide to positive behind the scenes management.* San Francisco: Jossey-Bass.

Kaiser, R. (2009). *The perils of accentuating the positive.* Tulsa, OK: Hogan Press.

Richo, D. (1999). *Shadow dance: Liberating the power and creativity of your dark side.* Boston, MA: Shambala Publications.

Van Velsor, E., & Leslie, J. B. (1995). Why executives derail: Perspectives across time and cultures. *Academy of Management Executive, 9,* 62–72.

References

Burke, R. (2006). Why leaders fail: Exploring the dark side. *International Journal of Manpower, 27*(1), 91–100.

Dotlich, D., & Cairo, P. (2003). *Why CEOs fail: The 11 behaviors that can derail your climb to the top—and how to manage them.* San Francisco, CA: Jossey-Bass.

George, B., & Sims, P. (2007). *True North.* New York, NY: John Wiley & Sons.

Goldsmith, M., & Reiter, M. (2009). *Mojo: How to get it, how to keep it, how to get it back if you lose it.* NY: Hyperion.

Grant, A. (2013). *Give and take: A revolutionary approach to success.* New York, NY: Viking Press.

Hazy, J. (2008). Patterns of leadership: A case study of influence signaling in an entrepreneurial firm. In M. Uhl-Bien & M. Russ (Eds.), *Complexity leadership Part I: Conceptual foundations* (pp. 379–415). Charlotte, NC: Information Age Publishing.

Hogan, R. (2007). *Personality and the fate of organizations.* New York, NY: Psychology Press.

Hogan, R. (2011). *The ambiguities of effectiveness.* Tulsa, OK: Hogan Assessment Systems, Inc.

Hogan, J., & Hogan, R. (2002). Leadership and sociopolitical intelligence. In R. E. Riggio, S. E. Murphy, & F. J. Pirozzolo (Eds.), *Multiple intelligences and leadership.* Mohawk. NJ: Lawrence Erlbaum.

Kaplan, R., & Kaiser, R. (2013). *Fear your strengths.* San Francisco, CA: Berrett-Kohler.

Kegan, R., & Lahey, L. (2001). *How the way we talk can change the way we work: Seven languages for transformation.* San Francisco, CA: Jossey-Bass.

Kegan, R., & Lahey, L. (2009). *Immunity to change.* Cambridge, MA: Harvard Business Press.

Kotre, J. (1999). *Make it count: How to generate a legacy that gives meaning to your life.* New York, NY: Free Press.

Kouzes, J., & Posner, B. (2006). *A leader's legacy.* San Francisco: Jossey-Bass (Quote on p. 8 used with permission from John Wiley & Sons, Inc published by Jossey-Bass, A Wiley Imprint.)

Kovach, B. E. (1989). Successful derailment: What fast-trackers can learn while they're off the track. *Organizational Dynamics, 18*(2), 33–47.

Leslie, J. B., & Van Velsor, E. (1996). *A look at derailment today: North America and Europe.* Greensboro, NC: Center for Creative Leadership.

Lombardo, M. M., & McCauley, C. D. (1988). *The dynamics of management derailment: Technical Report Number 34.* Greensboro, NC: Center for Creative Leadership.

Maccoby, M. (2003). *Narcissistic leaders: Who succeeds and who fails.* Boston, MA: Harvard Business School Press.

McCartney, W. W. (2006). Leadership, management, and derailment: A model of individual success and failure. *Leadership & Organization Development Journal, 27*(3), 190–202.

Miller, W. (1981). *Make friends with your shadow.* Minneapolis, MN: Augsburg Fortress.

Patterson, K., Grenny, J., Maxfield, D., McMillan, R., & Switzler, A. (2008). *Influencer: The power to change anything.* NY: McGraw-Hill.

Pesut, D. (2001). Healing into the future: Recreating the profession of nursing through inner work. In N. Chaska (Ed.), *The nursing profession: Tomorrow and beyond* (pp. 853–867). Thousand Oaks, CA: Sage.

Pesut, D. J. (2007). Leadership: How to achieve success in nursing organizations. In C. O'Lynn & R. Tranbarger (Eds.), *Men in nursing: History, challenges and opportunities* (pp. 153–168). NY: Springer Publishing.

Pesut, D. (2013). Evolving awareness. In C. Coleman (Ed.), *Man up: A practical guide for men in nursing* (pp. 181–202). Indianapolis, In.: Sigma Theta Tau International.

Peterson, C., & Seligman, M. (2004). *Character strengths and virtues: A handbook and classification.* New York, NY: Oxford University Press.

Quinn, R. (1996). *Deep change: Discovering the leader within.* San Francisco: Jossey Bass.

Rath, T., & Conchie, B. (2008). *Strengths based leadership.* New York, NY: Gallup Press.

Richo, D. (1991). *How to be an adult.* New York: Paulist Press.

Secretan, L. (2010). *Spark, flame, torch.* Ontario, Canada: Secretan Center.

Smith, K., & Berg, D. (1997). *Paradoxes of group life: Understanding conflicts, paralysis and movement in group dynamics.* San Francisco: Jossey-Bass.

Sullivan, E. (2013). *Becoming influential: A guide for nurses* (2nd ed.). Boston, MA: Pearson Education.

Sutton, R. I. (2007). *The No asshole rule: Building a civilized workplace and surviving one that isn't.* New York, NY: Warner Business Books.

Values in Action Institute. Retrieved 2 November 2013 from <http://www.viacharacter.org/www/>.

Wilber, K., Patten, T., Leonard, A., & Morelli, M. (2008). *Integral life practice: A 21st century blueprint for physical health, emotional balance, mental clarity and spiritual awakening.* Boston, MA: Integral Books.

Yount, S. (2007). *Leaving your leadership legacy: Creating a timeless and enduring culture of clarity, connectivity, and consistency.* Richmond, VA: Oaklee Press.

INDEX

Page numbers followed by 'f' indicate figures, 't' indicate tables, and 'b' indicate boxes.

CPSIA information can be obtained
at www.ICGtesting.com
Printed in the USA
BVHW010507120322
631111BV00002B/2

9 780729 541534